Shulamit Reinharz, Ph.D., is Associate Professor of sociology at Brandeis University. Currently she is a Research Scholar at the Brookdale Institute of Gerontology in Jerusalem where she is completing a monograph, *Aging on the Kibbutz* (University of Chicago Press). For the last 5 years, she was the co-editor of the journal *Qualitative Sociology* as well as producing two special issues, one concerning the use of computers in qualitative research, and the other concerning the development of qualitative sociological research in 10 different countries. Previous publications include *On Becoming a Social Scientist, Psychology and Community Change*, and numerous articles and chapters in the fields of qualitative methodology, social gerontology and women's studies.

Graham D. Rowles, Ph.D., is Associate Director of the Sanders-Brown Center on Aging and Associate Professor of Geography at the University of Kentucky. A native of Carshalton, England, Dr. Rowles received his B.A. and M.Sc. degrees from the University of Bristol, England, and his Ph.D. from Clark University in Massachusetts. His research over the past fifteen years has focused on the environmental experience of the elderly in urban, institutional and, most recently, rural settings. Dr. Rowles is a Fellow of the Gerontological Society of America and serves on the Editorial Board of *The Gerontologist*. His publications include *Prisoners of Space? Exploring the Geographical Experience of Older People* and a co-edited volume, *Aging and Milieu: Environmental Perspectives on Growing Old*, in addition to numerous articles and book chapters on the relationship between aging and environment.

Qualitative Gerontology

Shulamit Reinharz, Ph.D.
Graham D. Rowles, Ph.D.

Editors

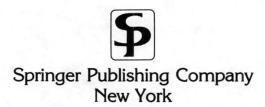

Springer Publishing Company
New York

Springer Publishing Company, Inc.
536 Broadway
New York, NY 10012

87 88 89 90 91 / 5 4 3 2 1

Library of Congress Cataloging-in-Publication Data

Qualitative gerontology.

  Includes bibliographies and index.
  I. Aged—Health and hygiene.   2. Aged—Care.
3. Gerontology.   I. Reinharz, Shulamit.   II. Rowles,
Graham D.
RA564.8.Q35   1987   362.6   87-20636
ISBN 0-8261-5230-9

Printed in the United States of America

Contents

Part III Commentary

Contributors

Harry J. Berman, Child, Family and Community Services Program, Sangamon State University, Springfield, Illinois.

J. Kevin Eckert, Department of Sociology, University of Maryland, Baltimore County, Catonsville, Maryland.

Betty Friedan, University of Southern California, Los Angeles, California.

Christine L. Fry, Department of Sociology and Anthropology, Loyola University, Chicago, Illinois.

David Gutmann, Department of Psychiatry and Behavioral Sciences, Northwestern University Medical School, Chicago, Illinois.

Charlotte Ikels, Department of Anthropology, Case Western Reserve University, Cleveland, Ohio.

Boaz Kahana, Department of Psychology, Cleveland State University, Cleveland, Ohio.

Eva Kahana, Department of Sociology, Case Western Reserve University, Cleveland, Ohio.

Robert Kastenbaum, Adult Development and Aging Program, Arizona State University, Tempe, Arizona.

Sharon R. Kaufman, Institute for Health and Aging, Department of Social and Behavioral Sciences, University of California–San Francisco, San Francisco, California.

Kathleen Kautzer, Department of Sociology, Regis College, Weston, Massachusetts.

Jennie Keith, Department of Sociology and Anthropology, Swarthmore College, Swarthmore, Pennsylvania.

Helen Q. Kivnick, California School of Professional Psychology, Berkeley, California; private-practice psychologist.

Kathleen I. MacPherson, School of Nursing, University of Southern Maine, Portland, Maine.

Aluma K. Motenko, Department of Sociology and Graduate School of Social Work, Boston University, Boston, Massachusetts.

Karl Pillemer, Family Research Laboratory and Department of Sociology, University of New Hampshire, Durham, New Hampshire.

Kathryn P. Riley, Department of Psychology, Cleveland State University, Cleveland, Ohio.

Robert L. Rubinstein, Philadelphia Geriatric Center, Philadelphia, Pennsylvania.

Phyllis R. Silverman, Department of Psychiatry, Massachusetts General Hospital, Harvard Medical School, Boston, Massachusetts.

Anselm Strauss, Department of Social and Behavioral Sciences, University of California–San Francisco, San Francisco, California.

Mary Ann Wilner, Massachusetts Federation of Nursing Homes, Dedham, Massachusetts.

Preface

The genesis of this book lay in an exchange of correspondence, two subsequent face-to-face meetings, and a flurry of phone calls that seemed to propel us inexorably toward a venture we hope will stimulate and enhance the use of qualitative approaches in gerontology. It all began in 1982 when we sent one another some of our writings. Subsequent correspondence quickly revealed that although our origins as social scientists lay in different traditions—geography and sociology—both of us were wrestling with issues of "being" and "knowing" and how these related to the dominant paradigm in gerontology.

At the time, we had not yet met. Indeed, it was not until we both presented papers in a special session on "Qualitative Research in Gerontology: Methodological Issues and Findings" at the 1983 Gerontological Society of America meetings in San Francisco that our mutual concerns brought us together. This session, chaired by Bernice Neugarten, a long-time advocate for diversity in gerontological methodology, was a follow-up to a similar symposium held in Boston the previous year. Like its predecessor, the session drew a standing-room-only crowd. The large attendance and enthusiastic reception suggested that our concerns were shared by many other people. In the session we discussed approaches to gerontology that emphasized the humanity of people as they age; that sought to break down barriers between researchers and subjects; that sought liberation from the constraints of exclusive reliance on a positivist view of science; and that sought to recast the role of the researcher by challenging distinctions between private and professional ways of knowing. The session, and similar symposia held at subsequent Gerontological Society of America meetings, was testimony to what we now believe to be a significant opportunity for gerontological researchers. Simply put, there is growing recognition that some important questions demand a qualitative approach and that the study of aging and the aged is enriched by the insights of such scholarship. The time seemed right for a book on qualitative gerontology.

In collaboration with our distinguished contributors, each of whom was asked to prepare an original manuscript, our goal was to provide a statement on the role and status of qualitative research in gerontology. Obviously, we could not hope to cover the whole array of methods in a single volume. For example, we would have liked to include a community study, a study that used the Human Relations Area Files, a study employing conversational analysis, or a study demonstrating focus group interviews. There simply was no room to do so. Nevertheless, we believe we have drawn attention to the range of qualitative methods and hope this book will encourage people to explore these methods and others.

An additional goal was to provide a resource for researchers and graduate students of gerontology that would transcend disciplines. We hope to reach people working in psychology, sociology, anthropology, geography, social work, public policy, and health sciences. To achieve this goal we have organized the book in terms of three objectives. First, although there is a growing literature on qualitative research in the social and behavioral sciences, and there are an increasing number of gerontological case studies, to our knowledge there is no comprehensive overview of qualitative research in gerontology. Thus, in Part I, we provide a rationale and an overview of the strengths and weaknesses of this type of research and discuss its relationship to other research approaches. Our hope is that this section will enable the reader to avoid viewing qualitative gerontology as a new orthodoxy. Rather, we would like readers to see it as a set of opportunities, an integrated way of "doing" and "being" that deepens our understanding of our own and others' aging experience.

Neither theoretical nor methodological justification is a substitute for the power of illustration. Consequently, the objective in Part II is to provide an array of exemplars of qualitative research. Our contributors were asked to focus on the *substance* of qualitative research and the insights it yields. At the same time, they have sought to convey the *process* of qualitative research and share what is most important about the specific methods they use.

Finally, in Part III, we have included an innovation in order to generate debate about qualitative gerontology. Three eminent scholars— Betty Friedan, David Gutmann, and Anselm Strauss—agreed to provide commentaries on qualitative gerontology (i.e., Parts I and II). These commentaries not only provide a perspective on the preceding chapters but also indicate some directions in which qualitative gerontology might usefully proceed. We believe our commentators have indeed sparked the dialogue with their colorful, engaging essays.

Our primary gratitude clearly goes to the contributors and commentators who graciously tolerated two independent and occasionally conflicting editors' suggestions for revisions with considerable equanimity.

And we are also conscious of and appreciate the forbearance of our spouses and families.

Three individuals deserve special comment. We would like to thank Bernice Neugarten and Richard A. Kalish, whose enthusiastic reading of our completed manuscript gave us that last burst of energy we needed to complete our work. Finally, we would like to acknowledge the contribution of Shirley W. Wilson at the University of Kentucky, who is personally responsible for your being able to read these words. Shirley typed, retyped, retyped, and retyped again, version after version of the manuscript and handled the plethora of thankless chores associated with producing an edited volume. Moreover, she did this with a grace, skill, and good humor that are unsurpassed in our experience. Shirley, we thank you.

SHULAMIT REINHARZ
Newton, Massachusetts

GRAHAM D. ROWLES,
Lexington, Kentucky

PART 1

Introduction

1

Qualitative Gerontology: Themes and Challenges

Graham D. Rowles
Shulamit Reinharz

Jennifer-Rose, a seventy-two-year-old widow, lived alone in a two-bedroom house on a particularly isolated stretch of the road between Queensglade and Colton, in rural northern Appalachia. She had high blood pressure and a colostomy resulting from surgery for cancer of the colon. After her husband died and her two children moved some distance away, she had to become self-reliant in the house where she had lived for 42 years.

Concern with the quality of housing and living arrangements of the rural elderly has led to surveys of the residential circumstances of individuals like Jennifer-Rose. One can imagine a survey researcher, let's call her Harriet, arriving on Jennifer-Rose's porch, clipboard and pencil in hand, to conduct an assessment. What might we expect from her visit? Certainly, there would be much useful data. Her report would probably document the poor condition of the dwelling—the leaky porch roof, the creaky wooden floor boards, the cracked steps that are so treacherous in winter, the peeling paint, and the drafty windows that send her fuel bills soaring. The report would inform us of Jennifer-Rose's excess living space and the rooms she had closed off. We might learn that ever since her surgery she had not been able to tend her yard, and as a result it had become overgrown and unkempt.

The report might also describe some of the problems Jennifer-Rose faced as a consequence of living alone, far from neighbors and from the center of Colton. Indeed, after a short visit, a conscientious survey researcher, such as Harriet, would have been able to provide a clear account of Jennifer-Rose's housing situation and might have concluded that to continue functioning effectively, she should relocate to "better housing."

It is likely that Harriet would not feel that she, personally, had been an important influence on the assessment. Since the research dealt with objective information, it could have been carried out by anyone carefully trained by the project director. Harriet would probably have discouraged Jennifer-Rose from getting started on too many stories, since she had several houses to assess that day if she was to complete her quota of randomly selected individuals. Harriet would also have avoided interjecting any of her own questions into the carefully prepared and pretested survey instrument. On the other hand, she would have been careful not to alienate Jennifer-Rose because the worst outcome of the encounter would have been to lose her as a respondent.

Interestingly, Harriet's assessment that Jennifer-Rose's housing was deteriorating, that it exceeded her ability to maintain it, and that she required some immediate change in her living situation would have been inconsistent with Jennifer-Rose's insistence on remaining in her home. Such insistence was more than residential inertia or capriciousness. Rather it represented a fundamental divergence of their perspectives: a contrast between assessment of her *house*, a physical structure providing a place of residence, and assessment of the same dwelling as her *home*, the locus of her identity.

Focusing on this second assessment, we might envision a second researcher, Mary, perhaps carrying a tape-recorder rather than a clipboard, adopting an entirely different methodology, obtaining different data, and producing a different report. Instead of completing a predesigned survey using questions derived from the researchers' *a priori* concerns, this interviewer might have attempted to establish rapport with Jennifer-Rose and to provide her with a context in which she could articulate and reveal the meaning of her dwelling. As she began to talk of her reluctance to leave and of her memories of building the house with her husband back in the 1930s, Mary would begin to understand Jennifer-Rose's definition of the situation. The aura of the "home place" would become apparent as, sitting on the swinging seat on her porch, she would stare out past the tree that had once supported her children's swing to the area where they had played in the sandbox. Jennifer-Rose might have explained to Mary how she would often muse on the yard as it had once been. In fact, precisely because there had been so much change in her life—what with her husband dying, her children moving away, and her surgery—she could maintain a sense of continuity only by remaining in the "home place." She was proud of her ability to stay.

Inside the house, Jennifer-Rose would redefine what Mary saw—the jumbled mustiness and disarray of the rooms, with the window light obstructed by the plant stands and hanging baskets of dusty African violets. Instead, Mary might see vibrant images of major events that had taken place within these walls: the joy of a celebration; the anguish of death and illness; the implicit, taken-for-granted sense of affinity resulting from the reinforcing routine of everyday use over more than four decades. Mary would come to realize how Jennifer-Rose's home had come to be worn like a glove, to be a central part of her identity, far more than the seemingly dilapidated structure that could be viewed from the road.

Mary would begin to look at the house the way Jennifer-Rose viewed it. She would probably find that she could understand much of what Jennifer-Rose was saying; but some of it would be unclear, so she would ask questions spontaneously as they went along. Mary would find different ways of putting things to make sure Jennifer-Rose knew what she meant by her questions. Most important, she would listen and try to be receptive to the ambience of the exchange. In this book it is our intention to focus on Mary's perspective, which we have termed "qualitative gerontology."

In our view, each scenario derives from a distinct epistemology, involves separate methods, and provides different kinds of information. Both are legitimate, either alone or in combination, as ways of enhancing our understanding of the aging process and the lives of the elderly (see also Loomis & Williams, 1983, p. 497). Alone they provide distinct perspectives on understanding aging; together their complementarity allows us to see how each perspective is only a partial view. Since knowledge always reflects the methods by which it was obtained (Reinharz, 1984), knowledge derived from one method exclusively is necessarily partial. Diversity in methods affords a more diversified understanding of any subject matter, including gerontology.

There is a plethora of writings that provides a philosophical rationale for qualitative research (see, for example, Blumer, 1969; Gadamer, 1975; Maslow, 1966; Reinharz, 1984; Rowles, 1978a; Schwartz & Jacobs, 1979; Silverman, 1985). It is not our intention to repeat such justifications but rather to demonstrate their use in gerontology (see also Fry & Keith, 1986; Neugarten, 1985). To introduce this book, our opening chapter discusses the perspective of qualitative gerontological research. We (1) identify characteristics of such research; (2) explore the relationship between qualitative and quantitative research; (3) describe alternative forms of qualitative gerontological research;

and (4) discuss special issues in qualitative research involving the elderly. In Chapter 2, by Robert Kastenbaum, many of the ideas discussed formally in this introduction are embedded in a lively, imaginative drama.

WHAT IS QUALITATIVE GERONTOLOGY?

Qualitative gerontology is concerned with describing patterns of behavior and processes of interaction, as well as revealing the meanings, values, and intentionalities that pervade elderly people's experience or the experience of others in relation to old age. In addition, qualitative gerontology seeks to identify patterns that underlie the lifeworlds of individuals, social groups, and larger systems as they relate to old age. A primary focus is on understanding and conveying experience in "lived" form with as little *a priori* structuring as possible. Qualitative gerontology attempts to tap the *meaning* of experienced reality by presenting analyses based on empirically and theoretically grounded descriptions.

Qualitative gerontological research requires careful attention to the data collection process to make sure the data supply the foundation for an analysis of meaning. The process of gathering data for qualitative research has special properties (Reinharz, 1983b; Rowles, 1978a). It usually requires *personal interaction* with the individuals and contexts under study so that the researcher can hear people's language and observe behavior in situ. Face-to-face interaction and careful observation enable the researcher to discover contradictions and ambivalences within what on the surface may seem to be a simple reality. For example, in Chapter 9 of this book, Kathleen Kautzer explains how meetings of an activist organization for nursing home residents contradicted her expectations.

Personal interaction and observation also facilitate description of the quality of relationships and processes of change as they unfold (Bigus, Hadden, & Glaser, 1982). In this volume, Chapter 7, by Robert L. Rubinstein, shows how qualitative methods uncover processes of change. He found that his assessment of the loneliness of the men he interviewed was revised during each succeeding interview. In addition, he was able to see how changes occurred when he conducted a second long-term series of in-depth interviews with elderly men and women.

In quantitatively oriented studies, there may be a single data collection period in which contact time is reduced to a minimum, or in the case of longitudinal studies, data are collected at intervals in order to monitor change. In these longitudinal studies, however, processes of change are not generally studied *during* the time lapse. Thus, characteristically, one finds notations such as $t(1)$, $t(2)$, $t(3)$. Time functions differently in qualitative studies. In these it is not unusual to read that the researcher was "in the field" for a year or more and was able to trace the evolution of events as they unfolded in situ. In this volume, Kathleen I. MacPherson's study (Chapter 10) is based on approximately four years of participant observation. On the other hand, some types of qualitative research do not require such a lengthy time investment. Several studies in this book, in fact, are based on continuous data collection over a period of only a few months.

In qualitative gerontological research, behaviors, attitudes, and beliefs are not considered as discrete entities. Rather, they are conceptualized as interacting and embedded in specific contexts. Thus, to understand one aspect of a situation, many others need to be known. This "awareness of context" sometimes occurs on the part of more quantitatively oriented researchers who recognize that their attempt to conduct a controlled experiment was actually part of a larger social system affecting the experiment in many important ways. A discussion of this issue can be found in Chapter 11, by Eva and Boaz Kahana and Kathryn P. Riley.

Because of this holistic perspective, qualitative gerontological researchers recognize that they are part of the phenomenon being studied and use their experience as data (Reinharz, 1984; Neugarten, 1985; Rowles, 1978a). Thus qualitative research frequently includes a reflexive attitude during data collection and interpretation (Emerson, 1983). Because of this reflexivity, qualitative studies tend to include detailed description of the research process in its mundaneness (Reinharz, 1984; Rowles, 1978a). Presenting a project in terms of its "natural history" or process, rather than simply in terms of its findings, is a characteristic of qualitative research (Becker, 1958). Since the researcher is intimately involved in relationships with research subjects, and since qualitative research is a process in which the researcher learns about others through the data she/he is gathering, the report necessarily includes discussion of the researcher's experience. In this book, Mary Ann Wilner (Chapter 8) and Phyllis R. Silverman (Chapter 12) present their projects within a reflexive framework. Wilner discusses the impact on her study groups of her attempt to collect data in two different ways. Silverman discusses how her data collection and analysis processes were affected by issues in her own life over an extended period.

In addition, qualitative researchers usually recognize the extent to

which their interviews and observations are opportunities for "cooperative dialogue" in which the subject (in tandem with the researcher)
learns new things about him/herself.

> Not only does the subject studied receive valuable feedback from the
> observer but the observer also obtains valuable clarifying knowledge re-
> garding what he observed from the experiential report of the person
> studied regarding his own experience. Both the person researched as well
> as the research person are thus being changed through the existential
> research method—they change each other (Von Eckartsberg, 1971,
> pp. 75–76).

The outcome is a "text" of the encounter that transcends the experience of both participants.

Just as different aspects of a phenomenon can be uncovered by
quantitative or qualitative research approaches, so, too, different
layers of consciousness are accessible to different qualitative methods. Harry J. Berman's contribution to this volume, Chapter 3, elabo-
rates on this theme. Starting with Freud's tripartite division of intrapsychic consciousness, Berman suggests that people act and interact
on numerous levels, including the interpersonal, preconscious, and
unconscious (clearly, one could add more levels). Given that there
are different modes of existence, Berman suggests that alternative
types of research methods are needed to gain access to each of these
realms.

In quantitative studies, random statistical sampling is usually desirable so that results can be generalized to the universe from which the
sample was drawn. In qualitative studies it is more likely that a small
purposive sample will be drawn. A purposive sample seeks cases that
represent specific *types* of a given phenomenon. The resulting sample
allows the investigator to study the range of types (Trost, 1986) rather
than determine their distribution or frequency.

Demonstrating that much can be learned even from an *n* of 1, Chapter 4, by Helen Q. Kivnick, offers new definitions of a late life stage
based on thorough analysis of one man's attitudes and behaviors as a
grandfather. In other cases, a small *n* represents the universe. An
example in this book is Aluma K. Motenko's study of six men (Chapter
6) who constitute the universe of accessible cases of men caring for
disabled wives and using the respite services of a particular social
service agency.

Hendricks and Hendricks (1986) offer a useful perspective on generalizability when nonrandom samples are used in social gerontology:

Generalizability in statistics refers to whether a relationship or trait is characteristic of a population as a whole, or whether it is particular to some part of it. . . . Generalizability in qualitative research should be considered differently. Rather than dealing with what is generally the case, we are looking at what might more generally be the case. Qualitative research explores the ways in which people interpret and negotiate the circumstances in which they find themselves; it seeks to penetrate the causal web and see just what it is that makes a situation or event as it is and not otherwise. It may thus uncover a variety of understandings of and reactions to essentially similar circumstances. . . . In saying that an approach to a problem is generalizable, we are saying that an approach may be applied, perhaps with some modifications, in circumstances other than the ones where we found it. Thus, quantitative methods might be used to identify widespread conditions (the structural constraints) that impinge on the lives of the elderly; qualitative methods may be used to identify creative and varied approaches to those conditions. Both approaches can shed light on the ways in which people age (pp. 13–14).

Kai Erikson has taken an interesting divergent stand on generalizability. He argues that:

the search for generalization has become so intense in our professional ranks that most of the important events of our day have passed without comment in the sociological literature. . . . There are times when the need for generalizations must yield to the urgency of passing events, times when the event must tell its own story (1976, p. 12).

In this vein, the chapters by Kathleen I. MacPherson (Chapter 10) on a menopause collective and Kathleen Kautzer (Chapter 9) on "Living Is For the Elderly" are case studies informed less by the need for generalization than by the "urgency of passing events."

Another characteristic of qualitative research is its *emergent* nature. Data are analyzed while they are being collected, and the evolving analyses are used to focus the collection of additional data. The process of seeking cases is guided by the search for contrasts that are needed to clarify the analysis and achieve the "saturation" of emergent categories through a process of constant comparison (Glaser & Strauss, 1967; Charmaz, 1983).

Qualitative gerontology is also characterized by its use of participants' everyday language and its emphasis on the description of natural settings. Everyday language is interactive and different from written texts, formal speeches, or responses to questions posed by a stranger. The former is characterized by the more spontaneous expression of narratives rather than by the deliberate declaration of rationalized answers. Qualitative gerontology is thus likely to capture and present the meanings embedded in the language of everyday life.

Description in qualitative gerontology also has special characteristics. First, according to Clifford Geertz (1973), it may provide an end in itself. His notion of thick description—of specific individuals, situations, or social settings—has become a goal of many qualitative researchers. Second, it differs from the aesthetically oriented account of the novelist or the information-packed report of the journalist, important as these contributions are (Mendelson, 1975; Sheehan, 1984). Rather, it is concept-rich because the qualitative social scientist's work is informed by and oriented toward theory. As Robert Emerson put it: "an ethnographic description is always a theory-informed representation of that thing, a rendering of the event that transforms it in particular ways" (1983, p. 21). Sometimes research reports hover between the aesthetically moving and the conceptually rich. This occurs frequently in collections of life histories containing little coding or conceptual analysis that could be used for hypothesis generation or theory building. An example would be Thomas J. Cottle's *Hidden Survivors: Portraits of Poor Jews in America* (1980). The word *portrait* nicely expresses Cottle's aim (see also Maas, 1980).

Qualitative description is necessary when studying individual and social situations that are unique, relatively unknown, or have become stereotyped. An excellent example of the power of qualitative interviews to examine stereotyped ideas is Smith and Bengtson's (1979) study of families in which one member has been institutionalized in a nursing home.

> Open-ended interviews were held over a period of two years with resident-patients of an institutional setting and with the child who was most involved with the parent at the time of entrance to the facility. . . . The findings of this study do not perpetuate the sterotype that elderly persons in institutions are abandoned by and isolated from their families. . . . The most predominant patterns were that of renewed and strengthened closeness and a continuation of family closeness (p. 439, p. 444).

To record everyday language in use and to describe conceptually situations as they are lived require that one conduct research in natural settings. Indeed, naturalism is a core characteristic of qualitative research that, in sociology, can be traced back at least as far as Harriet Martineau (*Society in America*) and Alexis de Tocqueville (*Democracy in America*), who in the mid-1830s traveled from their native England and France respectively to study the way Americans had attempted to embody a particular set of ideas in their new nation. A distinctive feature of their portraits of America was that they were grounded in a physical, sociopolitical, and historical context.

Qualitative gerontology is frequently characterized by this sort of immersion in context. It provides ethnographic detail that enables readers to gain a sense of the lives of the elderly by preserving individual uniqueness. The specific context compels us to see human life as fragments embedded in the passage of time and space. Because qualitative research tends to occur in natural settings, the researcher is in a good position to take into account the environmental influences surrounding that which is being studied—the architecture, other people, economic conditions, patterns of decoration, and myriad other cultural characteristics. Thus ethnographically oriented community studies are ideally suited for assessing the needs of a particular group so that services can be designed in ways that are sensitive to the environmental context and hence conducive to their actual use (Carp & Kataoka, 1976).

In qualitative research, the logic by which conceptual descriptions are formulated from data is usually inductive inference and synthesis, rather than formal hypothesis testing. This logic is used by anthropologists, psychologists, sociologists, historians, and other social scientists; it is not confined to one discipline. Consequently, the contributions to this volume represent a broad spectrum of disciplines.

Some qualitative researchers, insofar as they are able, attempt to divest themselves of all preconceptions; others proceed with a broad repertoire of concepts to draw on when needed. As many of the contributions in this volume illustrate, the process of drawing conclusions characteristically involves the painstaking and critical sifting and sorting of data from detailed field notes or transcripts of tape-recorded interviews. In this process, the researcher endeavors to stay as close as possible to the data themselves. Sometimes this entails developing an elaborate coding system, such as that described by Charlotte Ikels, Jennie Keith, and Christine Fry (Chapter 15). In other cases, such as the one described by J. Kevin Eckert (Chapter 13), it involves alternating phases of field research and reflection. In this process, concepts gradually emerge and are refined over time through reflexive interaction with research participants.

Since quantitative research within a positivist paradigm is characterized by formal rules of procedure and the constraints of particular forms of verification, it is presented in standardized, formatted ways. Qualitative research, on the other hand, tends to be personal or idiosyncratic in both procedure and presentation, limited only by the researcher's creativity in locating unconventional data sources (Gould, 1985) and developing and utilizing methods that will reveal the meaning permeating the world of lived experience.

Despite this variability, qualitative research possesses numerous characteristics on which methodologists agree (e.g., Agar, 1980; Bogdan & Taylor, 1975; Burgess, 1982; Emerson, 1983; Lofland & Lofland, 1984; Miles & Huberman, 1984; Schwartz & Jacobs, 1979; Silverman, 1985; Van Maanen, 1983, among others). Table 1-1 offers a summary of some of these characteristics.

Qualitative research, then, produces conceptually grounded descriptions of empirical events as lived. Because of this purpose, qualitative

TABLE 1-1 Attributes of Qualitative Research

Units of study	Experienced reality
Sharpness of focus	Broad, inclusive, exploratory
Data type	Feelings, behavior, thoughts, insights, actions as witnessed or experienced
Topic of study	Unlimited range
Sample size	Likely to be small
Role of researcher	
In relation to environment	Openness to environment, immersion, being shaped by it
In relation to subjects	Involved, sense of commitment, participation, sharing of fate
As a person	Relevant, expected to change during process
Impact on researcher	Anticipated, recorded, reported, valued
Implementation of method	Method influenced by unique characteristics of field setting
Validity criteria	Completeness, plausibility, illustrativeness, understanding, responsiveness to readers' or subjects' experience, study not necessarily replicable
The role of theory	Used in interpreting data and emerges from data
Data analysis	Undertaken during the study, relying on inductive logic and locating comparisons
Manipulation of data	Creation of gestalts and meaningful patterns
Research objectives	Development of understanding through grounded concepts and descriptions; development of hypotheses and theory
Presentation format	Description of emergent concepts plus documentation of process of discovery and presentation of subjects' everyday language
Failure	Failures, pitfalls documented
Values	Researchers' attitudes described and discussed, values acknowledged, revealed, labeled
Audience	Both scholarly and user community likely to be addressed

Adapted from S. Reinharz, *On Becoming a Social Scientist*. New Brunswick, NJ: Transaction Books, 1984, pp. 14–15.

research is frequently presented in language that combines the speech of the research subjects with the abstractions of social science. Such description has produced many of the most powerful images we draw on to understand aging—the image of injustice and despair in Jules Henry's *Culture Against Man* (1963) and the ambience of Jaber Gubrium's *Living and Dying at Murray Manor* (1975), both based on participant observation research in nursing homes; the particular American cast of Jeannie Kayser-Jones's (1981) study of nursing home life; the image of the "empty-nest" in Pauline Bart's content analysis of psychiatric records (1975); the displaced homemakers defined by Tish Sommers (1976) and Laurie Shields (1981); Susan Sontag's concept of a double standard of aging for women and men (1979); the idea of *ageism*, a term coined by Robert Butler (1969); the multiple stereotypes of old women in the work of Ruth Jacobs (1976); the image of a community of working-class widows in senior housing as portrayed by Arlie Hochschild (1973) and Jennie Keith Ross (1977); the sense of engagement among the elderly described by Barbara Myerhoff (1979); the effect of ethnic community on the process of aging as revealed by Margaret Clark and Barbara Anderson (1967); the stages of dying as delineated by Elizabeth Kübler-Ross (1969); the image of old, poor men deriving benefits from the city and avoiding services in J. Kevin Eckert's (1980) study of single room occupancy hotels; the portrayal of deinstitutionalized elderly mental patients in Nancy Scheper-Hughes's work (1981); the image of empty lives in Jerry Jacobs's study of a retirement community (1974); and the discovery of extremely large, highly permeable, amorphous, and spatially transcedent social worlds among the elderly in David Unruh's (1983) study of social integration, to name only a few.

RELATIONS BETWEEN QUANTITATIVE AND QUALITATIVE RESEARCH

The division of research into quantitative and qualitative domains has led to a state of affairs in which, unfortunately, proponents of each seem oblivious to the other's merits, despite the utility of each perspective. As a result, unexamined myths and metaphors—such as soft and hard data—abound that confuse rather than clarify (Goodwin & Goodwin, 1984). One myth is that qualitative and quantitative research are mutually exclusive; another is that qualitative methods are always subjective, whereas quantitative methods are always "uncontaminated" by context and are objective; and a third is that qualitative researchers are unconcerned about issues of generalizability, validity, and reliability, whereas quantitative researchers are satisfied with superficial insights.

It is certainly not our intention to polarize and exacerbate mistrust between the two research styles. However, in our view, these myths are fed by differences in power. Since quantification is associated with a reified view of science, which is dominant in the ethos of Western culture, and description is associated with literature, journalism, and the world of everyday interaction, quantifiers have the upper hand in a kind of power struggle in universities and research centers. Some have argued that this epistemological struggle ultimately rests on the fact that science has become gendered; i.e., numbers are defined as hard data, which are equated with reason and masculinity; language is defined as soft data, which are equated with emotion and femininity (see Keller, 1985; Reinharz, 1983a).

When, as is frequently the case, power resides in the hands of those engaged in quantitative research, people wishing to engage in qualitative scholarship may be denied publication opportunities, research funding, or jobs. By excluding qualitative research, quantitative researchers limit competing viewpoints. As a result, the quantitative paradigm is reinforced, reproduced in succeeding generations of researchers, and further institutionalized. Researchers who use qualitative methods become obliged to present extraordinary justification for their choice (Kanter & Stein, 1980). They may also be forced to work within a milieu in which their research is viewed as inferior or peripheral to the core scientific enterprise.

Others see separation between the two research styles not as competition but as a kind of "separate cultures" phenomenon. In a study of methodological trends in sociology publications, for example, Wilner (1985) found a sharp decline in qualitative studies published in a major journal between 1936 and 1982, while at the same time there was a predominance in the use of qualitative methods by authors of prize-winning books (see also Becker, 1977).

The preceding discussion of qualitative research has highlighted its distinctive characteristics. There are two ways in which the uneasy juxtaposition of the two paradigms may be reconciled. We call these alternatives "separate but equal" and "integrated."

By "separate but equal" we mean that different research approaches may be suitable for different types of research questions. Studies of meaning require qualitative research, studies of distribution or correlation require quantitative research. Second, qualitative and quantitative research methods may be used in tandem, with qualitative strategies appropriate for generating hypotheses and quantitative strategies appropriate for testing them. Alternatively, quantitative results may be interpreted or elaborated with qualitative follow-up. Third, qualitative methods may be useful in constructing instruments that can be used in quantitative research. For example, open-ended questions can be used to develop valid instrumentation for later large sample studies. A good example of this procedure is Bernice Neugarten and her associates' (1968) study of woman's attitudes toward menopause. In this study, exploratory interviews were used to develop an attitude checklist that was pretested with a larger sample. The instrument was then revised and subsequently incorporated within a lengthy interview protocol. This approach is especially important when conducting research on groups with which the researcher is unfamiliar (Jackson, Tucker, & Bowman, 1982).

"Integrated" implies triangulation or multiple operationism (Webb, Campbell, Schwartz, & Sechrest, 1966). This involves combining different methods in the same project to reveal different dimensions of the same phenomenon, to shore up the shortcomings of each method, or to double-check findings by examining them from several vantage points. Three chapters in this book demonstrate this process—those of Karl Pillemer (Chapter 14); Charlotte Ikels, Jennie Keith, and Christine L. Fry (Chapter 15); and J. Kevin Eckert (Chapter 13).

When studies are neither exclusively quantitative nor exclusively qualitative, and collect many different types of data, they are using a "flexible strategy of discovery" (Lofland, 1971). Flexibility may be particularly important when studying groups with communication difficulties, such as the frail elderly (Streib, 1983). The integration of different methods also makes it possible to weave back and forth between different levels of meaning (Connidis, 1983) and to provide contexts to make data meaningful. For example, in a needs assessment study in Chinatown, historical material about the conditions under which different subgroups of elderly Chinese arrived in this country were combined with health scores and correlated with income levels (Carp & Kataoka, 1976).

Triangulated studies may also be more pleasant for respondents. Gibson and Aitkenhead found that:

a mix of open-ended questions amid sets of structured items led to more enjoyable and hence more productive interviews. In particular, consistent batteries of multiple-choice questions led to rapid tiring and loss of interest by respondents (1983, p. 292).

Because of the numerous assets of triangulation, we are now in a period when researchers are conducting more studies employing this approach and theorists are attempting to develop logical models that integrate causal and interpretive analyses (Hayes, 1985).

FORMS OF QUALITATIVE GERONTOLOGICAL RESEARCH

Qualitative research in gerontology draws on a variety of procedures. Primary among these are content analysis of documents and artifacts, including historical archival material; in-depth interviews; and ethnographic research based on participant observation. The chapters in this book illustrate these methods (with the exception of historical analysis). Here we will briefly discuss some literature in these categories, beginning with a brief mention of historical work on aging.

Nearly three decades ago Shanas (1960) called for empirical studies of family relations in the "good old days." Her call brought forth a spate of studies and stimulated interest in this subject. For example, Engler-Bowles and Kart (1983) showed that elderly people in colonial times were advised by clergy "to retain sufficient holdings to ensure their security in old age rather than depend on the benevolence of their children" (p. 167). Their presentation of a set of testaments challenges the stereotype of family relations in America's past (see also Haber, 1983). On the other hand, Arnett's (1985) study of historical records revealed Middle Eastern societies viewed old age as a reward for righteousness and piety, a belief that protected people in their old age. Such research requires empathy with the experience of deceased individuals in order to understand the meaning of their lives and the values of the world in which they lived.

Interpretive content analyses of contemporary sources include images of aging and the elderly in humor (Nahemow, McCluskey-Fawcett, & McGhee, 1986; Weber & Cameron, 1978), poems (Sohngen & Smith, 1978; Wilson, 1986), adolescent literature, prescription advertisements, and essays (Blythe, 1979; Hellebrandt, 1980; Saul, 1974). Individual experiences of old age have been explored in personal journals (Berman, 1985; see also Chapter 3 in this volume), letters, autobiographies, and memoirs (Macdonald & Rich, 1983; Straus, 1974). May Sarton's journals (1973, 1977, 1980, 1984), Alan Olmstead's (1975) account of retirement, and Joyce Horner's (1982) description of life in a nursing home are also useful exemplars (see also Scott-Maxwell, 1968; Straus, 1974; Truitt, 1982; and Vining, 1978). John Clausen (1986) offers an excellent discussion of ways to evaluate these materials and assess the influence of "retrospective falsification" (pp. 12–14).

A second procedure, the in-depth interview, has been popular in qualitative gerontology. Eva Salber's (1983) interviews of poor, rural elderly in North Carolina and Robert Coles's (1973) interviews of the elderly of New Mexico explore the meaning of these people's lives in their particular environments. Robert Rubinstein (1986) employed in-depth interviews to build a image of elderly men living alone. In this book, in addition to Rubinstein's contribution (Chapter 7), Helen Q. Kivnick (Chapter 4), Aluma K. Motenko (Chapter 6), and Sharon R. Kaufman (Chapter 5) rely heavily on interviewing individuals separately.

A major focus of many gerontological in-depth interview studies is recording life histories that place elderly people's experiences in holistic context (Frank & Vanderburgh, 1986). In a classic study based on group interviews, Barbara Myerhoff (1979) created living history "classes" so that elderly Jews at the Aliyah Senior Center in Venice, California, could teach her and each other about the meaning of their lives. In each of these studies the interviewer was able to act as a translator of the frequently taken-for-granted understanding of his or her subject and to communicate it to a larger audience. Great skill is needed to preserve not only the substance of what was communicated but also the aura of the context in which it was communicated.

A third procedure—ethnography—is based on participant observation supplemented by other methods. Ethnographic research requires that the researcher immerse him- or herself in the environment being studied, choosing from a continuum of options ranging from complete participant to complete observer (Gold, 1958). There has been an outpouring of ethnographic studies of aging since 1974, when Jerry Jacobs contended that:

> participant observer studies of the life styles of the aged, in conjunction with interviews of the aged in various social settings over time, are conspicuously absent. Without such descriptive material we cannot proceed scientifically, that is, describe and classify phenomena by their common characteristics so as to be able to link them conceptually into a consistent and parsimonious system of explanation that will provide for understanding, prediction and control (1974, pp. 72—73).

A complete participant design was undertaken by Adshead (1972), who pretended that he was a nursing home patient, and by Moore (1985), who disguised herself as an elderly woman. Some studies have had greater emphasis on *observation* than participation, e.g., Gubrium's

(1975) study of a nursing home and Matthews's (1982) of a transportation system for the elderly. Others have involved a greater degree of *participation*. These include ethnographic studies of senior centers, senior housing, retirement hotels (Stephens, 1976; Teski, 1979), retirement communities (Marshall, 1981), mobile home parks (Angrosino, 1976), urban neighborhoods (Rowles, 1978b; Vesperi, 1985; Zube, 1980), and rural settings (Lozier & Althouse, 1974, 1975; Rowles, 1980, 1983a, 1983b; Yearwood & Dressel, 1983).

This book includes examples from both ends of the observational continuum. Mary Ann Wilner's chapter on two support groups (Chapter 8), one for elderly persons and the other for caregivers in families with a member afflicted by Alzheimer's disease, is based exclusively on observation. Indeed, when at the end of her study she attempted to assume a more active participant role, she discovered that her involvement was disruptive. On the other hand, J. Kevin Eckert, in Chapter 13, explains how he became an active participant in the single room occupancy milieu he was studying, even working for a period as a desk clerk in one of the hotels. Perhaps the most intense form of participation is found in Kathleen I. MacPherson's chapter, where she describes her active involvement as a member of a menopause collective from its origins to the present (Chapter 10).

J. Kevin Eckert's chapter exemplifies yet another important characteristic of ethnographies—combining observation with other methods, such as interviews, surveys, and archival analysis. This integrated approach is apparent in Masako Osako's study of adjustment to old age of Japanese Americans living in Chicago. The study was based on:

> structured interviews of 46 Issei, questionnaire surveys with 50 Nisei, unstructured intensive interviews with 18 Japanese Americans from various age groups, and the author's participant observation in the community (Osako, 1979, p. 448).

Because of this approach, the author was able to support a conclusion that contradicted expectations. Middle-class, American-born children of Japanese parents did *not* become alienated from their lower-class, Japanese-born parents, who in turn did not suffer lowered status and reduced authority.

Some ethnographic studies have made a major contribution to theory building because they have incorporated a comparative design. These include Jules Henry's (1963) comparison of a nursing home with other institutions; Lee Bowker's (1983) comparison of four different nursing homes in the framework of Erving Goffman's work on total institutions and Abraham Maslow's work on the hierarchy of needs; Jeannie

Kayser-Jones's (1981) comparison of nursing homes in Scotland and the United States; and Nancy Foner's (1984) analysis of conflict between age groups. Perhaps the most ambitious use of ethnographies for comparative purposes is Donald Cowgill's *Aging Around the World* (1986). On the basis of his categorization of all the cultural descriptions at his disposal, he concluded that "demographic aging is correlated with other aspects of modernization, the combined effect of which is a lower value of elderly persons" (1986, p. 194). In this volume, Charlotte Ikels, Jennie Keith, and Christine L. Fry's contribution (Chapter 15) exemplifies this comparative ethnographic approach.

Our summary of qualitative procedures would not be complete if it did not mention the use of photography to capture and present vivid images of the aging experience (Sanderson, 1971; Jury & Jury, 1976). The Jurys' study of the aging and final days of their grandfather provides an extraordinary record of their encounter with the reality of dying.

Finally, although the focus of this book is on studies that deliberately set out to uncover aspects of aging and old age for theory development or for practice (Rouse, Griffith, Trachtman, & Winfield, 1986), useful material is sometimes embedded in research about other topics. This material may possess even greater validity than deliberate research on aging since no particular expectations about aging guided the researcher. In order that these serendipitous opportunities be utilized, it would be helpful if researchers developed an awareness of age and aging in whatever subject matter they study (Reinharz, 1987). For example, in Laud Humphreys's (1970) study of anonymous homosexual sex in public bathrooms, he noted that the relative age of the partners affects the role they play in the sexual activity, demonstrating a diminution of power with age. Similarly, Colin Turnbull's study of *The Mountain People* (1972) revealed what occurs in societies with extremely limited resources: adults with a greater potential for surviving abandon the elderly who are more likely to die, and they, in turn, being fully acculturated, expect this differentiation. They step aside, leaving room for others, perhaps as some retirees step aside for younger workers.

SPECIAL ISSUES IN QUALITATIVE RESEARCH INVOLVING THE ELDERLY

Although most of the illustrations in this chapter pertain to studies of the elderly, the themes developed apply to qualitative research with any age group. In this section we briefly discuss the relationship between gerontology and qualitative research (see also Covey, 1985). To what extent are qualitative studies particularly appropriate for studying the elderly? Does qualitative research generate any special practical problems when undertaken with the elderly? What, if any, are the ethical dilemmas when qualitative research is undertaken with the elderly? In answering these questions it is important to acknowledge the diversity of the elderly. The majority of old people are relatively healthy, alert, and active. However, particularly among the oldest old, increasing frailty becomes an important consideration in conducting qualitative research. Our focus in this discussion is on in-depth interviews with the frail elderly.

There are both advantages and difficulties in conducting in-depth interviews with elderly people. Advantages stem from the congruence between the aspirations of the qualitative researcher to develop rapport and the apparent psychological needs of many older people to review their lives, to educate the young, and to find companionship, particularly when significant others are no longer available. The interest older people have in recounting important experiences and lessons has been defined by Erik Erikson as a distinct psychosocial stage and elaborated by Robert Butler in his concept of the "life review" (Butler, 1963). Even without the presence of researchers, elderly people might write their memoirs either for family use or for publication (Baycrest Terrace Memoirs Group, 1979). Involvement with a qualitative researcher may reinforce this inclination. Indeed, elderly research participants may find special pleasure in examining photographs, treasured personal possessions, and other objects that remind them of the past and in sharing these with researchers interested in their lives (Sherman & Newman, 1977; Boschetti, 1984; Rowles, 1978b). If the older person has a less rigid schedule than do younger people, arrangements for such time-consuming interviews are facilitated. In addition, as noted earlier, older people seem to enjoy this type of interviewing. Similarly, many interviewers derive pleasure from this type of work and find that it reduces or eliminates prior negative conceptions about older people.

These positive aspects of qualitative research with the elderly are counterbalanced by a number of difficulties in undertaking such research, particularly with the frail elderly. First, it is now understood that there are numerous problems in obtaining samples of older research participants, regardless of whether the quest is for a random or purposive sample of older people (see Ward, 1984, pp. 16–17). For example, poverty affects the availability of telephones, and institutionalization affects the likelihood of organizational membership—both of which are typical sources of names for sampling. Zimmer, Calkins, Hadley, Ostfeld, Kay, and Kaye, (1985, p. 281) found that:

the older the group to be recruited, the less success can be expected. The National Center for Health Statistics reports participation rates of about 97% for children, 75% for persons aged 21 through 60, and less than 60% for persons over 60. The success of recruitment efforts, however, can be enhanced. Newspaper articles describing the project and its staff—with pictures if possible—often assure elderly persons that the project is sound and reputable. Older people often need time to decide to participate. Potential participants may be uncertain and often will refuse if pushed. Patience and explanation of the importance of the potential subject's specific contribution may yield positive results.

Reluctance to participate in qualitative research may be reinforced by practical constraints. If the research requires travel, lack of transportation may be an impediment. Elderly people who are incontinent or who have difficulty sitting for extended periods may be cautious about participating in studies that require lengthy time commitment.

Psychological barriers to participation may also be encountered. Some elderly people are uncomfortable with signed consent forms. Indeed, in his work with the Appalachian elderly Rowles (1980, 1983a, 1983b) found that elaborate explanation of human subjects protections and formal consent forms were confusing and apparently extraneous. The interpersonal orientation of Appalachian culture was such that characteristics of the researcher's lifestyle and family were far more important considerations in obtaining participation and gaining entry to the lifeworlds of the elderly than the provision of formal assurances (necessary as these may be).

Other elderly people may be reluctant to participate because they fear that they have nothing "scientific" to contribute. Indeed, the aura of formality implicit in the initial contact with an elderly research subject—the necessity of explaining the project in terms that may appear technical, the level of commitment implied in signing a consent form, and the fact that for many elderly participants, raised in a culture with a "white-coated scientist" image of research, this may be their first contact with investigators from a university or research institute—may serve as barriers to participation.

After elderly people have been recruited for research, there may be problems of comprehension if they are unfamiliar with qualitative research techniques. Since traditional surveys and standardized techniques are more familiar, the older person may feel uncomfortable and disconcerted by the risk of "exposure" implicit in an open-ended interview. Because of suspicion or closeness, there may be difficulties isolating the interviewee from co-residents, such as a spouse, offspring, or roommate (Gibson & Aitkenhead, 1983, p. 294). When the elderly person is poor or relatively powerless, "fear of revealing personal information may make the individual reluctant to answer questions" (Zimmer et al., 1985, p. 282) and may accentuate this problem.

Comprehension problems may occur because the researcher and the interviewee have different native languages or dialects and different levels of education. When interviewing a frail elderly subject, additional time must be allowed so that there is ample opportunity to respond in terms of language that is mutually understood and reflects a shared definition of the situation under study. The researcher may also have trouble understanding respondents whose health affects their speech. In her study of aging on the kibbutz, for example, Reinharz (in press) found that some elderly people had weak voices that did not register on a conventional tape-recorder. Similarly, the frail elderly research participant with vision, hearing, or cognitive deficits may have difficulty comprehending the researcher.

Problems can also occur on an emotional level. A young or middle-aged interviewer may feel reluctant to ask questions directly about a stigmatized identity—old age—in a conversational format. Asking the same questions formally might pose less difficulty (Covey, 1985). Some material is difficult to elicit from older people because they are ashamed of revealing it. For example,

> Because the issue of educational background was a sensitive one, we did not question the peer educators about their formal schooling, but through interactions with them during the program we learned that their education ranged from as little as five years of elementary school to completion of four years of college (Shannon, Smiciklas-Wright, Davis, & Lewis, 1983, p. 124).

On the other hand, if the elderly person has a great deal of prestige, the younger interviewee may feel intimidated and unable to sustain an in-depth interview.

Rapport may be difficult to establish because the interviewee sees the interviewer as "too young" or because the interviewer feels uncomfortable with the appearance of the old person. If the interviewer is young, fears may be evoked about his or her own aging. The loneliness of an elderly male interviewee may be expressed in advances of a sexual nature to a young female researcher. Transference and countertransference—for example, the interviewer's seeing the respondent as a parent or grandparent—may also complicate the interview process.

Interviewers of elderly people frequently find that contact and questions stir up emotions, both in themselves and in the person being interviewed.

A question such as "How are you today?" may be answered with an episode of crying or the response "How should I be?" followed by comments about a child or associate. Elderly subjects must be allowed to express themselves, although this may lengthen the schedule that the investigator has set. If the interview takes too long, the subject may have lapses in attention and difficulties in recall and may become disinterested (Zimmer et al., 1985, p. 282).

Other investigators have not found this to be the case (Gibson & Aitkenhead, 1983, p. 293; Rowles, 1978b). While elderly interviewees can be expected to tire more quickly than do younger people, fatigue may be an even greater problem for the qualitative interviewer who is likely to find "overcooperativeness" among elderly interviewees (Gibson & Aitkenhead, 1983, p. 294). In fact, Rowles (1978b, p. 62) found that one of his major field problems was extricating himself from interviews:

Time was precious. She had to tell all; and there was so much to tell. Leaving came to be quite a problem. There was always just one more story, one more anecdote, one more incident to recount. Sometimes I was obliged to beat a rather embarrassed undignified retreat. Four hours was all I could take.

Maintaining an adequate number of study participants is an issue of increased significance when studying the elderly because of increased morbidity and mortality. In addition to the emotional strain on the investigator who must adjust to the death of subjects (Myerhoff, 1979), research problems are intensified when, as in much qualitative research, the population studied comprises a small number of individuals or a small group. Emotional issues are heightened. Rowles described his torn feelings in such a situation:

I was embarrassed and I did not know what to say. I had not bargained for this kind of experience when my research started. As I sat by his bed, my mind would be a confusing welter of thoughts and emotions. Sometimes I experienced anger. "Damn it. You can't die now. I haven't finished my research." Immediately I would be overtaken by feelings of self revulsion. Did our friendship mean only this? Another time I toyed with the idea of continuing the research in the hospital—a tape from his bedside! For an instant it seemed an exciting possibility. Thus would I engage in the conflict between my human sensibilities and my scholarly purpose. The surprising outcome of this internal dialogue was that my work seemed less important, less significant in the overall scheme of things. I began to realize that my association with Stan had, in itself, been as important as the data I had derived from it (1978b, p. 19).

This example introduces an ethical dilemma, one of many that confront the qualitative researcher. In recent years increasing concern has been expressed about the ethics of clinical research with elderly subjects (Ratzan, 1980; Cassel, 1985a, 1985b; Melnick, Dubler, Weisbard, & Butler, 1984; Dubler, 1984; Reich, 1978). These dilemmas are accentuated in qualitative research. In particular, ethical issues are intensified in studies that focus on developing interpersonal relationships with elderly individuals.

If the researcher attempts to develop rapport so that the elderly person reveals his or her lifeworld, there is a danger of exploitation in a variety of guises. Many elderly persons are trusting and vulnerable, particularly in circumstances where the interview relationship appears to be reciprocal. One manifestation of exploitation is the implication that the research can be of assistance to the elderly interviewee. It is unethical to pretend or imply that one is offering support or therapy, or that participation in the research will somehow "help" the elderly person or her peers, when one is committed primarily to basic research (Butler, 1981; see also Ratzan, 1980, and Butler, 1980). On the other hand, it is possible to exploit a relationship by never allowing research participants to contribute without direct financial compensation or some other reward (Rowles, 1978a; Cassel, 1985a). As Cassel notes, in discussing the ethics of research with vulnerable institutionalized elderly populations:

> One of the problems of chronic and incurable disease is that we really don't have an existential explanation that gives people a meaning to their suffering if we can't cure it. One of the ways to give meaning to an experience is to make a person feel that he or she is participating in a human endeavor in which they are not alone. Many of the people who are resident in long-term care facilities like to feel that they are making some contribution to the future, to society, and give meaning to their remaining lives in this way. By refusing to do research in those settings, we deny them that option (1985a, p. 798).

The real dilemma here, of course, is making the judgment of what is exploitation and what is simply the expression of an authentic relationship. Ultimately, this is an issue of personal conscience and judgment.

The difficulty of making such judgments can be somewhat alleviated by an attitude of scrupulous honesty:

There is no place even for benign pretense. The purposes of the research, even if (to the researcher's embarrassment) they can be only vaguely articulated, must be communicated to prospective participants in language they have some likelihood of comprehending. Because such expression may be perceived as threatening or may result in failure to live up to the image of an "all-knowing" social scientist, this may mean difficulty in securing participants. But being honest extends beyond this. It involves developing authentic, often extremely complex, relationships in which mutual dependency may develop. In such relationships reciprocally expressed emotions ranging from love to disdain, from sympathy to anger may be manifest at various times (Rowles, 1978a, p. 189).

Problems of confidentiality are also exacerbated in qualitative interview research because of the intensity of the exchange. Indeed, its very success is likely to encourage the elderly participant to divulge information that might not otherwise be obtained. This increases the burden of responsibility on the researcher, particularly in situations where respondents are part of small and strongly interrelated networks. A seemingly minor indiscretion in inadvertently revealing information that was given with the implicit understanding of confidentiality can seriously jeopardize the integrity of a study and compromise the researcher.

Ethical dilemmas are compounded by the necessity for eventual withdrawal from relationships that may have become close. The problem may be particularly acute with regard to elderly people who have been discovered to have unmet needs or who may have come to rely upon the researcher as an integral component, perhaps the primary one, of their support network. This problem of "phasing" (Janes, 1961) is well illustrated in this volume in Robert L. Rubinstein's account of his ongoing relationship with one of his research participants following the completion of his scheduled interviews (Chapter 7). The demands and obligations of the relationship do not cease once the data have been obtained.

Significant ethical issues are also involved in the use and publication of the findings. These extend beyond questions of confidentiality. Clearly, a degree of anonymity can be preserved through employing pseudonyms, as the authors in many chapters in this volume have done. But there is danger as well in romanticizing the research relationship and thereby distorting the "text" of the exchange.

A particularly difficult aspect of the publication of findings is connected to the issue of representativeness. It is difficult to ascertain the degree to which the results of research represent the elderly population or merely a component of this population (Levine, 1982). The ethical dilemma here lies not merely in the degree to which the studied population is representative in a statistical sense, but rather in the degree to which readers of the report will attribute the findings to the elderly population in general, regardless of technical caveats included in the text. Stereotypes about the homogeneity of the elderly may stand in the way of interpreting qualitative data. As Zimmer and associates found (1985, p. 281):

> The elderly consist of a heterogeneous population (more so than other age groups) with great differences in physical and mental status. Therefore, unless investigators carefully define the study population, the many variables among the elderly population will make interpretation of data difficult.

Serious ethical dilemmas may also result from accurate portrayal. To be truthful may be harmful when it exposes individual vulnerability or when it results in insights that may be disadvantageous to respondents (for example, if research reveals that particular benefits accruing to an elderly population are, in fact, unnecessary). Here we confront the dilemma of reconciling what is desirable on a macro or policy level and what is optimal from the perspective of individual study participants. As Becker (1964) has noted, there is always a measure of "irreducible conflict." In qualitative research this conflict is intensified by the intimacy of relationships with research participants. The ambiguity of roles as both researcher and confidant, scholar and friend, is a price that must be paid.

QUALITATIVE GERONTOLOGY IN PERSPECTIVE

With the increase in the aged population of the United States, it is not surprising that social gerontological research has flourished (Shock, 1982). Drawing on the major paradigms of social science, this research has been conducted within the entire gamut of research strategies and the entire range of disciplines. It is our contention that to improve our understanding of the aging process and the lives of the elderly, we must draw on the widest possible array of methods and disciplines. To highlight this point, we have invited chapters from sociologists, anthropologists, psychologists, nurses, policy analysts, and social workers, as well as people who identify themselves as gerontologists. Our own training is in geography and in sociology.

Surprisingly, although there is a strong and long tradition of qualitative research (Tesch, 1985), the distinctiveness of this methodology in gerontology has not yet been discussed in depth. In some instances, when the methodology of gerontological research is defined, qualitative methods are completely overlooked. For example, an excellent classic article on research methods in gerontology, James E. Birren's "Principles of Research on Aging" (1959), contains no suggestions concerning qualitative research. It has almost been necessary for each cohort of social scientists to rediscover the qualitative tradition anew.

Our intent is to fill this gap and draw attention to the potential of qualitative gerontology. To achieve this objective we have collected a set of highly diversified original chapters that present examples of this type of research. The chapters are arranged in the order that parallels the increasing set of cases the author studied. In addition, we have asked three distinguished individuals to comment on issues raised in the chapters to take us one stage further. In a sense, each of these people is a pioneer. Anselm Strauss, a pioneer in defining the inductive method in social research and providing a theoretical framework for qualitative research, stresses the need for emphasis upon qualitative data analysis and theory development. David Gutmann, a pioneer in doing cross-cultural developmental research and in understanding the potential for change in elderly people, focuses on legitimacy and the role of the stranger in qualitative research. Betty Friedan, a pioneer in defining women's experience who has now turned to studying the elderly, considers the potential of qualitative gerontology for confronting the "age mystique."

Neither the authors nor the commentators subscribe to a uniform point of view. They illustrate that qualitative gerontology has a wide range of practitioners who have not adopted a rigid set of methodological criteria. In part, this is because these researchers are highly attuned to the way their research topics affect the methods they use. For many of them qualitative research is a personal style, an attitude, a way of being in which the boundary between self and scholar is blurred. We, too, are not interested in creating a new orthodoxy for qualitative gerontology. Instead, we hope that this book will give added impetus to the tradition and resurgence of qualitative gerontological research and will serve as a resource both to new researchers and to other more experienced scholars. Most important, we hope that future qualitative gerontological research will lead to a deepening understanding of the lifeworlds of individuals like Jennifer-Rose and of the social and political processes that condition their experience.

REFERENCES

Adshead, F. (1972). *Patient life in a nursing home: An experiential study*. Unpublished doctoral dissertation. University of Southern California, Los Angeles.

Agar, M. (1980). *The professional stranger: An informal introduction to ethnography*. New York: Academic Press.

Angrosino, M. (1976). Anthropology and the aged: A preliminary community study. *The Gerontologist, 16*(2), 174–180.

Arnett, W. S. (1985). Only the bad died young in the ancient Middle East. *International Journal of Aging and Human Development, 21*(2), 155–160.

Bart, P. (1975). Emotional and social status of the older woman. In *No longer young—The older woman in America. Proceedings of the 26th Annual Conference on Aging, Institute of Gerontology, Ann Arbor, MI* (pp. 3–21). University of Michigan/Wayne State University.

Baycrest Terrace Memoirs Group. (1979). *From our lives: Memoirs, life stories, episodes and recollections*. Oakville, Ontario: Mosaic Press.

Becker, H. S. (1958). Problems of inference and proof in participant observation. *American Sociological Review, 23*, 652–660.

Becker, H. S. (1964). Problems in the publication of field studies. In A.J. Vidich, J. Bensman, & M.R. Stein (Eds.), *Reflections on community studies* (pp. 267–284). New York: John Wiley and Sons.

Becker, H. S. (1977). On methodology. In *Sociological work: Method and substance* (pp. 3–24). New Brunswick, NJ: Transaction Books.

Berman, H. J. (1985, November). *Admissible evidence: Geropsychology and the intimate journal*. Paper presented at the 38th Annual Scientific Meeting of the Gerontological Society of America, New Orleans, LA.

Bigus, O. E., Hadden, S. C., & Glaser, B. G. (1982). Basic social processes. In R. B. Smith & P. K. Manning (Eds.), *A handbook of social science methods: Vol. 2. Qualitative methods* (pp. 251–272). Cambridge, MA: Ballinger.

Birren, J. E. (1959). Principles of research on aging. In J. E. Birren (Ed.), *Handbook of aging and the individual* (pp. 3–24). Chicago: University of Chicago Press.

Blumer, H. (1969). *Symbolic interactionism: Perspective and method*. Englewood Cliffs, NJ: Prentice-Hall.

Blythe, R. (1979). *The view in winter: Reflections on old age*. New York: Harcourt Brace Jovanovich.

Bogdan, R., & Taylor, S. J. (1975). *Introduction to qualitative research methods*. New York: Wiley Interscience.

Boschetti, M. A. (1984). *The older person's emotional attachment to the physical environment of the residential setting*. Unpublished doctoral dissertation, University of Michigan, Ann Arbor.

Bowker, L. (1983). *Humanizing institutions for the aged*. Lexington, MA: Lexington Books.

Burgess, R. (Ed.). (1982). *Field research: A sourcebook and field manual*. Boston: George Allen and Unwin.

Butler, R. N. (1963). The life review: An interpretation of reminiscence in the aged. *Psychiatry, 26*, 55–76.

Butler, R. N. (1969). Age-ism: Another form of bigotry. *The Gerontologist, 9*, 243–246.

Butler, R. N. (1980). Protection of the elderly research subject. *Clinical Research,* *281,* 3–5.

Butler, R. N. (1981). What's best for the elderly research subject? *The Hastings Center Report,* Volume 15, p. 45.

Carp, F. M., & Kataoka, E. (1976). Health care problems of the elderly of San Francisco's Chinatown. *The Gerontologist, 16*(1), 30–38.

Cassel, C. K. (1985a). Research in nursing homes: Ethical issues. *Journal of the American Geriatrics Society, 33*(11), 795–799.

Cassel, C. K. (1985b). Research in geriatrics. *Generations, 8,* 45–48.

Charmaz, K. (1983). The grounded theory method: An explication and interpretation. In R. Emerson (Ed.), *Contemporary field research* (pp. 109–126). Boston: Little, Brown.

Clark, M., & Anderson, B. (1967). *Culture and aging: An anthropological study of older Americans.* Springfield, IL: Charles C. Thomas.

Clausen, J. (1986). *The life course: A sociological perspective.* Englewood Cliffs, NJ: Prentice-Hall.

Coles, R. (1973). *The old ones of New Mexico.* Albuquerque: University of New Mexico Press.

Connidis, I. (1983). Integrating qualitative and quantitative methods in survey research on aging: An assessment. *Qualitative Sociology, 6*(4), 334–352.

Cottle, T. (1980). *Hidden survivors: Portraits of poor Jews in America.* Englewood Cliffs, NJ: Prentice-Hall.

Covey, H. C. (1985). Qualitative research of older people: Some considerations. *Gerontology and Geriatrics Education, 5*(3), 41–50.

Cowgill, D. (1986). *Aging around the world.* Belmont, CA: Wadsworth.

Dubler, N. N. (1984). The ethics of research. *Generations, 8,* 18–21.

Eckert, J. K. (1980). *The unseen elderly.* San Diego, CA: Campanile Press.

Emerson, R. (Ed.). (1983). *Contemporary field research.* Boston: Little, Brown.

Engler-Bowles, C. A., & Kart, C. S. (1983). Intergenerational relations and testamentary patterns: An exploration. *The Gerontologist, 23*(2), 167–173.

Erikson, K. (1976). *Everything in its path.* New York: Simon and Schuster.

Foner, N. (1984). *Ages in conflict: A cross-cultural perspective on inequality between old and young.* New York: Columbia University Press.

Frank, G., & Vanderburgh, R. M. (1986). Cross cultural use of life-history methods in gerontology. In C. L. Fry & J. Keith (Eds.), *New methods for old age research* (pp. 185–207). South Hadley, MA: Bergin and Garvey.

Fry, C. L., & Keith, J. (1986). *New methods for old age research.* South Hadley, MA: Bergin and Garvey.

Gadamer, H. G. (1975). *Truth and method.* New York: Seabury Press.

Geertz, C. (1973). *The interpretation of cultures.* New York: Basic Books.

Gibson, D. M., & Aitkenhead, W. (1983). The elderly respondent: Experiences from a large-scale survey of the aged. *Research on Aging, 5*(2), 283–296.

Glaser, B. G., & Strauss, A. L. (1967). *The discovery of grounded theory.* Chicago: Aldine.

Gold, R. L. (1958). Roles in sociological field observations. *Social Forces, 36,* 217–223.

Goodwin, L., & Goodwin, W. (1984). Qualitative vs. quantitative research or qualitative and quantitative research? *Nursing Research, 33*(6), 378–380.

Gould, M. (Ed.). (1985). *Innovative sources and uses of qualitative data* (Special Issue). *Qualitative Sociology, 8*(4).

Gubrium, J. F. (1975). *Living and dying at Murray Manor*. New York: St. Martin's Press.

Haber, C. (1983). *Beyond sixty-five: The dilemma of old age in America's past*. New York: Cambridge University Press.

Hayes, A. (1985). Causal and interpretive analysis in sociology. *Sociological Theory, 3*(2), 1–10.

Hellebrandt, F. A. (1980). Aging among the advantaged: A new look at the stereotype of the elderly. *The Gerontologist, 20*(4), 404–417.

Hendricks, J., & Hendricks, C. D. (1986). *Aging in mass society: Myths and realities*. 3rd ed. Boston: Little, Brown and Company.

Henry, J. (1963). *Culture against man*. New York: Random House.

Hochschild, A. R. (1973). *The unexpected community*. Englewood Cliffs, NJ: Prentice-Hall.

Horner, J. (1982). *That time of year: A chronicle of life in a nursing home*. Amherst, MA: University of Massachusetts Press.

Humphreys, L. (1970). *Tearoom trade: Impersonal sex in public places*. New York: Aldine.

Jackson, J. S., Tucker, M. B., & Bowman, P. J. (1982). Conceptual and methodological problems in survey research on black Americans. In W. T. Liu (Ed.), *Methodological problems in minority research* (pp. 11–39). (Occasional Paper No. 7). Pacific/Asian American Mental Health Research Center.

Jacobs, J. (1974). *Fun city: An ethnographic study of a retirement community*. New York: Holt, Rinehart & Winston.

Jacobs, R. (1976). Typology of older American women. *Social Policy, 7*(3), 34–39.

Janes, R. W. (1961). A note on the phases of the community role of the participant observer. *American Sociological Review, 26*, 446–450.

Jury, M., & Jury, D. (1976). *Gramp*. New York: Grossman.

Kanter, R., & Stein, B. (1980). *A tale of O*. New York: Harper & Row.

Kayser-Jones, J. (1981). *Old, alone and neglected: Care of the aged in Scotland and the United States*. Berkeley, CA: University of California Press.

Keller, E. F. (1985). *Reflections on gender and science*. New Haven, CT: Yale University Press.

Kubler-Ross, E. (1969). *On death and dying*. New York: Macmillan.

Levine, E. K. (1982). Old people are not all alike: Social class, ethnicity/race, and sex are bases for important differences. In J. E. Sieber (Ed.), *The ethics of social research surveys and experiments* (pp. 125–143). New York: Springer-Verlag.

Lofland, J. (1971). *Analyzing social settings*. Belmont, CA: Wadsworth.

Lofland, J., & Lofland, L. (1984). *Analyzing social settings: A guide to qualitative observation and analysis*. Belmont, CA: Wadsworth.

Loomis, M., & Williams, T. F. (1983). Evaluation of care provided to terminally ill patients. *The Gerontologist, 23*(5), 493–499.

Lozier, J., & Althouse, R. (1974). Social enforcement of behavior toward elders in an Appalachian mountain settlement. *The Gerontologist, 14*(1), 69–80.

Lozier, J., & Althouse, R. (1975). Retirement to the porch in rural Appalachia. *International Journal of Aging and Human Development, 6*(1), 7–15.

Maas, J. (1980). *Fifteen past seventy: Counsel from my elders*. Berkeley: Shameless Hussy Press.

MacDonald, B., & Rich, C. (1983). *Look me in the eye: Women, aging and ageism*. San Francisco: Spinsters, Ink.

Marshall, V. W. (1980). Participant observation in a multiple methods study of a retirement community: A research narrative. *Mid-American Review of Sociology, 11,* 29–44.

Maslow, A. H. (1966). *The psychology of science: A reconnaissance.* Chicago: Henry Regnery.

Matthews, S. (1982). Participation of the elderly in a transportation system. *The Gerontologist, 22*(1), 26–31.

Melnick, V. L., Dubler, N. N., Weisbard, A., & Butler, R. N. (1984). Clinical research in senile dementia of the Alzheimer's type: Suggested guidelines addressing the ethical and legal issues. *Journal of the American Geriatrics Society, 32*(7), 531–536.

Mendelson, M. A. (1975). *Tender loving greed.* New York: Vintage Books.

Miles, M. B., & Huberman, A. M. (1984). *Qualitative data analysis.* Beverly Hills, CA: Sage.

Moore, P. A. (1985). *Disguised.* Waco, TX: Word Books.

Myerhoff, B. (1979). *Number our days.* New York: Dutton.

Nahemow, L., McCluskey-Fawcett, K. A., & McGhee, P. E. (Eds.). (1986). *Humor and aging.* New York: Academic Press.

Neugarten, B. L., Wood, V., Kraines, R. J., & Loomis, B. (1968). Women's attitudes toward the menopause. In B. L. Neugarten (Ed.), *Middle age and aging: A reader in social psychology.* (pp. 195–200). Chicago: University of Chicago Press.

Neugarten, B. (1985). Interpretive social science and research on aging. In A. Rossi (Ed.), *Gender and the life course* (pp. 291–300). New York: Aldine.

Olmstead, A. (1975). *Threshold: The first days of retirement.* New York: Harper & Row.

Osako, M. (1979). Aging and family among Japanese Americans: The role of ethnic tradition in the adjustment to old age. *The Gerontologist, 19*(5), 448–455.

Ratzan, R. (1980). Being old makes you different: The ethics of research with elderly subjects. *Hastings Center Report, 44,* 32–42.

Reich, W. T. (1978). Ethical issues related to research involving elderly subjects. *The Gerontologist, 18*(4), 326–336.

Reinharz, S. (1983a). Experiential analysis: A contribution to feminist research. In G. Bowles & R. Duelli-Klein (Eds.), *Theories of women's studies* (pp. 162–191). Boston: Routledge and Kegan Paul.

Reinharz, S. (1983b). Phenomenology as a dynamic process. *Phenomenology and Pedagogy, 1*(1), 77–79.

Reinharz, S. (1984). *On becoming a social scientist: From survey research and participant observation to experiential analysis.* New Brunswick, NJ: Transaction Books.

Reinharz, S. (in press). *Aging on the kibbutz.* Chicago: University of Chicago Press.

Reinharz, S. (1987). The embeddedness of age: Toward a social control perspective. *Journal of Aging Studies, 1*(1), 77–93.

Riley, M., Johnson, M. M., & Foner, A. (Eds.). (1972). *Aging and society: Vol. 3. A sociology of age stratification.* New York: Russell Sage.

Ross, J. K. (1977). *Old people, new lives: Community creation in a retirement residence.* Chicago: University of Chicago Press.

Rouse, D., Griffith, J., Trachtman, L., & Winfield, D. (1986). Aid for memory impaired older persons: Wandering notification. *Report of a Needs Assessment and Feasibility Study.* Research Triangle Park, NC: Research Triangle Institute.

Rowles, G. D. (1978a). Reflections on experiential fieldwork. In D. Ley & M. Samuels (Eds.), *Humanistic geography: Prospects and problems* (pp. 173–193). New York: John Wiley.

Rowles, G. D. (1978b). *Prisoners of space? Exploring the geographical experience of older people.* Boulder, CO: Westview Press.

Rowles, G. D. (1980). Growing old 'inside': Aging and attachment to place in an Appalachian community. In N. Datan & N. Lohmann (Eds.), *Transitions of aging* (pp. 153–170). New York: Academic Press.

Rowles, G. D. (1983a). Place and personal identity in old age: Observations from Appalachia. *Journal of Environmental Psychology, 3,* 299–313.

Rowles, G. D. (1983b). Between worlds: A relocation dilemma for the Appalachian elderly. *International Journal of Aging and Human Development, 17*(4), 301–314.

Rubinstein, R. L. (1986). *Singular paths: Old men living alone.* New York: Columbia University Press.

Rybash, J. M., Roodin, P. A., & Hoyer, W. J. (1983). Expressions of moral thought in later adulthood. *The Gerontologist, 23*(3), 254–260.

Salber, E. (1983). *Don't send me flowers when I'm dead: Voices of rural elderly.* Durham, NC: Duke University Press.

Sanderson, C. A. L. (1971). The week after next . . . *The Gerontologist, 11*(2), 1–58.

Sarton, M. (1973). *Journal of a solitude.* New York: Norton.

Sarton, M. (1977). *A house by the sea: A journal.* New York: Norton.

Sarton, M. (1980). *Recovering: A journal.* New York: Norton.

Sarton, M. (1984). *At seventy: A journal.* New York: Norton.

Saul, S. (1974). *Aging: An album of people growing old.* New York: John Wiley and Sons.

Scheper-Hughes, N. (1981). Dilemmas in deinstitutionalization: A view from inner city Boston. *Journal of Operational Psychology, 12*(2), 90–99.

Schwartz, H., & Jacobs, J. (1979). *Qualitative sociology: A method to the madness.* New York: Free Press.

Scott-Maxwell, F. (1968). *The measure of my days.* New York: Penguin.

Shanas, E. (1960). Family responsibility and the health of older people. *Journal of Gerontology, 15,* 408–411.

Shannon, B. M., Smiciklas-Wright, H., Davis, B., & Lewis, C. (1983). A peer educator approach to nutrition for the elderly. *The Gerontologist, 23*(2), 123–126.

Sheehan, S. (1984). *Kate Quinton's days.* New York: New American Library.

Sherman, E., & Newman, E. S. (1977). The meaning of cherished personal possessions for the elderly. *International Journal of Aging and Human Development, 8,* 181–192.

Shields, L. (1981). *Displaced homemakers: Organizing for a new life.* New York: McGraw-Hill.

Shock, N. (1982). Historical perspectives: United States. In W. Edwards & F. Flynn (Eds.), *Gerontology: A cross-national core list of significant works* (pp. 27–39). Ann Arbor, MI: Institute of Gerontology, University of Michigan.

Silverman, D. (1985). *Qualitative methodology and sociology.* Brookfield, VT: Gower.

Smith, K., & Bengtson, V. (1979). Positive consequences of institutionalization: Solidarity between elderly parents and their middle-aged children. *The Gerontologist, 19*(5), 438–447.

Sohngen, M., & Smith, R. J. (1978). Images of old age in poetry. *The Gerontologist, 18*(2), 181–185.

Sommers, T. (1976). *Aging in America: Implications for women* (Report No. 9). Washington, DC: National Council on Aging.

Sontag, S. (1979). The double standard of aging. In J.H. Williams (Ed.), *Psychology of women: Selected readings* (pp. 462–478). New York: Norton.

Stephens, J. (1976). *Loners, losers, and lovers.* Seattle: University of Washington Press.

Straus, R. (1974). *Escape from custody.* New York: Harper & Row.

Streib, G. (1983). The frail elderly: Research dilemmas and research opportunities. *The Gerontologist, 23,* 40–44.

Tesch, R. (1985). *Human science research bibliography.* Santa Barbara, CA: Dr. Renata Tesch, P.O. Box 30070.

Teski, M. (1979). *Living together: An ethnography of a retirement hotel.* Washington, DC: University Press of America.

Trost, J. E. (1986). Statistically nonrepresentative stratified sampling: A sampling technique for qualitative studies. *Qualitative Sociology, 9*(1), 54–57.

Truitt, A. (1982). *Daybook.* New York: Penguin.

Turnbull, C. (1972). *The mountain people.* New York: Simon and Schuster.

Unruh, D. R. (1983). *Invisible lives: Social worlds of the aged.* Beverly Hills, CA: Sage.

Van Maanen, J. (1983). Epilogue: Qualitative methods reclaimed. In J. Van Maanen (Ed.), *Qualitative methodology* (pp. 247–268). Beverly Hills, CA: Sage.

Vesperi, M. D. (1985). *City of green benches: Growing old in a new downtown.* Ithaca, NY: Cornell University Press.

Vining, E. (1978). *Being seventy: The measure of a year.* New York: Viking Press.

Von Eckartsberg, R. (1971). On experiential methodology. In A. Georgi, W. F. Fischer, and R. Von Eckartsberg (Eds.), *Duquesne studies in phenomenological psychology* (Vol. 1). Pittsburgh, PA: Duquesne University Press/Humanities Press.

Ward, R. (1984). *The aging experience* (2nd ed.). New York: Harper & Row.

Webb, E. J., Campbell, D. T., Schwartz, R. D., & Sechrest, L. (1966). *Unobtrusive measures: Nonreactive research in the social sciences.* Chicago: Rand McNally.

Weber, T., & Cameron, P. (1978). Comment: Humor and aging—A response. *The Gerontologist, 18*(1), 73–79.

Wilner, P. (1985). The main unit of sociology between 1936 and 1982. *History of Sociology, 5*(2), 1–20.

Wilson, R. N. (1986). Review essay: For which the first was made? Poetic reflections on the last of life. *The Gerontologist, 26*(4), 457–458.

Yearwood, A., & Dressel, P. (1983). Interracial dynamics in a southern rural senior center. *The Gerontologist, 23*(5), 512–517.

Zimmer, A., Calkins, E., Hadley, E., Ostfeld, A., Kay, J., & Kaye, D. (1985). Conducting clinical research in geriatric populations. *Annals of Internal Medicine, 103,* 276–283.

Zube, M. (1980). Outlook on being old: Working class elderly in Northampton, MA. *The Gerontologist, 20*(4), 427–431.

2

(Exit with Thunder)

Robert Kastenbaum

Which door shall we enter? The Laboratory of Extremely Scientific Gerontology is on our right (stage left), just past the bulletin board dressed with notices for technical conferences and impending grant deadlines. Down (up stage) the poorly lit stairs a faded sign confesses that here is to be found the Lost Souls Repertory Theater. Not much of a choice, is it? Drama has had its long day in the sun. Waste no tears for its present stumbling-fumbling-in-the-dark status. Sophocles, Shakespeare, and Company provided quite a diversion and something of an education for people denied the blessing of science and technology. Now, however, drama must be content with the bit role of entertainer. The new day belongs to Science, that laser-eyed deity whose mainframe never sleeps.

The choice becomes even more obvious if our mission is to seek knowledge of a gerontologic kind. Multivariate statistical techniques appear so much better suited to examining the complexities of age-related phenomena than, say, some old-timer careening through a fake storm and shouting: "Rumble thy bellyful! Spit, fire! Spout, rain! Nor rain, wind, thunder, fire, are my daughters; I tax not you, you elements, with unkindness; I never gave you kingdom, call'd you children" (*King Lear*, Act II, Scene II).

And so we enter the Laboratory of Extremely etc. Here refuge shall be found from rant and rhetoric. Here shall be found—but soft! The door slides open, the electronic sentry encodes us, and we are whisked silent inside.

TOUR #7

I am, like, your guide, like. This is Tour #7, isn't it? Professor Numba is still at crunch, so I'll sort of show you around. You have any questions, just—oh, by the way, don't touch anything that's purple or vibrating, OK?

This here's the library. Huh? *This.* Yeah, this computer display. We had some books once. Well, anyhow, when you need the lit review section for a grant proposal or manuscript, you just cue up anything you need. It's real keen. Anybody wanna suggest a topic? Exercise? Sure. Zippo—"McDonald, R., Hegenauer, J., & Saltman, P. Age-related Differences in the Bone Mineralization Pattern of Rats Following Exercise," *Journal of Gerontology,* (July), 1986, Vol. 41, No. 4, 445–453." How do you—what? Get the article itself? I don't know about that. All we usually need is the reference for where you need references. But you *can* get the abstract, if you're a real fanatic about reading and all.

Now this is something real interesting. Before we go in, let me ask you: anybody here have strong feelings about nuclear disarmament? You all do, huh? That's great. No—I don't want to hear them. OK. Now I'll open it up and you can step inside, one at a time, and just for a moment, OK? Watch your head. Yeah, it buzzes some, but don't worry. OK, everybody's been in who wants to go in? OK, now let me ask you again: what do you think about nuclear disarmament? Really? You don't much care? You, too? How about global meltdown? Doesn't mean a thing to any of you, one way or the other! Well, so that's our little Objectification Chamber. Not the latest model, but it does the job. Yeah, the effects wear off, that's why we quantitates have booster shots on a regular basis. I put it on the lowest setting for you, so you'll probably have all your raging and irrational opinions back before you leave.

You've heard about this next one, huh? I can't let you in the main chamber—strict rule. But just a sec, let me check the schedule. Yeah, OK. There'll be a "procedure" in a moment. We can all go up to the Observers' Ring. Step over here. Now everybody bunch up inside the red circle. Here we go—up and up! Just scrunch a little to the left and you'll find a place to sit in the OR. It's OK to talk; we're soundproofed up here. Here come the subjects. A lot of them, yeah. You wouldn't believe how many we can squeeze in. And here comes their furniture. Their dogs, their cats . . . that's right, everybody's making themselves real comfortable, just like in their own homes. I guess in the old days, before the Lab, gerontologists would have to deal with all this slop. Watch the big dial, the countdown, 5-4-3-2-blippo! Really something, huh? What? No, that sound's normal. Guess you never heard real number-crunching. The people? Yeah, they're gone all right! And all the sloppy-glop with them. Our computers don't care much for nuances, interactions, expectations, intentions, and all that gunk that holds individual lives together. You know what this computer operation costs and you don't want to cause indigestion! OK, everybody out! Bunch together in the circle, down we go!

So what did you think of the Decontextualization Chamber? Makes people subjects, then sort of harvests the data from them—only, by the time the computer starts crunching, there's no "them" left, just shiny, clean little bitties. But my favorite is down that corridor. I don't know if I'm supposed to show it to you, but what the—hey! Didn't I tell you not to touch anything that's purple or vibrating! Just leave the body there; the crew will sweep through in a few minutes . . . OK. There's no procedure right now for the FNTM Chamber, but you can see it and I'll try to cue up some data for you . . . Now this is just standard archival data. Nothing special is happening here; we're just watching some subjects grow up and grow old and at this check point—and this one— and this—we do a data harvest. OK. I'll keep that sequence going and add this one. You recognize it, huh? Another cohort, moving through its ordinary time line. Pretty boring, right? But, as you can see, we have the makings here of a time-lag design.

The fun begins when we make the first transformation. Here, why don't one of you give one of these lower dials a twist, not much. Zowie! Yeah, that's the technical name for it, a Zowie, the basic, most primitive FNTM. Sort of like the old graces, cherubims, seraphims, whatevers on their own little celestial levels. You can see the Zowie is a first-order product. It emerges from a statistical interaction between subjects in Sequence A and subjects in Sequence B. Sometimes I get blank looks when I explain this. But you follow, right? The Zowie is what you get when you take the *differences* between one cohort and another in a time-lag type of design. You don't need the real subjects much after that; it's like a further step in decontextualization, first the person is gone— foof!—and then even the isolated, quantified, worked-up data are replaced by a something that never was. It's only the very best and most expensive research that can accomplish this. Almost every gerontologist's ideal—every *real* gerontologist's ideal—is to replace people with subjects and subjects with Zowies, if not with even more evolved FNTMs. Anybody here can't see the advantage? The Zowie overcomes the limitations of ordinary people who either are harvested cross-sectionally or longitudinally, and therefore vulnerable to time-sensitive errors. Time of birth. Time of measurement. All that stuff. The Zowie moves through time, uhm, more purely, real delicate . . . like a phantom.

The more advanced stuff—oh-oh, is that Professor Cruncher coming? Maybe I shouldn't be telling you all this. Well, real quick—look here. Nesselchaie and those guys left off with the Zowie. We do them a lot better with the FNTM Chamber. Objectification, Decontextualization, and the creation of the Zowie still leave some contingencies uncontrolled. Like take for example the direction of time. How do we know if from 40 to 80 is aging, or just 40 years? What you need to do is get another group going from 80 to 40. This idea sounds real obvious now, but it was a long time in coming, and then designing the chamber was just technicalities. We can now create all kinds of FNTMs. They can be custom-designed to overcome any time-sensitive problem. What freedom! Gerontological science is no longer dependent upon actual people mucking along on a single track through their lives. Here at the Lab we can create, raise, and harvest FNTMs like you wouldn't believe.

You wanted Science? I've shown you Science! Oh, good morning, Professor. The tour was just leaving!

THE LOWER DEPTHS

Impressive, no? A courtesy call upon the Lost Souls Repertory Theater might not be amiss, however. The contrast can only heighten our appreciation for the Lab of Extremely etc., and those forsaken wretches in the theater dote upon any company. Watch your step, please, the stairs are not in the best of repair.

Ah! Lear, the King?

"Ah, quite! Quite mistaken, most excellent rogue."

But I saw you as Lear, the King!

"Sir Toby, the Belch this day or, rather, this *Twelfth Night*. The emblem a tilt yon door does bespeak a repertory company, or I am bond-slave to a turnip and consanguineous with an ass."

You mean that yesterday's tragic king is today confined to—

"Confine! I'll confine myself no finer than I am: These clothes are good enough to drink in; and so be these boots too; and they be not, let them hang themselves by their own straps."

Belch, then. We are seekers of gerontologic truth and fresh from an enlightening tour of the Laboratory. Admittedly, we were much impressed. No doubt you have a more critical view, so we would like to give you the opportunity to—

"Reason, you rogue, reason! The Laboratory of Extremely Scientific Gerontology is neither a sword to this tender throat nor a foul vapor to this fair nose. A brave frolic, think ye instead!"

You actually *like* the Lab?

"Like? Where is the like to be discovered? Certainly not in our dottering scripts, mincing pantomimes, and creaking stage-craft. Science has become the very monster of sweet intervention! Look ye beyond the Bard, past Ibsen, below Beckett, above Albee, aslant Ionesco! Tell me who whence and where looms the like in bold dramatic conception? Off and off and yet off Broadway spy unto me a theater so absurdist, so bizarred, so brutish that it holds to the glory of the Laboratory the frailest taper?"

You see gerontologic science, then, as having some theatrical aspects?

"O peace, little villain. It *is* theater. A world to and of itself, substituting for quality, number; for continuity, correlation; for the free play of passion and intellect, the vise of experimental control which is nought but the versa of life untrammeled. Screw your own brain-pan to the test: reflect upon the selectivity of dramatic representation, unless the bowels of your mind be constipated by the feckless ingestion of inert facts."

Well, yes, dramatic representation *is* selective. We are shown only a few moments, a few situations. The rest we take on faith. A messenger rushes in to announce that the ship has been lost at sea. We assume the ship, the sea, and the bubbles rising. But we also assume that a multitude of prosaic events occur off-stage. The governor's wife sleeps off the night before. The dashing lieutenant takes a leak. The prime suspect has a continuous existence between Acts I and III, although we see him only on widely scattered occasions.

"A fine simmering indeed! From the most unlikely pans may issue the most savory stews! How now does gerontologic science raise to a new height the principle of selectivity?"

I guess that's really what the Lab is all about. The Decontextualization Chamber reduces people to vapors that are then distilled and quantitated. The process is taken even further in the FNTM Chamber, where vapors are so transformed and mixed that the original subject becomes a most distant ancestor to the data. By this point, the abstracted numbers no longer have much relationship to "real people." From the most sophisticated, rigorously controlled, and ingeniously analyzed studies emerge data that are not about real people at all. I must agree, this is a stroke of dramatic genius: a script without characters! A tale told by a—

"Enough! That's one of my lines! More to the nub, the Laboratory does *not* tell a tale 'full of sound and fury.' Where, pray tell, is the impulse? The struggle? The conflict? The situation and the stake?"

You've got me there. Situationality is ignored by most gerontologic research of a quantitative persuasion. The curtain does not rise on people embedded in the particularities of their own lives. We do not see them jockey for advantage and attempt to balance one need or motive against the other. There is no drama at all unless there is something at stake, and there is little drama unless there is strife and complexity between characters as well. We, the audience, get hooked on a real drama because it speaks to our own wishes, fears, and conflicts. The most banal claptrap claims our attention if only it offers a dash of menace, a clash of will, a tensioning toward climax and resolution.

"Cheap-penny indeed are the dramatical devices set to snare the all-too-eager prey. But in Science what majesty! In this lofty realm—two floors up, as it were—there is no petty play of passing passions, nor plodding plots with prattle pleated. Here, indeed, drama has its own head o'er leaped, becoming more than its self, or Self self-transcendentalified! Tragedy and Comedy, the twinned masks, slip away. We behold the naked visage of—ah!—Disinterest. The drama resides precisely in the triumph *over* drama."

So, Belch, Science welcomes us to the other side of drama, representations of life liberated from the impurities. Untidy life was once shaped and heightened by drama. Our esteem was flattered by all this attention to the creatures of our ego. Skilled actors and sly devices further aggrandized our every quirk and folly. Now the time has come for drama itself to be shaped and heightened. The stuff of human drama is purified, objectified, quantified, and decontextualized. In time, a more perfect universe replaces both mundane life and its distorting mirror, the theater. Ourselves to blame if we insist on expecting this new realm to resemble its inferiors, or advanced knowledge to be issued in convenient tubes for application to our dreary little individual lives. A pure theater of the mind! But what does this mean for the construction of gerontologic truth?

"Though not clean past your youth, there is yet some smack of age in you, some relish of the saltness of time."

The "saltness of time," Belch?

"Sir John Falstaff to thee now—are you afflicted with the disease of not listening, the malady of not marking? Go ye hence to a secluded bower and find in the saltness of time a seasonable employment for your sweet pretty wit."

No more counsel, good Sir John?

"If I had a thousand sons, the first humane principle I would teach them should be, to forswear thin potations and to addict themselves to sack."

THE SALTNESS OF TIME

And so we reflect a moment, here in this secluded bower, as in the nearby Interstate stream traffic plays and sports.

The "saltness of time" is experiential or it isn't anything at all. A literal interpretation of Sir John's words would lead us to such sources as "Taste Intensity Perception in Aging" (Weiffenbach, Cowart, & Baum, 1986). This well-controlled experiment takes us right to the uneasy border between objectivism and subjective experience. The men and women participating in the study are required to enact the role of assessment devices in a series of taste threshold tests. Age and sex are abstracted as relevant variables; all else has been carefully decontextualized. The response measure is particularly revealing. Participants were not asked to say anything, nor were they trusted to place a numerical value upon their perceptions. Instead they were asked to make "cross-modal matches of linear extent to perceived taste intensity" (Weiffenbach et al., 1986, p. 466). This was accomplished by manipulating a retractable metal tape measure along a laminated board. The participants' actual experiences of sodium chloride, citric acid, and other substances never entered into the study and will probably go as secrets to their graves. The basic "stuff" of the article is numbers derived from manipulations of the retractable metal tape measure and then transformed and analyzed in a variety of moderately entertaining ways (linear regression of log response magnitude on log stimulus strength, monotonic trend, etc.). The study is a little gem on its own terms. These terms, however, do not include trust in human experience and the ability to articulate this experience. Precautions are taken to avoid contaminating the study by opening it to the qualities of subjective experience, even though qualitative factors are introduced on the stimulus side (the various substances to be tasted). Quality is acceptable only when it can be transformed into quantity. (Why, at least, couldn't the participants have been allowed to stick out their own tongues as a form of cross-modal matching? Never mind: I know why.)

The objective, quantitative, decontextualized approach provides unique and sometimes indispensable information. It has the habit, however, of asking only those questions that can be answered with both feet on the safe side of the boundary.

To understand "the saltness of time" seems to require other methods, and, therefore, other ideas about what comprises legitimate and productive methodology. This quest might even require other ideas about the relationship between knowledge and the human condition. But for now, after those exhausting adventures up and down stairs, we make do with just a few simple thoughts:

1. *Ordinary life can be understood as drama.* Indeed, we understand very little if motivation, conflict, and, above all, at-stakeness are ignored.

2. *When ordinary life is formulated it becomes narrative drama.* This happens every time we attempt to explain our lives to ourselves or others. In a sense, our lives become the stories we tell. An incipient dramatic structure takes shape as we construct (and reconstruct) the story of our lives. Secondary plots and cirumstances may be pruned away to allow certain events to stand tall and alone; momentous forebodings are chalked in with primary colors; overarching themes are embroidered upon for heightened aesthetic satisfaction.

3. *The drama is enriched by multiple and interactive stories.* Our version is supported or challenged by other narrative constructions. Among the most vicious and delicious conflicts is the competition for the "real" or "best" version. (Science and professional expertise may intrude, but these versions must compete along with the others.)

4. *Dramatic structure encompasses both the relationships among people in the present situation (vertical structure) and relationships over time (horizontal structure).* The unit of study, then, includes social interaction as well as individual action. (Analyze *King Lear* without respect to his daughters, the military situation, etc.!)

5. *Time is truly of the essence.* Although time is an elusive and irksome variable in much objectivistic research, experiential time is critical to development and aging. During the course of adult life, has this person developed, aged, or recycled certain roles and postures again and again? Has the sense of time's passage contributed to a glow of satisfaction, or a glower of fury? Have the "days dwindled down to a precious few," or has one slyly "turned off the meter" and scripted a new life for every dawn? Has something of fresh-water youth been preserved in old age, or must all tastes filter through the salty residue deposited by the stream of time?

It is doubtful that questions of this kind can be answered by manipulating a retractable metal measure on a laminated board—and so gerontology is free to develop concepts and methods more suited to the subject matter.

There are beginnings. *Number Our Days* (Myerhoff, 1979) is the ironically quantitative title for a pioneering work that reveals some of the potential inherent in qualitative gerontology. Sensitive to the implicit dramatic structure in ordinary human lives and to the story-telling process, Myerhoff has opened one promising path. Concepts originating with both Freud and Piaget are integrated by Fast (1985) in her *event theory* (yet to be applied to gerontology, as far as I know). Here also is potential for disciplined, systematic research into time-sensitive processes that does not rush to quantify all observations. Still another approach awaiting exploration is that offered recently by Prado. In *Making Believe: Philosophical Reflections of Fiction*, Prado (1984) first suggests a somewhat different way to look at narrative fiction. Perhaps the most significant contribution is the respect with which story-telling is treated by a philosopher and how much emphasis is given to the creative impulse in developing narrative structure and substance. *Rethinking How We Age* (Prado, 1986) offers a stimulating interpretation of cognitive processes in later life from the standpoint of plot conceptualizations. Creating dramatic narratives from the material of our lives continues to be a major cognitive activity. Further, Prado suggests that

> . . . impending death may cast us more as authors of our narratives than protagonists in them. Perhaps we recede from our narratives in beginning to see them as continuing without us. . . . Some distance themselves from life through the conceit of trying to manipulate it, by trying to determine the course of events after their death. It may not be too much to say that the naive tendency to narrate, to produce stories, is enhanced in old age as compensation for impending death. In a way it is all we have left, our last opportunity to determine reality for ourselves and others (Prado, 1986, pp. 143–144).

There are, then, some thought-provoking approaches already available to guide qualitative research in the world beyond the Laboratory for Extremely etc. Additional concepts and methods are likely to arise should more gerontologists choose to pursue enticing questions wherever they lead. One certainly discovers the problems soon enough, even if the solutions are not immediately forthcoming. Part of my current research, for example, approaches the phenomenon of "Music Composed in the Shadow of Death" (Kastenbaum, 1986). The possibility of creativity and the certainty of death are in contention while the last grains of sand slip to the bottom of the hourglass. What happens? How? And why? There is no ready-made methodology for this kind of investigation, nor is it adequate to apply concepts taken off the shelf. What one learns quickly is that each composer's life and work must be examined on its own terms and yet somehow balanced within an overall structure. In this sense the research project itself becomes an emergent dramatic structure that continues to interact with its subject matter. The blurring of fixed boundaries that troubles some people in qualitative research does not necessarily result in a loss of objectivity. Lear, Belch, or Falstaff might have added that Drama is coldly experimental, just as Science is rhapsodically dramatic. If a dramatic element doesn't ring true or make its contribution, out it goes! The laws of exclusion have not been precisely formulated, but they are applied to scripts and productions every day. Similarly, qualitative research must also pass muster. Schubert's *Schwanengesang*, for example, seems to offer a clear example of music composed in prospect of death—until inquiry reveals that the title was invented posthumously by an opportunistic publisher. Experience with qualitative research hones one's awareness of error and "not rightness."

(SOUND: Thunder rolling nearer, topped by eerie voice-like winds . . .)
GUIDE: The Zowies! They've escaped!
FALSTAFF: They are fairies; he that speaks to them shall die . . .

Pardon: I see we've just slipped into the wrong script—

(*Exit with Thunder*)

REFERENCES

Fast, I. (1985). *Event theory*. Hillsdale, NJ: Lawrence Earlbaum Associates.
Kastenbaum, R. (1986, November). *Music composed in the shadow of death: Analysis of 25 composers*. Paper presented at the annual meeting of the Gerontological Society of America, Chicago.
McDonald, R., Hegenauer, J., & Saltman, P. (1986). Age-related differences in the bone mineralization pattern of rats following exercise. *Journal of Gerontology, 41*, 445–452.
Myerhoff, B. *Number our days*. (1979). New York: Simon & Schuster.
Prado, C. G. (1984). *Making believe: Philosophical reflections on fiction*. Westport, CT: Greenwood Press.
Prado, C. G. (1986). *Rethinking how we age*. Wesport, CT: Greenwood Press.
Weiffenbach, J. M., Cowart, B. J., & Baum, B. J. (1986). Taste intensity perception in aging. *Journal of Gerontology, 41*, 460–468.

PART 2
Contemporary Practice

3

Admissible Evidence: Geropsychology and the Personal Journal

Harry J. Berman

PERSONAL JOURNALS AND GEROPSYCHOLOGY

The idea that what is admissible as evidence in geropsychology[1] is too narrowly defined is not new. Neugarten (1985), Kastenbaum (1973), Gutmann (Gutmann, Griffin, & Grunes, 1982), and Poon (1980) have all argued for adopting methods that allow the subjects in our research, whether interviewees or clients, to inform us more fully about the experience of aging.

Our limited knowledge of the inner lives of older people and the judgment that evidence about aging that is informative, genuine, and helpful is actually unscientific can be attributed to the hegemony of early twentieth-century positivism over late twentieth-century behavioral and social sciences. As a result, acceptable data, scientific evidence, and, in the extreme, knowledge itself, are confined to that which has been generated from potentially replicable public operations using measured concepts (see, for example, Bridgman, 1927).

The underlying metaphor here is that knowledge is *drawn out* of the objects of research by researchers. This intrusive, extractive metaphor is worth noting for two reasons. First, it establishes a dominant–subordinate relationship between the researcher and the object of research, which may be appropriate in the investigation of molecules but is problematic in the study of human beings. Second, it predisposes psychological researchers to discount freely given, rather than extracted, evidence about psychological processes. The purpose of this chapter is to reflect on one source of such freely given data, the personal journal, and to consider how its use as evidence about psychological processes would necessitate revisions in our thinking about knowledge.

Prior to World War II psychologists expressed substantial interest in personal documents. Charlotte Buehler (1935), Else Frenkl-Brunswik (Frenkl, 1936; Frenkl-Brunswik, 1939); Jerome Bruner (Allport, Bruner, & Jandorf, 1941) Gordon Allport, Alfred Baldwin (1940, 1942), and others used diaries, life histories, and autobiographical material to investigate responses to catastrophe, mechanisms of self-deception, and changes over the life cycle (Wrightsman, 1981). After World War II interest waned, an outstanding exception being Gordon Allport's *Letters from Jenny* (1965). As Wrightsman (1981) noted, the "state of the art" regarding the use of personal documents in psychology had not advanced—until very recently—beyond Gordon Allport's monograph, written over 40 years ago (Allport, 1942). The recent change was provoked by critical examinations of the assumptions that underlie the behavioral and social sciences (Gergen, 1982; Neugarten, 1985; Runciman, 1983). These psychologists have established the epistemological grounds for a reassessment of personal documents, in general, and personal journals, in particular, as psychological data.

The personal journal or diary[2] is a distinct literary form (Fothergill, 1974; Matthews, 1970). Such journals consist of regular entries in which people recount events and reflect on their reactions to those events. Following Fothergill (1974), the term *personal journal* is used here to designate journals in which the life of the author is the prime subject. These may be distinguished from diaries, in which the author is involved only indirectly. Examples of journals that are not personal are travel journals, diaries of expeditions or military campaigns, diaries of public or political affairs, or diary records of special interests, such as fishing or gardening. Although personal journals may include descriptions of travels, political events, or special interests, such descriptions serve primarily as material for personal reflection.

The personal journal as literary form has evolved over the past three centuries. Although many examples of diaries in English exist from the fifteenth century on (Matthews, 1950), the first journal that could be called personal is that of Samuel Pepys (Pepys, 1970–1976), written more than 200 years later in the middle of the seventeenth century.

By the beginning of the nineteenth century diary writing was beginning to be recognized as a literary activity open to both established and nonestablished writers. The writing in these diaries was characterized by immediacy, self-reflection, and authenticity. In nineteenth-century French diaries, known as *journaux intimes*, these qualities were carried to an extreme. The writers of *journaux intimes* demonstrated their cultivated capacity for passionate responses to music and literature and their unusual sensitivity to all kinds of stimuli (Fothergill, 1974). By the nineteenth century the personal journal was adopted as a presentational strategy for fiction (Abbott, 1984), a style continued to this day (Walker, 1982; Updike, 1975).

The task of evaluating the utility of personal journals as sources of evidence about the process of aging rests on the clarification of the criteria for evaluating journals. Personal journals vary in their quality. As Fothergill (1974) has noted, the great mass of diary writing is poor from the perspective of literary merit. His comment applies equally well to diaries' potential contribution to geropsychology. Nevertheless, I suggest three provisional criteria for evaluating the potential of personal diaries to contribute to our understanding of aging.

First is the balance between events and reflections on those events. Diaries that focus exclusively on one or the other are less likely to yield useful information about development than are those in which there is movement back and forth between inner and outer events. Second is the heterogeneity of the entries. Instead of linear development, as in a story, a "good" journal contains a miscellany of entries that give a sense of the "almost infinite number of things that flow through the consciousness" (Barbellion, 1984, p. 210). Virginia Woolf put it thus: "a diary should be so elastic that it will embrace anything solemn, slight or beautiful that comes into my mind. I should like it to resemble some deep old desk, or capacious hold-all, in which one flings a mass of odds and ends without looking them through" (1953, p. 13). Third is the age of the author. An "older" person is likely to confront developmental issues of later life.

Publication does not establish a journal's worth; it is only a factor in its accessibility. Some diaries now published had remained unpublished for centuries. Pepys's journal, for example, written between 1660 and 1669, was first published in part in 1825 and was not published in its entirety until the 1970s.

Publication might actually lessen the value of the personal journal, since the possibility of publication might have influenced the writer in some way. This is a complex matter if a criterion for a good diary is unpremeditated sincerity. Some believe that in diaries everything

should be "forthright and without subterfuge . . . spontaneous, unpremeditated and completely convincing" (Untermeyer, 1957, p. v). However, it is important to recognize that sincerity and premeditated utterance are not mutually exclusive. In addition, because many diaries *have*
been published, serious diarists cannot be certain that theirs will not be
published, too. Thus, the presence of an imagined audience (see below)
or the thought of potential publication does not necessarily undermine
the journal's authenticity.

It is naive to think that people keep journals just for themselves and
that there is no censoring and no imagined audience present. After
analysing 150 published journals, Mallon (1984) concluded that though
the diarist's "you" may not be palpable, there is an implied "you." As
Dinnage (1984, p. 3) has noted: "there is no diary writer including
ourselves and Uncle Henry who never imagines the other person reading the page." However, unlike responding to a structured interview,
writing a journal is not literally a social act, and journals are not as
likely to be suffused with the attempts to make socially desirable statements as are other forms of publications and interviews.

Recently published journals that meet the provisional criteria for use
by geropsychologists are Florida Scott-Maxwell's *The Measure of My Days*
(1979); Elizabeth Vining's *Being Seventy* (1978); a series of four journals
by May Sarton (1973, 1977, 1980, 1984); Ann Truitt's *Daybook* (1982);
Alan Olmstead's *Threshold: The First Days of Retirement* (1975); and Joyce
Horner's *That Time of Year* (1982). Scott-Maxwell's journal describes the
day-to-day experience of a 70-year-old woman; Sarton's *Journal of a
Solitude*, the day-to-day experience of a 58-year-old woman.

In these journals the authors' purpose was not to answer questions
posed by psychologists. Rather the authors dealt with issues that
emerged in their day-to-day experiences. The content, form, and conceptual schemata they employed belonged to them rather than to us as
researchers. This is not to say that these journals are oblivious to
formal psychological perspectives. Educated people are aware of psychology and psychoanalysis (Sarason, 1977; Ricoeur, 1979). Scott-Maxwell, Vining, and Sarton make explicit reference in their journals to
works of Jung and Erikson without trying to provide a Jungian or
Eriksonian interpretation of their lives. Rather, ideas of psychological
theorists and others are places to begin reflections. The point is to
recognize what the journals are not: they are *not* attempts to prove,
validate, or illustrate any particular psychological theory. Nor are the
entries shaped by a research perspective the way responses to a structured interview or questionnaire or even a Thematic Apperception Test
card would be. Rather, the entries in the journals are freely given, as

opposed to extracted by an instrument, and therefore have a form natural to the person who provided them.

Authors are conscious of their reasons for engaging in journal writing. For example, in *Being Seventy*, Vining says that she wants to record "the things I do for the last time or enjoy less keenly" (1978, p. 5). At the end of *Journal of a Solitude*, Sarton (1973) states her purpose:

> This journal began a year ago with depression, with much self-questioning about my dangerous and destructive angers, with the hope that self-examination would help me to change (pp. 206–207).

Elsewhere in *Journal of a Solitude* she makes a simple comment that applies generally to conscious reasons about why established writers keep journals. She says: "My business is the analysis of feelings" (p. 44). For Sarton, and presumably for other established writers, the analysis of feeling can take a variety of forms: poetry, fiction, or journal writing.

Established writers also keep journals to refresh themselves. In a review of Woolf, Rosemary Dinnage (1984, p. 3) wrote: "The diary is the spontaneous overflow of a committed writer's tremendous energy; as she breathed she wrote." Dinnage finds that the diaries served to liberate, freshen, and uncramp Woolf. Journals may serve for writers as muscle stretches and deep breathing do for athletes: as a means of preparing for the main event or of recovering from sustained expenditure of imaginative effort.

The encounter of the geropsychologist with personal journals resembles—but is not identical to—the encounter between clients and therapists. The journals are a continuing report of life in the present—regardless of when that present was. The reader sees the days unfold much as a therapist would during a year of therapy. Also, like a therapist, a geropsychologist brings to these texts empathy, developmental theories, and psychological concepts. The analyst of texts depends on being open to the feelings aroused by the texts as a basis for grasping the world of the other.

The bidirectionality of this exchange is important. The author of a journal gives a geropsychologist a communication about some facet of experience that may not be expressed in available theory. At the same time, the geropsychologist's theories and concepts may provide a more encompassing perspective than was available to the author.

The analogy between the therapist and the client, and the geropsychologist and the writer of the personal journal, has limits that are instructive. The obvious difference is that the journal writer is not literally present for the reader, but is removed in time and space. The only means of communication is the written word. Another difference is that, unlike a therapist, the journal analyst cannot guide, probe, or ask for clarification. Whether these differences are bad or good depends on one's purposes. For purposes of understanding the experience of aging, it may be an advantage not to be present with the informant, and thus to avoid, in subtle or overt ways, shaping the report. Moreover, for research purposes, the journal has a distinct advantage over case material, which is not available to the public and is filtered through the eyes and ears of the therapist. The journal is therefore more authentic and compelling.

In order to illustrate the type of materials available in personal journals and to show the bidirectionality of the exchange between the journal writer and the geropsychologist, I present an analysis of excerpts from two personal journals, Scott-Maxwell's *The Measure of My Days** and Vining's *Being Seventy*** (Berman, 1985, 1986).

THE MEASURE OF MY DAYS

The Measure of My Days is a particularly rich source of inner experiences that parallel the outer changes occurring in later life. At the time of its original publication in 1968, Scott-Maxwell was 85 years old. Her life had been productive and varied. As a teenager, she had been a stage performer. At 20, she began a career as a writer of short stories and plays. She married at 27 and left the United States to live with her husband in his native Scotland. There she continued to write while raising a family and working for women's suffrage. In 1933, at age 50, she began training in analytic psychology, studying under Jung, after which she practiced psychology in clinics in Scotland and England.

The most striking and surprising element of the book is Scott-Maxwell's description of her passion for life, a passion that exists despite physical and social losses and that, if anything, is refined and sharpened by those losses. She begins her journal with the following:

> We who are old know that old age is more than disability. It is an intense and varied experience, almost beyond our capacity at times, but something to be carried high. (p. 5)

Elsewhere she writes:

> Age puzzles me. I thought it was a quiet time. My seventies were interest-
> ing and fairly serene, but my eighties are passionate. I grow more intense
> as I age. (p. 13)

In moving passages on the intensity of her feeling for life, she writes:

> Another secret we carry is that though drab outside—wreckage to the eye,
> mirrors a mortification—inside we flame with a wild life that is almost
> incommunicable.
>   It feels like the far side of precept and aim. It is just life, the natural
> intensity of life, and when old we have it for our reward and undoing.
> (pp. 32–33)

Scott-Maxwell's passion for life emerges out of her physical and
social world—a physical world dominated by her frailty, a social world
in which she feels out of place. Her description of her frailty, or more
accurately, her relationship with her frailty, is particularly helpful in
illuminating the experience of being old. She writes:

> I used to draw, absorbed in the shapes of roots of trees, and seed pods, and
> flowers, but it strained my eyes and I gave it up. Then ten years ago I
> began to make rugs. . . . But my hands were too arthritic, it had to end,
> and now only music prevents my facing my thoughts. (p. 13)

And:

> I long to laugh. I want to be enjoyed, but an hour's talk and I am exhausted.
> (p. 8)

And elsewhere:

> We old people are short tempered because we suffer so. . . . Little things
> have become big; nothing in us works well, our bodies have become
> unreliable. We have to make an effort to do the simplest things. We urge
> now this now that part of our flagging bodies, and when we have spurred
> them to further functioning we feel clever and carefree. (p. 35)

According to Scott-Maxwell, the twin issues faced by those who
become frail are thoughts of invalidism and thoughts of death. Of the
latter she writes:

> My only fear about death is that it will not come soon enough. (p. 75)

And:

> When a new disability arrives I look about to see if death has come and I
> call quietly, "Death is that you, are you there?" So far the disability has
> answered "Don't be silly, it's me." (p. 36)

She cannot treat the possibility of invalidism, of being a burden to
others, of losing her capacity to take care of herself, with the humor
present in the passages about death. Commenting on her feelings about
having surgery, she says:

> I had one fear. What if something went wrong and I became an invalid?
> What if I became a burden, ceased to be a person and became a problem, a
> patient, someone who could not die? (p. 91)

And later:

> I don't like to write this down, yet it is much in the minds of the old. We
> wonder how much older we have to become, and what degree of decay we
> may have to endure. (p.138)

A key point here is that this woman's increasing frailty and concomitant reduction of activities create the conditions for an intense involvement with the essence of life, with the nonphysical aspects of human-
ness, with ideas themselves. She says:

> Old people are not protected from life by engagements, or pleasures, or
> duties; we are open to our own sentience, we cannot get away from it, and
> it is too much. (p. 14)

And:

> To be dominated by abstract ideas is part of the helplessness of old age.
> (p. 58)

Scott-Maxwell's passion for life arises out of her relationship with the
social world. Near the beginning of the journal she writes:

> Being old I am out of step, troubled by my lack of concord, unable to like or
> understand much that I see. Feeling at variance with the times must be the
> essence of age. . . . (p. 5)

Later she writes:

We old people are not in modern life. Our impressions of it are second or third hand. It is something we cannot know. (p. 136)

As in the case of her frailty, the consequence for Scott-Maxwell of detachment from the social world is, paradoxically, not less involvement with life, but more. She is explicit on this point, asserting, "Now that I have withdrawn from the active world I am more alert to it than ever before" (p. 5). Also, far from not caring about the events of the world, she cares very deeply.

Old people have so little personal life that the impact of the impersonal is sharp. Some of us feel like sounding boards, observing, reading; the outside event startles us and we ask in alarm, "Is this good or bad? To where will it lead." (pp. 5—6)

These selections from Scott-Maxwell's journal illustrate the bidirectionality of the exchange between the geropsychologist and the journal writer.

A concept a geropsychologist might apply to this book is the idea of the individual life structure, as delineated by Daniel Levinson (Levinson, Darrow, Klein, Levinson, & McKee, 1978; Levinson, 1980). The individual life structure is the set of a person's attachments at a given moment and the priorities among them. Typically these consist of attachments in the domains of family, occupation, leisure roles, and religious activities. Levinson has also described how other types of attachments may become part of a life structure. Examples include an attachment to a house, a community, a geographic area. Understanding a life structure means understanding the meaning of attachments in the person's life. Such meanings are most clearly revealed when choices between alternatives have to be made, such as leaving a much-loved house for a new job or foregoing a new job in order to remain close to family.

Levinson and associates (1978) see the individual life structure undergoing change throughout adulthood. They discuss the timing of changes among mid-life men and the forces that bring about those changes. The passages from Scott-Maxwell suggest a revision of the life structure concept when applied to women in later life. Specifically, the passages cited above suggest that in later life attachments may be different from those formed earlier. Whereas attachments in younger years tend to be linked to specific roles or objects, a key attachment at the end of life may be to life itself, an abstraction that comes to replace more tangible attachments lost through diminished physical capacities, deaths, and the sheer passage of time.

BEING SEVENTY

Being Seventy: The Measure of a Year by Elizabeth Gray Vining presents a remarkably clear picture of the day-to-day life of a healthy, successful person in the year of her seventieth birthday, a decade birthday. There are entries on 143 different days between August 26, 1972, and October 5, 1973, the day before her 71st birthday. As we read her book, we are aided in seeing the world as she does because Vining is an experienced writer with a highly developed capacity for introspection.

Elizabeth Gray Vining was born in Philadelphia in 1902, the younger of two daughters. A graduate of Bryn Mawr College, she wrote books for adults and children under the names Elizabeth Janet Gray and Elizabeth Gray Vining. Vining married at age 26 and four years later was a widow when her husband died in a car accident. She never remarried. During and immediately after World War II she worked for the American Friends Service Committee and in 1946 was appointed tutor to Crown Prince Akihito of Japan. She later wrote the widely read *Windows for the Crown Prince*, based on her experiences as royal tutor. When she wrote *Being Seventy* she had completed 23 books, including novels, biographies, and her autobiography, *Quiet Pilgrimage*, published in 1970. She was living in an apartment in Philadelphia in reasonably good health. She had no immediate family, her older sister having died three years earlier.

The most striking initial impression from the journal is how busy this woman is. She travels: she spends one month in Japan participating in a writer's conference; another month at a writer's colony on Ossabaw Island off the coast of South Carolina; and two months on annual summer vacation in New Hampshire. She lectures: she mentions giving seven different speeches and presentations during the year, but it is not clear that all her talks are mentioned in the journal. She entertains: she hosts extended visits of friends from Japan and from Ireland. She is actively involved with friends: she visits friends, writes to friends, talks to friends. And she drives: up and down the East Coast. All the while she is diligently working on a biography of John Greenleaf Whittier, which she completes, types into final copy, and mails off to the publisher ahead of a September 1 deadline.

Clearly, this woman is highly engaged in the world. She has many connections to other people that occupy her time and attention; she has her work, her writing, which she calls the basis of her life (p. 83), "The soil out of which other things spring" (p. 128); she has a passionate interest in the events of the world in that momentous year that saw the bombing of Cambodia and the Watergate hearings.

The principal message Vining conveys about the thoughts and feel-ings of a woman her age center around the themes of culmination and impending change. She writes:

A door shuts. It is shut not in one's face but behind one. In front is a new landscape, bleak perhaps at times, lit no doubt at others by mysterious beauty, but cut off in the distance by a wall, which for the first time is close enough to be visible. One stands in a limited space, with the door behind and the wall somewhere in front. (pp. 4–5)

The sense of culmination can be seen in her reactions to attending her fiftieth college reunion:

I shall not attend any more. . . . It was a good reunion, perhaps the best we have had, and for that reason it is well to end on it. Later we shall be putting a brave face on age; now we are enjoying its rewards.
    From now on we live sub specie aeternitatis. We have made our contri-bution, whatever it is; whatever it may be. (p. 141)

The sense of culmination and impending change is bound up with her awareness of her age. The journal is particularly useful in clarifying the nature of that awareness.

I wish I could stop thinking about being old. It's not that I mind it so much or fear it; it's just that I am so aware of it all the time. (p. 2)

What she means by "all the time" is elucidated in several other entries. It is not that at every waking moment she thinks "I am old." On the contrary, "days go by and I scarcely think of it" (p. 132–133). It is more that the fact of her age enters into consciousness with what she feels is great and, generally, unwanted frequency.
    Sometimes the fact of her age enters into consciousness as an expla-nation for mishaps or failings:

I stumble on the stairs and think 'old and clumsy.' I suppose I'll get worse. A name or a word eludes my mind and I think, 'Losing my memory' . . . (p. 3)

On other occasions the fact of her age enters into consciousness as the shocking recognition that she is labeling or has labeled as "old" a person who is her present age.

When I was eight . . . we went next door to see [my friend's] grandparents. They both seemed to me incredibly old, he with his white beard and she with her black silk dress. I suppose they were no older in 1910 that I am now. (p. 7)

As I look forward to Kendal [the retirement community she plans to move to] . . . I sometimes catch myself thinking of all the nice things I am going to do for those old people there, and I remember that I am one of those old people myself. (p. 187)

The most disconcerting example of this recognition comes with the discovery of a journal she kept at 31. At that time she was surrounded by four women in their seventies, approximately Vining's present age. At age 31 she wrote:

I am sorry for old ladies. Failing faculties and failing looks must be a constant irritation to unfailing vanity. . . . One pities them, one loves them, one cherishes them, one can so rarely like them. (p. 136)

Part of what makes these moments of age awareness so shocking to her is the sense that she doesn't feel old, so how *could* she be the age she *knows* she is. She writes:

It isn't as if I felt old. I don't. Inside I feel often as gauche, as shy, as incapable of wise or effective action as I did at sixteen, or as surprised and delighted by unexpected beauty. (p. 4)

Thus she cannot help being aware of her age, being aware that she is now the age that she used to think of as old and that other people think of as old. Yet this awareness is coupled with what she senses as a contradictory awareness, the awareness that she doesn't feel old.

The sense of being on the brink of a major change in life is certainly not restricted to older people. Rather it can occur in earlier adult years and can be associated with a variety of events not necessarily tightly linked to chronological age—falling in love, starting graduate school, getting a new job, and being pregnant. However, the sense of being on the brink, the sense of culmination and impending change described by Vining, bears a striking resemblance to two earlier periods in people's lives that *are* age-linked. These are the transition from adolescence to young adulthood and from young adulthood to middle age.

Our understanding of this feeling of being on the brink, particularly as it relates to people around age 20 and around age 40, can also be interpreted in terms of Levinson's concept of the individual life structure that changes throughout adulthood. The change in individual life structure is neither uniform nor random. Rather Levinson sees change occurring in bursts. He presents a model of individuals passing through stable, structure-building periods succeeded by unstable, transitional, structure-changing periods. Furthermore, the progression of structure-building and structure-changing periods is set in a larger framework of what Levinson refers to as eras. The four eras—childhood, early adulthood, middle adulthood, and later adulthood—represent the overarching structure—Levinson calls it the anatomical structure—of the life course. Each era, according to Levinson, represents a distinct phase in biological, psychological, and social development.

Although all transitional, structure-changing periods carry with them the sense of being on the brink of great change, it is reasonable to think that those transition periods that bridge eras, the major units of life, would be accompanied by a more intense experience of culmination and impending change than intermediate transition periods. A vast professional and popular literature documents the attempts of adolescents to build a first adult life structure. This literature captures the accompanying feelings of culmination and new beginning. The fictional form that tells the story of coming of age is so common that, in German, a single word, *Bildungsroman*, designates this literature. The mid-life transition similarly involves a substantial disassembly of an earlier life structure, with concomitant feelings of culmination and new beginning, as reflected in both professional and popular literature. Although it presents a general view of development over the course of life, Levinson's book deals mainly with the mid-life transition: men in the age range of 35–45 years.

Thus we are moderately well acquainted with the era-bridging transitions between childhood and early adulthood and between early adulthood and middle adulthood. What it feels like to *become* an older person is relatively unknown. From this perspective, Vining's journal is a rare and valuable document. It is a rich description of the psychological landscape of the third cross-era transition, the transition between middle adulthood and later life.

WHAT CONSTITUTES KNOWLEDGE OF AGING?

The point of the study of personal journals is not to replace the standard sources of information about psychological functioning, but rather to expand the domain of admissible evidence and to complement data obtained from prevailing methodologies. But just what type of evidence or data is provided by journals?

One way to understand personal journals is to assume, as did Freud in his topographic model, that people function on three distinct levels: an interpersonal level, analogous to Freud's conscious functioning; a border or transitional level, analogous to Freud's preconscious; and a purely intrapsychic level, analogous to the unconscious. If people are viewed in this way, we could say that research on aging that uses interviews or looks at social behavior taps the interpersonal and conscious level of functioning; that research using projective tests to study aging (Gutmann, Griffin, & Grunes, 1982) taps the intrapsychic or unconscious level of functioning; and that the personal journal taps the border or transitional area between the two.

Journals vary in the extent to which they gravitate toward the conscious level, that is, the degree to which they put on a social face versus the degree to which they gravitate toward the unconscious level. But regardless of a particular journal's position on the conscious–unconscious continuum, personal journals share the characteristics of exposing conflict-laden feelings and permitting the reader to track those feelings over time. Journals allow us to glimpse inner conflict at different phases of later life and the natural courses along which such conflicts evolve. This is an aspect of knowledge of aging that journals are well suited to provide.

A second answer to the question of what type of evidence is provided by personal journals is to recognize, as the British philosopher of social science, Runciman, has done (1983), three modes of understanding. The first is the understanding necessary to provide a statement of what *has been observed* to occur. Runciman calls this reportage. The second is the understanding of what *caused* a situation to occur, or how it came about. He calls this explanation. And the third is the understanding necessary for what Runciman calls description. Description means addressing the question of what *it is like* to think, feel, say, and do something.

In gerontology there is a bias toward identifying the idea of knowledge of aging with Runciman's first category: reportage (knowledge of facts). This bias is reflected in the popularity of and research on Palmore's (1977, 1981) Facts on Aging Quizzes (Holtzman & Beck, 1979; Brubaker & Barresi, 1979; Monk & Kaye, 1982). In these studies the scores on the Facts on Aging Quiz are used to provide an operational definition of knowledge of aging. Under this definition subjects who score high on this test are presumed to have knowledge of aging. Although the value of Palmore's quizzes as a heuristic device and as a means of prompting discussion cannot be disputed, there is considerable question about using this test to represent the domain of knowledge of aging. Older people themselves may score low on Palmore's quiz, yet would we wish to assert, without qualification, that they are ignorant of aging?

Knowledge of aging consists not only of reports about facts and explanations of causes but also of descriptions of age-related experiences. Experiences may be age-related in that they typically occur to people of a certain chronological age and a particular gender in a given society. Once we acknowledge that descriptions of age-related experiences are a part of knowledge of aging, the value of personal journals as a source of such descriptions becomes readily apparent.

NOTES

1. Geropsychology is the subspecialty of developmental psychology that focuses on psychological development in later life. Clinical geropsychology is the subspecialty of clinical psychology that focuses on mental health issues in later life. Over the past decade these terms have gained acceptance and have been used in articles appearing in professional journals such as *The American Psychologist* (Smyer & Gatz, 1979), *Professional Psychology* (LeBray, 1979; Siegler, Gentry, & Edwards, 1979), *Educational Gerontology* (Hubbard, 1984), and *The Journal of Geriatric Psychiatry* (Lawton, 1976).

2. The terms *journal* and *diary* both express but are not strict about dailiness. Since there is no consistent difference in their use (Fothergill, 1974; Mallon, 1984), they are used interchangeably in this chapter.

REFERENCES

Abbott, H. (1984). *Diary fiction: Writing as action.* Ithaca, NY: Cornell University Press.

Allport, G. (1942). *The use of personal documents in psychological science.* New York: Social Science Research Council.

Allport, G. (Ed.). (1965). *Letters from Jenny.* New York: Harcourt, Brace and World.

Allport, G., Bruner, J., & Jandorf, E. (1941). Personality under catastrophe: An analysis of German refugee life histories. *Character and Personality, 10,* 1–22.

Baldwin, A. (1940). The statistical analysis of the structure of a single personality. *Psychological Bulletin, 37,* 518–519.

Baldwin, A. (1942). Personal structure analysis: A statistical method for investigating the single personality. *Journal of Abnormal and Social Psychology, 37,* 163–183.

Barbellion, W. N. P. (1984). *The journal of a disappointed man and a last diary.* London: Hogarth Press.

Berman, H. (1985, March). *On the brink: Elizabeth Vining's* Being Seventy. Paper presented at Humanistic Perspectives on the Aging Enterprise in America Conference, Center for the Study of Aging, University of Missouri, Columbia.

Berman, H. (1986). To flame with a wild life: Florida Scott-Maxwell's experience of old age. *The Gerontologist, 26,* 321–324.

Bridgman, P. (1927). *The logic of modern physics.* New York: Macmillan.

Brubaker, T., & Barresi, C. (1979). Social worker's level of knowledge about old age and perceptions of service delivery to the elderly. *Research on Aging, 1,* 213–232.

Buehler, C. (1935). The curve of life as studied in biographies. *Journal of Applied Psychology, 19,* 405–409.

Dinnage, R. (1984, November 8). Review of V. Woolf's diaries. *New York Review of Books,* pp. 3–4.

Fothergill, R. (1974). *Private chronicles.* New York: Oxford University Press.

Frenkl, E. (1936). Studies in biographical psychology. *Character and Personality, 5,* 1–35.

Frenkl-Brunswik, E. (1939). Mechanisms of self-deception. *Journal of Social Psychology, 10,* 409–420.

Gergen, K. (1982). *Toward transformation in social knowledge.* New York: Springer.

Gutmann, D., Griffin, B., & Grunes, J. (1982). Developmental contributions to late onset affective disorders. In P. Baltes & O. G. Brim (Eds.), *Life span development and behavior* (Vol. 4) (pp. 243–261). New York: Academic Press.

Holtzman, J., & Beck, J. (1979). Palmore's facts on aging quiz: A reappraisal. *The Gerontologist, 19,* 116–120.

Horner, J. (1982). *That time of year: A chronicle of life in a nursing home.* Amherst, MA: University of Massachusetts Press.

Hubbard, R. (1984). Clinical issues in the supervision of geriatric mental health trainees. *Educational Gerontology, 10,* 317–323.

Kastenbaum, R. (1973). Epilogue: Loving, dying and other gerontologic addenda. In C. Eisdorfer & M. P. Lawton (Eds.), *The psychology of adult development and aging,* (pp. 699–708). Washington, DC: American Psychological Association.

Lawton, M. (1976). Geropsychological knowledge as a background for psychotherapy with older people. *Journal of Geriatric Psychiatry, 9,* 221–233.

LeBray, P. (1979). Geropsychology in long-term care settings. *Professional Psychology, 10,* 475–484.

Levinson, D., Darrow, C., Klein, E., Levinson, M., & McKee, B. (1978). *The seasons of a man's life.* New York: Knopf.

Levinson, D. (1980). Toward a conception of the adult life course. In E. Erikson & N. Smelser (Eds.), *Themes of love and work in adulthood* (pp. 265–289). Cambridge, MA: Harvard University Press.

Mallon, T. (1984). *A book of one's own: People and their diaries.* New York: Ticknor & Fields.

Matthews, W. (1950). *British diaries: An annotated bibliography of British diaries written between 1442 & 1942.* Berkeley: University of California Press.

Matthews, W. (1970). The diary as literature. In R. Latham & W. Matthews (Eds.), *The diary of Samuel Pepys* (Vol. I) (pp. 7–14). Berkeley: University of California Press.

Monk, A., & Kaye, L. (1982). Gerontological knowledge and attitudes of students of religion. *Educational Gerontology, 8,* 435–445.

Neugarten, B. (1985). Interpretive social science and research on aging. In A. Rossi (Ed.), *Gender and the Life Course* (pp. 291–300). New York: Aldine.

Olmstead, A. (1975). *Threshold: The first days of retirement.* New York: Harper & Row.

Palmore, E. (1977). Facts on aging: A short quiz. *The Gerontologist, 17,* 315–320.

Palmore, E. (1981). The facts on aging quiz: Part II. *The Gerontologist, 21,* 431–437.

Pepys, S. (1970–1976). *The diary of Samuel Pepys* (Vols. 1–9). (R. Latham & W. Matthews, Eds.). Berkeley: University of California Press.

Poon, L. (1980). A last word. In L. Poon (Ed.), *Aging in the 1980s* (pp. 622–623). Washington, DC: American Psychological Association.

Ricoeur, P. (1979). Psychoanalysis and contemporary culture. In P. Rabinow & W. Sullivan (Eds.), *Interpretive social science: A reader* (pp. 301–337). Berkeley: University of California Press.

Runciman, W. (1983). *A treatise on social theory: Vol. I. The Methodology of Social Theory.* Cambridge, Eng.: Cambridge University Press.

Sarason, S. (1977). *Work, aging, and social change.* New York: The Free Press.

Sarton, M. (1973). *Journal of a solitude.* New York: Norton.

Sarton, M. (1977). *A house by the sea: A journal.* New York: Norton.

Sarton, M. (1980). *Recovering: A journal.* New York: Norton.

Sarton, M. (1984). *At seventy: A journal.* New York: W. W. Norton.

Scott-Maxwell, F. (1979). *The measure of my days.* New York: Penguin. (Original work published 1968)

Siegler, I., Gentry, W., & Edwards, C. (1979). Training in geropsychology: A survey of graduate and internship training programs. *Professional Psychology, 10,* 399–395.

Smyer, M., & Gatz, M. (1979). Aging and mental health: Business as usual? *American Psychologist. 34,* 240–246.

Truitt, A. (1982). *Daybook.* New York: Penguin.

Untermeyer, L. (1957). Introduction. In P. Dunaway & M. Evans (Eds.), *A treasury of the world's great diaries* (pp. v–vii). New York: Doubleday.

Updike, J. (1975). *A month of Sundays.* New York: Knopf.

Vining, E. (1978). *Being seventy: The measure of a year.* New York: Viking Press.

Walker, A. (1982). *The color purple: A novel.* New York: Harcourt Brace Jovanovich.

Woolf, V. (1953). *A writer's diary* (L. Woolf, Ed.). London: Hogarth Press.

Wrightsman, L. (1981). Personal documents as data in conceptualizing adult personality development. *Personality and Social Psychology Bulletin, 7,* 367–385.

4

Grandfather John Heller: Generativity Through the Life Cycle

Helen Q. Kivnick

As both a psychodynamic clinician and a qualitative researcher, I suggest that conducting qualitative, case-study research has a number of elements in common with clinical work. By discussing these similarities, I hope to enable the reader to draw on a general familiarity with the process of psychodynamic psychotherapy as a source of understanding for the often less familiar process of qualitative research. One way of describing my role as a psychotherapist is to say that I facilitate a patient's open-ended reflections and that I utilize theory from the fields of psychopathology, psychotherapy, and human development to interpret these reflections in a maximally therapeutic fashion. Throughout the treatment I may be viewed as proposing theoretical hypotheses and evaluating their adequacy on the basis of the patient's responses. That is, as a psychotherapist I engage in what amounts to an ongoing process of hypothesis testing and revising concerning theories of psychosocial development, psychopathology, and psychotherapy.

Of course, there are major differences between psychotherapy and qualitative, case-study research—differences in population, in goal and focus, and in interactional behavior. Those who seek psychotherapy have identified themselves as patients, as individuals who are in some way disabled in the process of living their lives. In contrast, qualitative research subjects are not selected on the basis of such difficulties, and they are therefore more likely to be representative of the population at large. Psychotherapy patients seek me out with the expectation that I will try to understand them, for *their* clinical benefit. Research subjects, in contrast, meet with me at *my* request, and they are clearly informed that I plan to use the information they provide in order to understand issues I have identified as important. These differences in goal and focus lead to major differences in interactional style and behavior between the clinical and the research practitioner. And it must be emphasized that the qualitative researcher is not necessarily trained as a clinician, and vice versa. Nonetheless, there are instructive similarities.

As a qualitative life-cycle researcher, I seek to facilitate an informant's reflections on his or her life cycle and to consider these reflections either as they contribute to existing theory or as they suggest the development of new theoretical hypotheses. The open-ended nature of this process encourages the informant, like the therapy patient, to provide all of the material that seems subjectively important. In both cases I have access to the vast quantity of events, observations, memories, and emotions that constitute an individual's experience of his or her own life. In both cases I also have the responsibility for making, from this material, a construction with demonstrable theoretical integrity.

LIFE-CYCLE THEORY

The clinical-like, life-history data for this chapter were collected as part of a study that integrated qualitative and quantitative research methods to explore various facets of the experience of grandparenthood (Kivnick, 1982a, 1982b). However, I am now shifting my interpretation of this material from a focus on grandparenthood alone to a consideration of the broader issue of generativity throughout the life cycle. This interpretation is grounded in the Eriksons' theory of psychosocial development, as summarized below (Erikson, 1982; Erikson, Erikson, & Kivnick, 1986).

Epigenetic theory describes the life cycle as comprising eight stages or periods. Each period is dominated by a tension between two opposing psychosocial tendencies, e.g., toddlerhood's tension between a sense of autonomy and an opposing sense of shame or doubt; early adulthood's tension between a sense of intimacy and an opposing sense of isolation. In each stage, the individual is challenged to bring these two opposing tendencies into dynamic balance with one another. However, at any point in life the individual is not wholly occupied with the psychosocial tension that is currently focal. In each period the individual is also involved in reviewing those tensions whose times of ascendancy have passed and in anticipating or "previewing" those tensions whose times of ascendancy are yet to come. Thus, the adolescent who is focusing on identity and identity confusion is also re-equilibrating feelings of autonomy and shame/doubt in newly age-appropriate terms, as well as previewing the feelings of generativity and stagnation that will not become focal for years to come. Effectively balancing any pair of opposing psychosocial tendencies requires the individual's participation in the world in which he or she is living. Although psychosocial development may be viewed as a complex of internal, psychological processes, these processes take place, at least in part, in terms of the individual's involvement with the surrounding society—involvement in relationships and exchanges with the people, the materials, the institutions, and the ideas that constitute that society.

The tension between generativity and stagnation has been described as dominating the period of middle adulthood. During this long period the individual participates in activities of procreativity, productivity, and creativity, fulfilling middle adulthood's imperative for "the maintenance of the world" (Erikson, 1980). Through all of these activities the individual ideally balances the capacity for generative caring and the tendency toward self-absorbed stagnation. However, this tension does not emerge, fullblown, with the onset of parenthood, responsible employment, reliable productivity, or any other social symbol of adulthood. Rather, it is anticipated throughout pre-adulthood, in the child's interactions with caring adults and in observation and experimentation concerning adult roles. In a parallel fashion, the balance between generativity and stagnation does not remain locked in time, disappearing when the individual moves beyond middle adulthood and into later life. Rather, these opposing tendencies continue to be expressed and equilibrated in terms that are appropriate to the relationships and activities that characterize "post-maintenance" adulthood (Kivnick, 1985), that is, that portion of adulthood during which the individual is no longer responsible for the maintenance of the world. We have referred to this later-life capacity for caring and nurturing as "grand-generativity" (Erikson, Erikson, & Kivnick, 1986).

METHOD

This chapter reconstructs the life cycle of a grandfather I shall call John Heller. First, it presents a brief chronology. Then, in a period-by-period fashion, it illustrates some of the ways in which generativity and themes of family caring are woven into the fabric of his psychosocial development, from early childhood through current grandparenthood. In so doing, I hope to use a particular theory of life-cycle development to gain a consistent understanding of the nature of this man's current experience of "grand-generativity."

LIFE CYCLE: JOHN HELLER

John Heller looks to be much older than his 63 years. His face is slack. His hair is white and thin, dampened and carefully combed across his head. He habitually dresses in a clean, wide-striped polo shirt and a pair of rough-woven Levi's—clothes that do little to conceal his developing paunch. His shoes have thick crepe soles; his step is light, but slow. His style of dress and his considerable height always suggest an athlete showered and cleaned up after a game, but his walk lacks the spring, his voice lacks the power, and his bearing lacks the readiness for action that go with this image. For all his height and his increasing girth, there is a surprising sense of translucent, almost ghostlike, insubstantiality about him.

John Heller and his wife Alice occupy the upstairs flat of a two-story house. Alice's brother lives downstairs. Theirs is a working-class neighborhood just north of San Francisco's Candlestick Park. The street is rather narrow, the houses are all close together, and there is no grass. During our interviews cars rev their motors outside the window and whizz down the street. Occasionally we are distracted by an automobile horn emulating a trumpet playing "La Cucaracha." Inside a protective iron gate, the stairway up to the Hellers' home is brightened by flowerpots filled with red geraniums. John and Alice Heller have been married for 40 years. They have one daughter, Marie. She and her husband Don live in Mountain View, about 35 minutes down the Peninsula. They have two children, Donnie, age 13, and Cindy, age 10.

The Hellers' living room is cheerful and airy, pleasantly crowded with plants, furniture, and knicknacks and dominated by a large television set on a portable stand. School photographs of the two grandchildren smile out from walls, shelves, and cabinet surfaces. Along one wall lies the bed of a small white poodle, Lolly, to whom Mr. Heller turns for relief throughout our interviews. Above Lolly's bed hangs a larger-than-life-sized picture of a dog like her, done in chips of glass.

I met with Mr. Heller for five open-ended interviews, conducted in his living room in the early afternoons. Approximately six months after these sessions I returned once more, to administer a quantitative questionnaire. Mr. Heller was extremely nervous throughout the interviews. I frequently had the feeling that he was not used to discussing feelings, experiences, or relationships at length and that in order to satisfy my insistent "Can you tell me any more about that?" he was saying whatever came into his mind. Each response became a series of associations, delivered rapidly and terminated abruptly in uncomfortable silence. While he spoke his hands wandered up and down the arm and the cushion of his chair. He seemed grateful to have Lolly pawing and sniffing nearby, and he frequently interrupted himself to tell her to get down, to sit still, or to come over to his lap.

In early response to my initial invitation to "Tell me about being a grandfather," Mr. Heller provided the following reflections on what dominates his current experience of grandparenthood:

> It's what I've always wanted, a grandchild. Now I end up with two of them—a girl and a boy. And I think it was more fun when they were smaller. You know, now since they're grown up they have their own ideas, and you go down to see them now, and they don't hang around you as much as they used to. You know, now they got other kids and they go out and play with them all the time. But they're—they're still friendly and they talk to us, you know, come around, call us up once in a while. We talk to 'em. We see them at least once a week, and it's just good, just fun.
>
> I just felt great that I was gonna be a grandfather . . . I'd have somebody down there to see and someone there to take out . . . to the park and to play ball with or something like that. I was just anxious to have . . . We just went to visit, and then when he was younger it was a great treat to go down there and take him out—watch him crawl; watch him walk. Watch him ride his bike for the first time. Stuff like that, you know.

John Heller strongly identifies with his grandchildren, as is indicated by his statement that when he watches Donnie play ball, "It's just like it was me." More important, he conveys a powerful sense of regarding them as validation of himself, his life, and his interests. When he speaks proudly of their love for him he is validating his worthiness as an object of love. When he speaks of their generosity and responsibility, he is validating himself as a generous, responsible grandparent. When he thinks of them as "somebody to take out to the park" he is validating his own interest in going out to the park. It is this need for validation that leads him both to blurt out his unhappiness with his grandchildren's growing network of activities and to interrupt his own complaining with such reassurances as, "They don't ignore us; nothing like that."

In considering John Heller's life cycle I am struck by the paucity of detail he can provide. In contrast to most other grandparents in the study, Mr. Heller discusses the major events of his own lifetime with no certainty about specific dates or even about the order in which events occurred. He knows almost nothing about his grandparents, and he tells little about his parents' lives before he was born. He does not seem to view his lifetime or his family history as an integrated sequence of events and experiences. In our sessions together, he mentioned events as they came to mind in his own assocations or in answers to my questions. Even when asked specifically to do so, he has difficulty placing events in historical time or considering experiences, one in terms of another.

John Heller was born in San Francisco, California, in 1916, the first of four children and his parents' only son. His father, Karl Heller, was a German citizen. At about 20, shortly after the turn of the century, he had ". . . left his people and hopped a boat, and worked on a merchant marine ship. And then he jumped ship over here and he stayed here." Karl Heller left behind a number of brother and sisters, in addition to his parents and other relatives, and he never saw any of them again. He landed on the East Coast and made his way across the country, ". . . working here and there." In San Francisco he attended the German Club, and it may have been there that he met the woman whom he married in 1912. John Heller's mother had come to the United States with her sister some time before. Mr. Heller knows nothing at all about his mother's family in Germany, and he can only speculate about her having left after the deaths of her parents.

Around the time of his marriage, John's father went to work as a waiter and bartender in a large Irish pub; he stayed in that job until he retired. John Heller was born in 1916, four years after his parents' marriage. He and his three younger sisters were all born at home. During his childhood the family moved three or four times, living in neighborhoods that were largely Italian and that have, in recent years, been torn down to make room for the freeway. John Heller describes his childhood as ". . . a lot of fun, with a lot of friends . . ." who went to school together and played sports together. "We was always together; it was one big bunch." Sometime between 1930 and 1933, in his mid-to-late teens, John and his friends organized themselves into the Knights. "A bunch of guys rented a big empty store and fixed it all up and made a club out of it." He says little about what the Knights' activities actually were, except that the group sponsored occasional dances. At one of these dances John's future wife Alice arrived with one of his friends. By the time the night was over John had taken her home, and they have been together ever since.

When John and Alice met in 1934 she was still in high school. He had left school after eleventh grade and was working at a series of odd jobs in wineries, canneries, department stores, and shipyards. Like all of his childhood friends, Alice was of Italian parentage. After dating Alice for nearly four years John was baptized as a Catholic. The next year, in 1939, they were married. At that time he was doing electrical work in a shipyard. He served in the navy from 1943 to 1945, continuing to do electrical work. After leaving the service he became an apprentice electrician in the same shop from which he would retire 27 years later. John and Alice postponed having children until after he had completed his military service, with the result that their daughter Marie was born in 1945.

In 1948 John Heller moved his family into the house where he and Alice still live. He and Alice were about 30 at that time; Marie was about three. During the years of active parenthood John and Alice were also actively involved with their siblings and with John's parents. They all saw each other frequently and seem to have functioned as an effective support network for one another. Although Marie was an only child, she spent a great deal of childhood time with her cousins, with one aunt babysitting for the children of all the working siblings.

John's parents both lived to be grandparents to Marie. His mother died in 1954, when Marie was nine or ten years old. His father died in 1968, when Marie was 22, approximately a year after the birth of her own son. Marie had been married around 1965. Donnie was born the next year and named after his father. Cindy was born three years later. She was given the first name of Alice's mother and the middle name of John's mother, the great-grandmothers she never knew. In 1974 John Heller retired from electrical work, and his life has remained rather stable since that time.

At this point I shall look more closely at Mr. Heller's life history, in terms of the Eriksons' eight periods of development. I shall consider his resolution of each psychosocial conflict and the role of generativity at each stage in his life.

John Heller's parents were both German immigrants whose families never left Europe. John never knew any of his grandparents. He knows nothing at all about his mother's parents, remembering no stories, no photographs, and no reminiscences on her part. John's father, on the other hand, corresponded with his family in Germany, exchanged photographs with them over the years, and shared this long-distance relationship with his son. Although as a child John could understand the German his parents spoke at home, he never learned to speak the language himself or to understand it in written form. Therefore his participation in his father's correspondence remained indirect. He had to rely on his father's translations in order to receive information, and it was only on the basis of his father's initiative that he could communicate in return. He seems to have no clear idea of who individual members of his German family were—or even who belonged to which generation. Such confusion is understandable in view of the fact that he never met any of these people and so had no personal points of reference among them. He also had no personal contact with multigenerational families, so he had no structural point of reference, either. Like John, all of his childhood friends were the children of immigrants who had left their parents in an Old Country. Like him, his friends had no personal contact with grandparents. Like him, they were forced to rely on their parents' correspondence for any contact at all with older, more distant generations. However, the nuclear family of John Heller's childhood was more isolated than were those of many of his friends in that neither of his parents had siblings to constitute a stable extended family.

During his childhood, then, John had no contact with grandparents (with *anyone's* grandparents) and no ongoing sense of what parental siblings might mean to him as aunts and uncles. His sense of lineage seems to have been largely geographical rather than generational, with all members of the family in Germany representing the forebears of his own small nuclear family in America. This childhood unfamiliarity with a generational hierarchy makes less surprising Mr. Heller's continual slips, during the interviews, from one generation to the next. In answering a question about his father as grandfather to Marie, for example, John skipped a generation and explained that his father had known Donnie (the grandson of John Heller himself) only as an infant, in the last year before he died. John demonstrates a rigid capacity to view people almost exclusively in terms of their relationships to him and to view kinship roles almost entirely in terms of the individuals who play these roles in his own life.

John Heller describes his childhood primarily in terms of his friends and the activities they shared. It is only with some effort that I can piece together an image of his family during these childhood years, and of his feelings within that family. He says that his father was a bartender and a waiter at an establishment he describes as ". . . the biggest bar in the city, in its day." Largely as a function of the people he met through work, his father attended meetings of the San Francisco German Club for many years, but John himself had no direct contact with this organization or the culture it represented. When I asked Mr. Heller about his father, during our discussion of his childhood, he explained that his father was ". . . always working at night and asleep during the day."

Mr. Heller's favorite activities as a child were the sports he used to play with his neighborhood friends, like ". . . street hockey, handball, and all that sort of stuff. . . . We used to go to the ball games all the time, just to keep score. . . . When we didn't go to the games we kept the scores at home." During childhood his neighborhood included a large Italian-owned vegetable garden and some small farms. In addition to playing city sports, John and his friends used to help cultivate the gardens and care for the farm animals. He remembers with more excitement than he displays concerning other topics, that when the circus came to town he and his friends would water the elephants and help with the tents in exchange for free tickets. All of these childhood activities took place outside John's family. His sisters stayed at home and had friends in the immediate vicinity; John's life always centered around the Italian families who lived a few blocks away.

About his own family during his childhood Mr. Heller says only that there were rules and routines to which adherence was unwaveringly demanded. "You had to come home for dinner. And whatever Mother made, boy, that's what you had. . . . Otherwise you didn't eat anything at all. . . . And you had to be in at a certain time at night." Parents were stricter and you obeyed them more. He went on to say about his mother that, "She was a very quiet mother. . . . A very clean mother. . . . Very neat about everything. . . . She talked a little broken English." He also says that she wore her hair in a bun and that she liked to listen to opera records.

The picture John Heller paints of his childhood family is of a unit in which his physical needs were met, in which he learned the social skills and values necessary to survive in the world outside, but in which he was emotionally hungry. Mother's interests were alien to his own; she could hardly speak his language. I am also led to believe that she was closer and more devoted than this to John's sisters—both because they were younger and needed more attention and because they were girls and were, by definition, more like her. Unfortunately, John's memories of his father as sleeping all the time and as having little interest or competence in arenas that were central to his son suggest that young John experienced his father as unavailable as well.

The paucity of information about John Heller's early years makes it extremely difficult to reconstruct his balancing of the earliest psychosocial tensions. Since he was the firstborn, it is likely that during infancy he received more concentrated care and attention from his mother than he remembers in later years. However, during the stages of early childhood and play age, when the radius of significant relations expands from Mother to include, first, Mother and Father, and then the basic-family, John seems to have experienced the negative impact of Father's unavailability and Mother's increasing busyness with new babies. Although John has no memories of this early period, his memories of later childhood reflect an individual with underdeveloped senses of will and, to a lesser extent, of purpose. Certainly in his later life he describes himself as behaving with what looks like a striking lack of determination. This deficiency may be traced back to the second and third psychosocial periods, and we may speculate that it results from a family environment that provided inadequate generative support for their son's robust development during these years.

I do not describe this deficiency as particularly pathological or regard John Heller's family life during this period as particularly pathogenic. His family does not appear to have been markedly different from hundreds of thousands of poor immigrant families whose struggles to survive left little parental attention or nurturance for children at certain developmental stages. In many families, however, grandparents, aunts, uncles, and older siblings were able to supplement parental efforts, both instrumental and affective, and thereby to enhance a particular child's chances of achieving optimal development at any period. In these other families the grand-generativity of family elders and the nurturance of other relatives often represented an important supplement to the care that struggling parents could provide. The relative isolation of John Heller's family left them on their own, forcing John to rely on his parents' caring alone, or to go outside the family altogether and find there what he could.

In later play age and throughout school age John turned to the neighborhood friends who were to be so important to him until after his marriage. At the time that the child's radius of significant relations expands to encompass neighborhood and school, John's environment provided considerable interpersonal richness in these arenas. These were the years in which he and his friends helped the circus get set up; helped feed, clean, and pasture the local farm animals; and scavenged the dumps for repairable bicycles and sports equipment. These were the years in which he became involved in sports, both as a participant and as an active observer.

As part of a group of neighborhood children John was welcomed into many homes, where he received a kind of parental attention that was appropriate to his needs and interests, and was strikingly absent from his own parents. Other children's parents took him to baseball games and eagerly discussed game scores and batting averages; his own parents did not. When he was young enough to be dependent solely on generativity within his own family, his psychosocial development suffered. When he grew old enough to be able to depend on relationships outside his own family, he began to thrive. The only unambivalently positive comment John Heller made about himself, to me, was that he had been "a great hero at baseball." The skills that were the seeds of that heroism germinated and firmly took root during latency, outside his family.

As has been noted earlier, none of John Heller's childhood friends had grandparents who had emigrated from the Old Country. His direct interpersonal experience has always been limited to his parents' generation, his own generation, and the generations that have followed. During late play age and latency John began to write occasional letters to his father's family in Germany. He was unable to describe to me what he wrote about, or what they wrote about in return. He wrote in English, relying on them to have his letters translated, and vice versa. Despite the somewhat indirect nature of this correspondence, it seems to represent a real effort by young John Heller to establish connection with the larger family from which his nuclear family was so painfully isolated.

During adolescence John and his friends formalized their group in becoming the Knights, in securing and renovating a clubhouse, and in maintaining their organization and its functions over a period of several years. This club seems to have been John's primary reference group—the group around which his identity centered and whose behavioral and attitudinal norms he adopted. It was here that he consolidated senses of fidelity and loyalty in companionship and mutual effort. It was here that he engaged in the clandestine smoking and drinking that represented the age- and culture-appropriate levels of rebellion in that era. His fellow Knights were the people with whom he left school after eleventh grade to spend the days fishing and, eventually, working at a series of manual jobs that reinforced his sense of himself as physically powerful and socially immobile. John's role in the Knights seems to have been that of "active follower," as opposed to that of leader or decision maker. He does not talk about having decided to leave school after the eleventh grade; he says only that he did so together with his friends. As an active follower in the Knights he consolidated a lifelong capacity to do well (to become skillful and to be faithful) on the basis of someone else's initiative, will, and purpose. This adolescent style is understandable in an individual whose earlier childhood provided the relatively weak senses of will and purpose described earlier for John Heller. (Also involved in John's adolescent consolidation of identity was his sense of fidelity to extended family. For all of its distance, John's correspondence with his German relatives offered him an important opportunity to participate in family-based caring outside the nuclear family unit.)

John Heller's young adulthood centered around his marriage to Alice. As noted earlier, he met her at one of the Knights' dances, where he demonstrated uncharacteristic initiative and will in wooing her away from one of his friends. He has not parted from her since. He portrays the period of his early marriage in terms of the partnership and cooperation appropriate to the intimacy of this developmental stage. It is striking, however, that his description of this period also conveys a generalized sense of purpose more powerful than that he had hitherto displayed. Not only did he very purposefully woo Alice away from his friend that first night. He and Alice quite deliberately decided to postpone the family they both wanted and expected until after his military service. He also describes having *chosen* to serve in the naval branch of the military, both because he thought he would enjoy the work and also because he wanted to establish that link with his father's history in the merchant marines.

John Heller's feelings about his father seem to have changed during this period. In contrast to the meager descriptions he provides of Father sleeping through his childhood, he remembers Father during this period of his own early marriage as ". . . very comical and full of life. He knew everybody and he was always full of jokes." These lively memories date to the period of John's early marriage and not back any earlier. When asked to describe his earliest happy memory of his father he tells of ". . . going down on Sundays and drinking beer with him. . . . I guess I was married by then." Clearly John Heller was able to flourish in his marriage, both personally and interpersonally, in ways that helped him strengthen earlier weaknesses.

I met John's wife Alice approximately six months after the completion of the life-history interviews, when a colleague and I came to administer quantitative questionnaires to the two of them. I was enormously surprised at her effervescence and her lively sense of humor. In contrast to her husband's uncomfortable diffidence and reticence, she was talkative and open, and she seemed to be completely at ease with the structured interview process. While I interviewed John in our accustomed seats in the living room, my colleague interviewed Alice in the kitchen, on the other side of a pair of sliding doors. Occasionally we would be interrupted from her side of the doors with a shouted question, such as, "Hey, John, exactly when was Donnie born? I can't remember. What did *you* say for that question?" Among 10 or 15 husband–wife pairs interviewed in this way, Alice was the only respondent to display such unabashed informality. Rather than inappropriate, her spontaneity seemed refreshing, playful, and, somehow, respectful. At the end of each quantitative interview, the respondent was asked if he or she was willing to participate in future research. Glancing at me and then quickly away, John demurred, saying he guessed he'd told me about all he had to say. When Alice finished with her interview she quickly sat beside John on the couch, squeezed his hand, and said, "I told 'em we'd both be glad to talk to 'em again. OK?" John laughed and replied, "I said I thought not." Alice turned to me and said sweetly, "Well, you can always call us. We'll see how we feel then."

Alice's unexpected exuberance, her interpersonal ease, and her striking social grace shed considerable light on John's psychosocial development from the time of their marriage. As an individual who does well on the basis of someone else's leadership John has been able to thrive, following along with and supporting Alice's initiative. As an example, in their current life Alice does not drive. When John describes her caring for a blind friend, caring for friends' children, visiting sick friends, or shopping for the grandchildren, it is with the knowledge that he makes all of this generativity possible by providing all of her transportation.

With their marriage John and Alice became increasingly close to her siblings, visiting frequently, babysitting, and gathering as a clan. From his own play age John had observed this kind of closeness and reciprocal involvement among the Italian families of his friends, and he had long been welcomed into various of these families. However this was the first time he himself really belonged to such a family, with all the rights and responsibilities of membership. In the presence of clearly established norms he was able to be an effective, responsible member of Alice's family and also to generalize these behaviors to his own family. He describes an ongoing reciprocal involvement with his own sisters but cannot talk specifically about his involvement at a period earlier than this one, of his early marriage. The structure and direction provided by his marriage to Alice seem to have enabled John to develop the multifaceted sense of love appropriate to this stage of development and, on the basis of this psychosocial strength, to begin engaging in effective reworking of earlier, inadequately balanced psychosocial tensions.

John Heller's middle adulthood seems to have been a stable, productive period in which he balanced capacities for generativity and stagnation to develop a real capacity to "care for"—a capacity that focused on his family. Unlike our stereotypical image of the work-oriented American male, Mr. Heller does not describe a passionate adulthood devotion to or ongoing excitement about either his work *per se* or his success and advancement in his field. In his 27 years as an electrician, working in a single shop, he performed competently under the direction of his bosses. He does not describe any particular skills he developed or any jobs of special interest. He does not speak with noticeable pride of the quality of his work. Instead he describes his good fortune in having had a steady position with a large company, in being sent each day to a job where there was work for him, and in having worked for several years each on jobs that kept him on, so that he could provide a steady income for his family. A member of the union for 27 years, he was never involved in union politics because "that's too much work. You have to be out most of the time, at meetings and all this stuff." True to the character style discussed throughout this chapter, he functioned effectively at work, accepting assignments and carrying out instructions. He viewed his job primarily as an activity through which he cared for his family. He did not display initiative; he does not regret opportunities not taken.

John Heller has developed his sense of generativity almost entirely within his nuclear family, and it is in his parenthood that he demonstrates pride in what he has created with the past 40 years of his life. When asked, generally, to discuss his early and middle adulthood, he speaks immediately of Marie's childhood, during which he thought a lot ". . . about giving her everything that we could give her—without spoiling her, you know. . . . Just giving her a good home, being good parents to her." He has difficulty articulating his feelings as a young parent with hopes for his small daughter. It is a struggle for him to find the words to tell me, "I just hoped she'd grow up to be something, grow up and get married, you know. We never bossed her much or tried to make decisions for her. No, we hoped she would grow up to be good." In this very general statement he expresses both his hopes for his daughter's life and also his feelings about how to be a good parent.

The extended family has been a constant source of support and a constant frame of reference for the adult John Heller. When Marie was a little girl and both Alice and John were working, Marie spent quite a bit of time at the home of one of Alice's sisters. In describing Marie's birth John noted that he and Alice were the first of all the siblings to marry and that Marie was the first child to be born. (Notably, he does not say that she was the first grandchild. He was not thinking in those terms then.) Within a year of Marie's birth Alice's sisters all had children. John described his nieces and nephews to me, with a striking, direct, and individualized knowledge and concern. Clearly these nieces and nephews are and have always been persons of real importance to him and for whom he has experienced some real sense of responsibility.

With Marie's birth John Heller had his first direct experience with grandparenthood: his parents were now grandparents to his daughter. Marie was the first grandchild in the extended family, and for John's parents her birth must have represented a major landmark. In Marie, these two familially isolated, immigrant parents had successfully created a third generation. Acknowledging Marie's intergenerational importance, John and Alice named their daughter after her two grandmothers.

John says that his parents were both good grandparents and that they enjoyed Marie a lot. He is particularly enthusiastic and specific about his father's pleasure and ease with children, saying, "He was very good with kids. He really liked them. . . . He used to show them puzzles and play games with them, stuff like that." We may speculate that in watching his father greatly enjoy playing with his young daughter, John Heller was able, indirectly, to appreciate the fun-loving adult attention that had been so conspicuously absent from his own childhood. In marriage John was able to develop a certain kind of new appreciation for his father; in parenthood he was able to deepen and enrich that appreciation. We may also speculate that John's appreciation contributed to his father's later-life sense of grand-generativity.

John Heller's parents saw their young granddaughter at least a couple of times a week. John himself was instrumental in all of this contact. Although his parents lived only 10 minutes away, they did not drive and were therefore dependent on him for transportation. Grandparent contact always involved three generations, regardless of whose home was the site of a given visit. It is striking that John's parents never spent time alone with Marie, without him and Alice. They were never asked to babysit. "If we went someplace, anyway, like the beach or something, we always took them along with us—the Palace of Fine Arts, go out there to feed the ducks, something like that." Clearly John Heller's burgeoning generativity extended to his parents. In encouraging them to care for their granddaughter he found himself caring for them, as well. This process enabled him to continue to renew his earlier-life, somewhat precariously balanced psychosocial tensions and, in so doing, to continue to strengthen his relatively weak senses of will and purpose.

In large part, the meaning of John Heller's own grandparenthood is tied up with his reviewing and revitalizing the themes of his whole lifetime. He says that he began to think about becoming a grandparent when Marie was married, in 1965–66. He was eager for this new role, explaining, "You always wish for grandchildren." When Donnie was born Mr. Heller was excited at the prospect of having someone to do things with. He articulates his hopes for his grandparenthood as, ". . . just to watch him grow up. Watch him play ball—something in athletics." For the first year of Donnie's life John's father was alive to be a great-grandfather to the child. Though Father's own immigrant background had deprived John of grandparents, John was able to give to this father a great-grandson who had a family link three generations back.

Much as John Heller describes himself as having cared for his own parents in his middle adulthood, he describes Marie as caring for him and Alice today. She buys them gifts on shopping trips. She invites them to visit so she can cook for them. John beams with pride as he talks about Marie in this way. He is proud of the large house she and her husband can afford, proud of the activities in which she participates, proud of her homemaking expertise, and proudest of all of her success as a parent. He seems to view this success as a validation of his own earlier generativity, which in turn he explains in terms of his father's skill. Since his description of his early childhood is strikingly devoid of examples of his father as a good parent, we may speculate that his own very rich, increasingly validated capacity for caring has contributed to his feelings of generational connectedness, to the extent that he seeks to place himself and his generative success in a generational line of similar success.

However, John is not as singularly dependent on Marie as he describes his parents having been on him. He is just now beginning the transition from generative responsibility into the period that calls for post-maintenance grand-generativity. This transition is a gradual one, and there is much in his relationships with Marie and with his grandchildren that continues to demonstrate active, direct generativity. He and Alice have a mobile home at Folsom Lake, where he is pleased to have the grandchildren spend two or three weeks of summer with them. He speaks with understated pride of his and Alice's buying the grandchildren their new school clothes and Alice's altering them to perfect specification. He is also proud about the friendly arguments between his daughter and himself; when he takes her food shopping before a meal they will be eating at her home, each of them insists on paying the bill. John does not always have the last word in these loving arguments. He often demonstrates an essential capacity of grand-generativity in deferring to Marie. That is, he accepts her care in a way that validates her own sense of caring.

For John Heller grandparenthood and grand-generativity are bound up with his concept of extended family in several ways. Earlier I speculated about the ways parenthood had contributed to his sense of an intergenerational family of which he was the center. As a grandparent he is involved in a different extended family, with his daughter and her husband at the center. In this new family he and Alice are one of two sets of in-laws, and his and Alice's siblings and their children represent only two of four family branches. John speaks proudly of Marie's capacity to sponsor holiday celebrations for this clan. He mentions the convenience for the grandchildren inherent in the fact that he and Alice live so close to their in-laws that the children can see all four grandparents on a single visit.

In sharp contrast to elders who view themselves as patriarchal founders of clans, John Heller accepts with apparent equanimity his membership in a family defined around his daughter. He does not seem to share the need demonstrated by these patriarchal elders for grand-generative power and control. Rather, in keeping with his own lifelong psychosocial processes, he is quite comfortable expressing post-maintenance caring without wielding power. As a child he neither had nor observed grandparents as patriarchs or matriarchs of clans. In his earlier-life experience it was the parents who were responsible; members of other generations were beneficiaries of parental responsibility. In addition, he has shown himself, throughout his lifetime, to function most effectively when he is implementing someone else's initiative. Although he blossomed in the period of his own generative responsibility, his dominant psychosocial style of effectiveness under instruction is particularly well suited to the grand-generativity of later life.

This style has led him to begin the psychosocial transition from middle adulthood to later life at a younger chronological age than do many other individuals. That is, his psychosocial age is greater than that of many chronological peers. For example, although all of the grandparents in this study were proud of the financial, professional, and marital achievements of their children, other than John Heller, only those informants well over the age of 75 spoke proudly and comfortably of being provided for by their children. The comfortable acceptance of being cared for certainly represents an aspect of old age's reworking of the middle-adulthood tension between generativity and stagnation. However, at 63, Mr. Heller has not yet reached what society—or the other respondents in this study—regard as old age. This discrepancy suggests both that psychosocial age is determined by an interaction between lifelong dynamics and chronological norms and that it is psychosocial, rather than chronological, age that determines the meaning any individual will find in a given experience.

The nature of John Heller's experience with generativity and grand-generativity throughout his life cycle, and the relative weakness of his own senses of will and purpose in comparison to love and care, seem to have propelled him into psychosocial old age chronologically earlier than many individuals enter this period. He retired from his profession early—as soon as he had secured his pension. In striking contrast to several informants more than 10 years his senior, he describes himself as pleased to be finished with his working life and as comfortable having little to do. He employs the professional skills he developed over the course of more than 30 years only under special circumstances, and with far more of a sense of caring for the individual for whom he is working than a sense of pride in his work. He displays no inclination to begin a new post-retirement career or to function as a consultant in the field of his adulthood career. His primary concerns are those of indirect, no-longer-responsible, post-maintenance generativity. He is focusing his current life on the grandparenthood role he created for his parents and into which he, himself, has been most eager to move.

REFERENCES

Erikson, E. H. (1980). On the generational cycle: An address. *International Journal of Psychoanalysis. 61*, 213–233.
Erikson, E. H. (1982). *The life cycle completed*. New York: Norton.
Erikson, E. H., Erickson, J. E., & Kivnick, H. Q. (1986). *Vital involvement in old age.* New York: Norton.
Kivnick, H. Q. (1982a). Grandparenthood: An overview of meaning and mental health. *The Gerontologist, 22*, 59–66.
Kivnick, H. Q. (1982b). *The meaning of grandparenthood*. Ann Arbor, MI: UMI Research Press.
Kivnick, H. Q. (1985). Intergenerational relations: Personal meaning in the life cycle. In J. A. Meacham (Ed.), *Contributions of human development: Vol. 14. Family and individual development* (pp. 93–109). Basel, Switzerland: Karger.

5

Stroke Rehabilitation and the Negotiation of Identity

Sharon R. Kaufman

The meaning of illness to the patient has emerged in the last decade as an important area of inquiry for anthropologists and sociologists studying medicine. Several goals can be accomplished by addressing and understanding patients' perspectives on health problems. First, the social, psychological and moral dimensions of illness can be delineated by eliciting the subjective response of a person to being ill.[1] This response includes the patient's view of the significance of the health problem, how it affects relationships, and the actions taken to ameliorate the condition (Helman, 1985). Second, focusing on the problems of those who experience illness can explain more behaviorally than can approaches focusing solely on "objective" disease entities or on a narrow medical understanding of disease processes and treatment (Reif, 1973; Strauss & Glaser, 1975). Conrad (1985) and others have noted that a patient-centered approach reveals that individuals, while experiencing illness, must also get on with the rest of their lives. Decisions they make and actions they undertake regarding their treatment reflect much more than the medical advice they are given: actions are influenced by the imperatives of daily life, personal priorities, and lifelong patterns of response to crisis and disruption. Patient behaviors may or may not be compatible with treatment regimens. Third, it is hoped that describing patients' experience will broaden providers' understandings of the meaning of illness so that treatment goals that are realistic for the patient can be designed and implemented. Ultimately, the effectiveness of treatment must be made on the basis of patients' perspectives as well as providers' knowledge (Maretzki, 1985).

This chapter seeks to contribute to our understanding of the meaning of illness to the patient by describing and analyzing the illness careers (Strauss, Schatzman, Bucher, Ehrlich & Sabshin, 1981) of two elderly individuals who have had strokes. In investigating individuals' choices and behaviors in the year following a stroke, I wish to draw attention to some of the differences between practitioner and patient approaches to treatment and care. My intent is to address the implications of this particular illness for the patient. It is hoped that these implications can ultimately influence the long-term care of stroke patients.

STROKE: REHABILITATION VS. RECOVERY

Stroke—the disruption of cerebral blood flow—is a medical crisis that affects mainly elderly persons. Recovery from this illness is characterized by slow and in most cases only partial return of function, a variable but usually lengthy period of work in rehabilitative therapy, and uncertainty as to final outcome. The process of rehabilitation from a stroke is mediated by several medical factors—including the site of lesion, the severity of neurological damage, and the patient's overall health. Recovery is influenced as well by numerous other factors, such as the patient's age, ability to pay for support services, and attitude toward therapy and health care. Because the rehabilitation process is long and is influenced by demographic, psychological, and sociocultural as well as medical variables, it affects all aspects of a person's life.

In following the illness careers of 102 stroke patients for one year from the time of the stroke, we found a divergence in practitioner and patient treatment goals, expectations, and strategies for improvement: as the year unfolded, patients and their caregivers approached the delivery of health care in different ways and sought to ameliorate different problems. Practitioners directed their efforts toward the *rehabilitation process* through the observation and measurement of discrete, physical tasks or behaviors on the part of the patient. Though patients participated in rehabilitation by performing tasks requested of them in therapy, they were not engaged in achieving the structured goals of rehabilitation medicine. Rather, patients directed their efforts toward *recovery*—a nonspecific, diffuse goal—which implies notions of normality, continuity, and identity. Patient concepts of recovery included dimensions of the person that usually are not included in the medical model. This chapter illustrates the divergent and sometimes contradictory responses of practitioners and patients to stroke and its aftermath.

METHODS

The findings and interpretations offered below are drawn from a three-year investigation of social and cultural factors that impinge upon the rehabilitation of persons over 50 who have strokes. Data were gathered by the traditional anthropological techniques of participant-observation and open-ended interviewing. Our goal was to collect qualitative data on practitioner and patient perspectives on the stroke rehabilitation process.

Field work consisted of initial, open-ended interviews with 32 health providers who work with stroke patients. These interviews provided information concerning stroke rehabilitation ideology and practice (see Kaufman & Becker, 1986, for details of these findings). Second, we observed 102 patients in the hospital setting, especially during therapy sessions. Specific attention was paid to patient interaction with therapists and responses of patients to therapy. Third, after discharge, we interviewed a subsample of 64 patients in the home, nursing home, and/or rehabilitation facility on the average of four times over the next 12 months. These interviews were one-half to two hours in length and focused on the patient's response to the stroke and therapy, medical concerns, reactions to disability, and plans for the future. Family members, friends, attendants and other caregivers were observed interacting with patients and were interviewed whenever possible. The patient interviews allowed us to gather rich information concerning the meaning of stroke, rehabilitation, and recovery for the patient.

DIVERGENCE IN PRACTITIONER AND
PATIENT PERSPECTIVES

The practitioner perspective centers on the observable tasks of rehabilitation that they have been trained to administer and evaluate. Their concern is primarily with patients' visible response to and performance in physical, occupational, or speech therapy. Practitioners set specific, measurable goals for patients—walking 50 feet, buttoning a shirt, reading out loud—based on the severity of the stroke and the resulting physical limitations. They focus on tasks patients can perform with unaffected body parts and on the ability of the patient to "make substitutions" and "compensate" for disabilities that do exist. The goal of all rehabilitation specialists, and indeed any health practitioner caring for a stroke patient, is "functional independence"—the ability of the patient to care for him- or herself as fully as possible with or without assistive devices. Degrees of functional independence are measured by physical, visible signs of self-care and behavior, known in the rehabilitation world as activities of daily living, or ADLs (Kaufman & Becker, 1986).

Implementing the goal of functional independence is one aspect of the stroke rehabilitation process. Following the careers of stroke victims as they leave the hospital and attempt to reorganize their lives revealed that their choices about therapy, problems of daily life, and the meaning of health care evolve as the illness career progresses and diverges from practitioners' concerns. To be sure, physicians' and therapists' goals are usually relevant and important to the patient, especially in the first few months following a stroke. However, as time passes, patients are ultimately engaged in a personal struggle for recovery. This goal is subjectively perceived and is not within the scope of physicians' or other providers' interventions or, indeed, frameworks of understanding.

When an individual is hospitalized, and later, when a person still thinks of him- or herself as a patient, effort and thought can be directed to the practitioners' goals. Most patients we observed wanted to be "good patients," that is, they wanted to follow doctors' orders and meet therapists' standards of performance. In the early stages of rehabilitation (which could involve several months), stroke patients look toward both medical stabilization and visible gains in therapy as keys to recovery. Their views are congruent with those of their caregivers. Eventually, however, the individual stops considering him- or herself solely as a patient. Perspectives of the self and of therapy widen, priorities change, and people reevaluate the notion of progress and their sense of future. Individuals move beyond professional frameworks for evaluating their needs and goals.

As patients talked about their strokes and their recovery, they described three problems that seem to characterize the poststroke experience: (1) the discontinuity of life patterns, (2) the failure to return to "normal," and (3) the redefined self. First, the patient discovers that he or she cannot take the patterns of life for granted anymore. The familiar daily, weekly, and seasonal routines are no longer possible and must be modified. Depending on the level of disability, changes in life patterns may be either drastic or subtle. In either case, the person knows that life has changed and that he or she must actively and consciously make choices about behavior that previously had been assumed. People must plan their days and their lives following a stroke—the long as well as the short term—instead of just living them. This is frequently frustrating, since the recovery process is slow and unpredictable. Also, patients know that the future is uncertain despite the apparent stabilization of the condition.

Second, one may never return to previous conceptions of "normal." When patients are asked, "Do you feel you have recovered from the stroke?" or "Do you feel your life is back to normal?" the answer is invariably "no." Even patients without a visible disability give this answer, for they believe that they are physically, emotionally, or cognitively different from their former selves, in spite of "perfect" performance in therapy. This may be surprising to practitioners who see that visible rehabilitation goals are being met.

Third, persons who have had a stroke need to learn whether they are the same as before the stroke. In the face of priorities imposed by practitioners, curtailed routines, and physical losses, and with so many outward signs of normality and consistency gone, individuals search for anchors of predictability. In addition, they seek to define and build links between the old self and the life ahead of them. The need to preserve continuity of self or reconstruct some semblance of continuity when dislocations or catastrophies interrupt the normal flow of life course events has been addressed in the literature (Clark & Anderson, 1967; Kaufman, 1986; Lifton, 1967; Myerhoff, 1979). Persons who have had strokes face the task of integrating the profound disruptions that have occurred into their self-image, so that a continuous sense of self emerges. These three problematic issues unfold in the lives of stroke patients and, we found, lie at the heart of recovery.

To illustrate the evolving divergence between practitioner and patient goals, expectations, and responses. I describe the illness careers of two women who suffered strokes, Mrs. Smith and Mrs. Jones.[2] Their strokes produced similar physical results: both women were left with weakness, stiffness, and sensory loss in their left arms and legs. The health care delivered to the two women was typical of the entire study group; for example, they both had physical and occupational therapy while in the hospital, they received the hospital's home care services for approximately two months following their discharge, they were then referred to outpatient and community and support services, which they used. For both women, as for all study participants, the continuity of health care and support services during the poststroke year was excellent. Both women appeared to me to be intelligent and articulate. They answered my questions thoughtfully. Throughout our interviews during the year following the stroke, both women tried to look at their situations with humor and equanimity.

Mrs. Smith was considered by those who treated her to be the ideal patient. There are several reasons for this characterization. She shared her caregivers' goals and she agreed with their methods of treatment. She was deeply invested in the ideology of stroke rehabilitation—the promotion of functional independence—and the fundamental American values of action, mastery of disease, and autonomy on which they are based. For the most part, she was highly motivated to do whatever her caregivers suggested, and she adhered precisely to their therapeutic prescriptives. Both her performance in therapy and her response to therapists' advice met her caregivers' highest expectations. Mrs. Jones, on the other hand, was described to me as a "difficult" and "demanding" patient because her behavior did not conform to her caregivers' expectations. She had no investment in the ideology of stroke rehabilitation, nor was she motivated to perform the therapeutic tasks so important to those who treated her. She did not place a high priority on following medical advice.

Practitioner attitudes toward the two women represented extremes, as one could expect. Mrs. Smith was described as a "good" patient for two reasons—she made "marvelous progress" in therapy and she was a cooperative, compliant patient. Except for one incident, which I will describe, she wanted and accepted both the degree and type of medical intervention she received. In the long run, her illness career exemplifies relative agreement between practitioner and patient modes of understanding the meaning of illness. Although Mrs. Jones's functional independence did improve over time, she generally did not follow the advice of her caregivers and her goals in no way corresponded with theirs. From the start, she believed there was too much intervention in her life. As time passed, the range of intervention increased. Her illness career demonstrates escalating and unresolved conflict between practitioner and patient modes of understanding.

The stroke was the central problem in Mrs. Smith's life. During the poststroke year she concentrated her full energy on reducing the limitations and frustrations it caused by voluntarily entering a relationship with her caregivers that was based on shared priorities, a willingness to follow physician and therapist suggestions, and an expressed need for their advice and physical presence. More often than not, she viewed herself as a patient in order to deal with the stroke. For Mrs. Jones, as we shall see, the stroke was one of many pressing uncertainties—medical and otherwise. After her hospital discharge, she focused her attention on personal goals aimed at reducing uncertainty and increasing control over her own life. Her goals had nothing to do with her residual limitations or, indeed, other physical health issues. She generally did not view herself as a patient.

Thus, an account of the illness careers of these two women illustrates several themes. (1) Practitioners strive for rehabilitation; patients strive for recovery. Their different perspectives emerge from their separate understandings of the illness and influence the nature of their respective health care decisions. (2) Regardless of whether patients agree with the goals of stroke rehabilitation, most hold onto a sense of self and a sense of progress that they refuse to have violated (Marshall, 1981). (3) A passive, compliant patient role is not a given in relationships between elderly individuals and their caregivers. Choices of passive versus active behavior in response to treatment and following or disregarding therapeutic regimens are continually negotiated within the context of responses to illness and medical intervention, conceptions of the self, and lifelong behavior patterns.

Mrs. Smith

Mrs. Smith is a petite, delicate-looking woman with a lot of energy. She is 66 years old and Caucasian. According to her doctor and the physical therapists who worked with her, Mrs. Smith suffered a mild stroke from which she made a "quick" and "remarkable" recovery. Indeed, compared with most other study participants, her disabilities were minor.[3] Prior to her stroke, she was an agile and active woman with no physical limitations or health problems. Divorced many years, Mrs. Smith lives alone. She worked all her adult life and retired nine months before the stroke from a demanding executive secretarial position she had held for 20 years. Mrs. Smith retired the day before her 65th birthday. She said she did not want to work anymore; she wanted time to relax, see friends, and maybe get a part-time job, "something fun," not high-pressure secretarial work. She wanted a new routine. At the time of her stroke, she was in a period of transition. Her life had not settled into any predictable pattern; she claims she was on the verge of deciding how to spend her time. She was active, walking around the city a lot, having lunch out with friends, going to the theater, but she felt she was in a period of limbo. Characterizing herself before her stroke, Mrs. Smith told me: "I've always been active and proud of my work, and I've always been in a hurry."

Following her hospital discharge, Mrs. Smith had the services of the hospital home care physical and occupational therapists. Mrs. Smith looked forward to their visits and was eager to make progress in her therapy sessions. She learned the exercises recommended to her and practiced them daily, without fail. Mrs. Smith firmly believed—as did her therapists—that if she performed the therapeutic exercises, she would regain strength, feeling, and dexterity and return to "normal." For six months, the exercises dominated her time. She focused on completing and perfecting each one; their achievement was the symbol of her recovery. When I asked Mrs. Smith to describe a typical day, she told me:

> After breakfast, I start with my exercises, and I have a program. I start down the walkway on the walker. I go right down to the end and go back and forth twice, and that's six times a day. Then I ride the bicycle; then it's the hand exercises. Really, it's amazing. The exercises take quite a good portion of the day; I have so many.

When the two months of home care services ended, the physical therapist arranged for Mrs. Smith to get continued physical therapy as an outpatient in the hospital where she had been a patient. The therapist who worked with her during this six-week period told me, "Everyone wants to have a patient like Mrs. Smith. Her gains are unusual, much faster and more far reaching than is normal. Her progress is fantastic." Mrs. Smith was fully committed to all her therapy sessions, first at home, and then as an outpatient. She remarked, "The therapy and exercises they give me are so important. The exercises are boring, but I feel they're good for me. I think if I do all the things I'm supposed to, the sooner I'll be getting back to normal."

At the suggestion of the outpatient physical therapist, Mrs. Smith then started an exercise class designed for stroke patients at a local community center. Deciding that the continuity of therapy was critical to her recovery, she let no time elapse; she arranged to start this class the week the therapy terminated. Mrs. Smith told me, "The classes are terrific. I feel I'm getting stronger, making progress. This is the most important thing I'm doing right now." At each transition point—the end of home care services and the end of outpatient therapy—Mrs. Smith agreed completely with the suggestions made by her health care team (which now included her physician, an occupational therapist, and two physical therapists) about the treatment of her residual disabilities. Her goals were the same as those of her caregivers: to become functionally independent.

Six months after the stroke, Mrs. Smith fell and broke her left hip.[4] When she returned home, she received the hospital home care services again for two months—this time the physical therapist and a home health aide. She had to resume her initial exercises to strengthen her weak side and regain her walking skills and confidence. Again, she performed the prescribed exercises, assuming they were essential to her recovery. At the time home care ended (eight months poststroke), Mrs. Smith told me, "Now I have a fear of falling that I never had before." She said that she needed a lot of "moral support" from the therapist and home health aide to take a shower by herself—she was terrified of falling in the shower. Mrs. Smith wanted the intervention of the health care team. She wanted their guidance for her exercise regimen, their physical presence when she showered, and their emotional support and encouragement for the difficult process of learning to do things by and for herself.

After the home care services terminated, Mrs. Smith had another fall. She did not break any bones or sustain any physical injuries this time. However, her sense of purpose and notion of progress were fundamentally shaken as she questioned, for the first time since the stroke—now 10 months ago—the value of all the therapeutic exercises and her assumed full recovery. For the first time since her stroke, she chose to disregard medical advice. She recalled:

The orthopedic surgeon (who performed the hip surgery) said I should have a brace for that weak knee, to keep if from buckling under. But I didn't want it. I decided against it. I didn't even go look at it. I just felt it would deter my walking even more—carrying around all this extra paraphernalia. And it would make me be an invalid. He said that exercises wouldn't help. He made me feel there was nothing I could do. He made me feel like I wasn't a person. So, then I decided to call my own doctor, and see what he thought. He recommended that I call the physical therapist (from home care) and ask her opinion. And I was thrilled that he recommended that. So I called her right away. She came out to the house, and said, "You don't need a knee brace, that knee is strong, a brace won't keep you from falling. You just need to work on making that knee and leg stronger." And she set up three outpatient visits at the hospital for me. Those sessions were marvelous. They were with A.—such a nice man, a fine man. He also said, I don't need the brace and it won't help me. He recommended that I keep up with some exercises, and that I have to pace myself. He knew that I did things very fast, that I've always moved fast, and that I just have to slow down. So, that's what I'm trying to do.

Though the orthopedic surgeon sought to treat only her physical limitations, Mrs. Smith interpreted his advice *in relation to* other dimensions of her life: her daily routine, her self-image, and her investment in therapy. Her choice, refusing the brace, demonstrates her rejection of health care that would impinge on anything more than her physical disabilities by opposing her values or threatening her self-image. More-over, her choice illustrates the way in which rehabilitative decision making is influenced by assumptions about recovery, the need to pre-serve a certain self-image, and notions of how one's life should be lived. Mrs. Smith had invested everything in the therapeutic exercises she had been performing for 10 months. To follow the orthopedic sur-geon's advice would have meant abandoning the tasks and goals she had created for herself in the past year. Exercises were her path to recovery from the stroke, and she planned to recover fully. In addition, the fact that she used the exercises to structure her days and months ensured routine and purpose in an otherwise unfamiliar life period. She knew, especially since her most recent fall, that the course of rehabilita-tion itself was uncertain, sometimes frightening, and full of setbacks. In addition, we recall that she had been in limbo before the stroke, in a period of no predictable daily round, no newly arrived at plan of action. In the past year, she had created a new career—doing rehabilitation exercises. She was actively engaged in recovery from a stroke *and* she had created a knowable, meaningful routine for herself. If exercises "wouldn't help," as she claims the orthopedic surgeon suggested, then her attempt to restore her full health and simultaneously create a meaningful daily round would be undermined. It is no wonder the surgeon's suggestion challenged her worth and made her feel that she "wasn't a person."

The physical therapist (*A.*), on the other hand, confirmed her self-image by acknowledging that she's "always moved fast." This trait is part of who she is, and it has been sustained through her long rehabili-tation. Not only does this therapist confirm that she is still a person, but also he emphasizes that *she is the same kind of person she's always been.* This reassurance is essential for someone who can no longer move in the same ways or maintain the same life as before the illness. His suggestion, to modify her actions by slowing them down, does not attack her self-image, routines, or future plans. On the contrary, his suggestion affirms Mrs. Smith's choice.

When I visited Mrs. Smith one year after her stroke, she was still doing the exercises prescribed by the physical therapist twice a day. She also had returned to the twice-weekly classes at the community center. Her primary concern was her commitment to the therapeutic exercises to ensure her recovery, and she was aided in this goal by continued support from both physical therapists at the hospital and exercise instructors at the community center. The agreement between the health care team and Mrs. Smith gave structure and meaning to her everyday life.

Mrs. Jones

At the time of her stroke, Mrs. Jones had more practitioners involved in her care and had more aspects of her life under surveillance than did Mrs. Smith. During the course of her illness career, "medicine's reach" (Arney & Bergen, 1984, p. 166) extended into many dimensions of her life. As a result, much of Mrs. Jones's behavior was subject to "treatment" and "management."

Many practitioners were involved in her care for three reasons: (1) According to her physician, she had five chronic conditions: hypertension, chronic obstructive pulmonary disease (COPD), arthritis, cataracts, and psychiatric illness. These were closely monitored by her physician. (2) She was an alcoholic residing in sheltered housing for senior alcoholics. She was supervised there by social service practitioners and mental health counselors. (3) After her hospitalization, she was discharged to a board-and-care home (personal care below the level of formal nursing care). This facility had a proprietor who was responsible for Mrs. Jones's care and behavior. Where Mrs. Smith's care was directed to only one dimension of her life, the functional disability following the stroke, Mrs. Jones's care, in contrast, was directed to a much larger range of what were considered "problem areas." She was treated for her chronic conditions, alcohol abuse, and her personal habits as well as for her functional disabilities following the stroke. In addition, the moral dimension of her life was "managed" because her attitudes and goals opposed those of her caregivers.

Sixty-eight and Caucasian, Mrs. Jones was living in sheltered, temporary housing for senior alcoholics when she had a stroke. She had been residing at this establishment for almost six months. According to her caregivers, Mrs. Jones was making good progress there and was about to move to an independent senior apartment. The stroke changed the course of her life.

Mrs. Jones's stroke resulted in limitations similar to those of Mrs. Smith. At the time of her discharge from the hospital, Mrs. Jones could not walk up or down stairs unaided, could not bathe alone, and could not dress without assistance. Following her hospitalization, Mrs. Jones was too disabled to return to the sheltered residence, so the hospital discharge planner arranged for her to be placed in a board-and-care home. In California, board-and-care homes accept people who are ambulatory and continent but who cannot provide for all their daily needs. Board-and-care homes are run by "proprietors" who are responsible for supervising all medications and therapeutic and recreational activities for the residents. Depending on an individual's personal history, cognitive abilities, and attitude toward independence, board-and-care can represent anything from the safety and comfort of a family home to the confinement of a prison. For Mrs. Jones, board-and-care was at best a school dormitory with rules she tried to ignore and at worst, a prison. Because she was disabled, had no privacy, and had her behavior monitored by the proprietor of the facility, Mrs. Jones lost whatever personal freedom and autonomy she previously had possessed. She hated being there. From the day she entered the facility, her overriding goal was to get out. I learned that, to her, recovery from the stroke meant moving out of board-and-care and into the senior apartment as previously planned.

The following conversation, which took place between one of the hospital therapists and the proprietor—in Mrs. Jones's presence—illustrates the type of surveillance to which Mrs. Jones was subject:

PROP.: She can smoke only four cigarettes a day. I am very firm about that.

THER.: I hope she doesn't smoke up here (upstairs in the bedroom).

PROP.: Oh, no. I don't let her smoke up here. I only let her smoke downstairs [in the sitting room].

THER.: Is it safe to have her smoking?

PROP.: Oh, yes, it's safe.

THER.: I mean, does she have to be watched?

MRS. J.: (Interrupting) I'm safe. It's perfectly safe. Nobody watches me.

THER.: (To proprietor) She isn't in any danger of burning down furniture, is she?

The therapist wanted to ensure the patient's and the facility's safety and survival, but, in the process, he was oblivious to his treatment of Mrs. Jones. She later told me, "They are always right there. They make me feel incompetent and inadequate."

Like Mrs. Smith, Mrs. Jones looked forward to the hospital home care therapists' visits, but there the similarity ends. Mrs. Jones enjoyed the therapists because they were lively, friendly, young, concerned about her well-being, and provided relief from an otherwise boring and meaningless routine. Mrs. Jones had no investment whatsoever in the ideology of rehabilitation—the promotion of functional independence. She seemed to place no value on performing the therapeutic exercises or on any activity designed to promote complete self-care. She never did her prescribed exercises. The following dialogue, which I observed between Mrs. Jones and the occupational therapist one month after her stroke, typified the type of encounters she had with the therapists during the home care period:

O.T.: You look good. Who put on your make-up?

MRS. J.: The proprietor did it.

O.T.: I want you to do as much for yourself as possible.

MRS. J.: (Laughing) Who said so?

O.T.: I did.

MRS. J.: But I don't want to. I don't like to and she does it so much better.

O.T.: But you are supposed to do things for yourself. Come on, I want to see you put it on yourself. Besides, holding the eyebrow pencil will be good for that hand.

The occupational therapist badgered her into applying more lipstick and eyebrow pencil by herself. Mrs. Jones completed the task, but protested throughout. The occupational therapist would not take "no" for an answer.

In some ways, it is ironic that Mrs. Jones did not participate willingly in therapy sessions or practice the exercises on her own, for accomplishing the therapeutic tasks would have given her, at the very least, some bodily freedom that the stroke had taken away. But to participate willingly in therapy would have meant succumbing to control by the therapists. Mrs. Jones would not give up her ability to make independent decisions without a fight. Besides, performing the therapeutic tasks as directed would signify that she supported her therapists' goals, and she did not. Functional independence, the essential goal of all rehabilitation specialists, reflects the fundamental and widely shared American values of personal autonomy, the importance of action (Hsu, 1972; Clark & Anderson, 1967), and mastery of disease (Pfifferling, 1980). As the dialogue between Mrs. Jones and the therapist illustrates, patients who are involved in the rehabilitation process must meet the expectations of practitioners by demonstrating, if not actually sharing, these values. Mrs. Jones was a "difficult" patient in part because she did not share these values and was simply unmotivated to perform the tasks so important to her caregivers. Apparently for much of her adult life, Mrs. Jones had never been fully "functionally independent" as measured by health care practitioners. She had not cooked, shopped, nor attended to all of her own daily needs for many years. She had not been demonstrating complete autonomy before the stroke. To attempt to express this value now through "therapeutic" tasks seemed irrelevant to her. Her attention and energy were focused on the new regulations and restrictions by which her life was controlled.

When the two months of home care services ended she was at a crossroads, a transition point in the delivery of care. The health care team (which consisted of a geriatrician, nurse, occupational therapist, physical therapist, and several social workers) had to decide how to "manage" her. Her limitations remaining from the stroke included a weak and stiff arm and hand and general unsteadiness when walking. But these concerns were dwarfed by what the health care team considered more important, all-encompassing problems. They believed her chronic conditions—especially hypertension and COPD—needed to be monitored. In addition, they did not trust her behavior. All in all, her caregivers felt it was unrealistic for her to attempt to live independently. They thought her health would deteriorate and she would begin drinking again if she lived in an unsupervised environment. They could not support her goal of leaving board-and-care. The health care team was concerned about managing a number of dimensions of her life. These included: (1) her drinking patterns, (2) her smoking patterns, (3) her compliance regarding prescribed medications, (4) her self-care behavior, and (5) the continuation of her stroke rehabilitation regimen.

To monitor all these dimensions, the team arranged for her to attend twice a week the adult day health center affiliated with the hospital. There she received occupational therapy, physical therapy, group and individual counseling, and physical exercise. In addition, she participated in a "creative writing workshop," where she wrote poetry. On two other days, she attended a community-sponsored "activity center" for alcoholics where she received counseling, support, and peer-group socialization. She liked going to the health and activity centers, both because she enjoyed the activities there and because she was out of the board-and-care facility for most of the day. She told me that the most important aspects of her "treatment" were the poetry workshop (where she was able to express her creativity), the group therapy sessions (where her self-esteem was bolstered), and the friendship developing between herself and one of her counselors. Though these activities were provided by her health care team to structure different aspects of her life, Mrs. Jones considered them domains in which she had the most autonomy.

After several months of contact with the health care team following her stroke, Mrs. Jones had acquiesced to their collective opinion—that she needed supervision. She had also agreed with them that professional help was good for her, and she accepted all aspects of her treatment regimen as productive and useful. However, her long-term goal of leaving board-and-care remained unchanged. As the months passed, Mrs. Jones's ability to tolerate her lack of autonomy in the board-and-care home deteriorated. The proprietor claimed that Mrs. Jones "disobeyed" her. From the start, the two women were having an escalating battle of wills. The proprietor wanted Mrs. Jones to get dressed and go downstairs every morning; Mrs. Jones wanted to stay in bed as long as she pleased. The proprietor brought the prescribed medications to Mrs. Jones several times a day; Mrs. Jones refused to take them or asked for more. The women exasperated each other.

Telling her caregivers she wanted to leave board-and-care had not brought about a change; neither had arguing with the proprietor nor refusing to follow the facility regimen. Mrs. Jones responded to the health care team's inertia over this issue by having a mental breakdown. Six months after her stroke, Mrs. Jones was admitted to the psychiatric unit of a local hospital. Her physician explained:

> Mrs. Jones was at the adult day health center and began hallucinating and talking nonsense. The social worker called her psychiatrist, who called an ambulance and admitted her.

Four days after she was hospitalized, Mrs. Jones explained:

> "I was going nuts at the board-and-care under the strain of it all. When I got to (adult day health center), I felt very dizzy, like something was wrong, and I felt like I was going crazy. . . . I expect now they'll try to find a place more compatible for me."

Talking with her further, I learned that the day before she was admitted to the hospital, her favorite counselor had informed Mrs. Jones that she was moving away. Mrs. Jones told me, "That really shook me up." Her strongest emotional support was disappearing from her life. That was "the last straw" and made life at the board-and-care home intolerable. Though her breakdown was not a conscious or deliberate choice, it seems that in order to effect a change in her situation, she had to take some action that would underscore her desperation. She had been a psychiatric hospital patient in the past—it seemed the best option to her now.

During her psychiatric hospitalization, Mrs. Jones told me she absolutely did not want to return to board-and-care. But she was overruled by the health care team and returned to the board-and-care home. From their perspective, her health could be "stabilized" best if she returned there. Five months later (13 months poststroke), she had a second, severe stroke and died.

To summarize, practitioner approaches to the care of stroke patients are represented by the ideology of stroke rehabilitation: patients should comply with physicians' and therapists' goals, demonstrate the fundamental American values of autonomy, action, and mastery of disease, and work toward "functional independence" through a prescribed and monitored therapeutic regimen. As the two case studies illustrate, patients do not necessarily share practitioner priorities or their underlying values. Patients attempt to create order in their lives following a stroke, but their attempts center on the subjective experience of recovery, which may or may not resemble the structured goals of stroke rehabilitation. For Mrs. Smith, recovery was characterized by two goals: (1) to return to her former way of moving and doing things by regaining her full range of physical ability and (2) to achieve both subjective knowledge and outside reassurance of continuity of self—that she was the same kind of person she had always been. For Mrs. Jones, recovery meant the ability to escape the intervention and surveillance that accompanied residing at the board-and-care home—even at the risk of further hospitalization and greater deviation from social norms. Her goal was to maintain continuity of purpose. She had been working toward independent living before the stroke; she desperately sought to achieve that goal afterwards.

IMPLICATIONS

These findings have a variety of implications for the delivery of health care, especially to older persons. Four issues that emerge from this research are discussed below.

The Importance of Biographical Knowledge

While a discussion of the life histories of Mrs. Smith and Mrs. Jones is beyond the scope of this chapter, it is important to recognize that neither woman responded to the stroke or the health care they subsequently received in a vacuum unaffected by biographical and cultural factors. Their behaviors during the poststroke year emerged from their pasts, their personal histories. In order fully to understand the meaning of stroke to the individual who experiences it, one needs to know who that person is. Clinically, in order to prescribe appropriate and relevant therapeutic goals for a patient, one needs to know the historical and social context of a person's life. To predict behavior, one needs to know the past.

Mrs. Smith has always been a perfectionist and conformist, "doing the right thing" in social interaction, maintaining order and cleanliness in her own home, and taking pride in the precise execution of her demanding secretarial duties over the years. She has always wanted to please others—her employers, her son and daughter-in-law, and friends. Two of her great frustrations since the stroke are her physical inability to clean her apartment as thoroughly as she would like and her inability to get out of the house to buy birthday presents for friends and family. Her behavioral responses to the stroke, therapy, and her caregivers are made in the context of her lifelong attention to detail, precision in carrying out instructions, and desire to please others and do what is socially correct.

Mrs. Jones had always been a nonconformist and free spirit. For much of her adult life, her behavior deviated from social norms. She managed to get along in the world by relying upon—and manipulating—the resources at her disposal, primarily the health and social services that were available and the individual service providers whom she befriended over the years. Her responses to the intervention in her life following the stroke derived from her long-term need and established pattern of maintaining a certain level of autonomy while being "medically managed."

The Issue of Compliance

In a recent review of selected compliance studies, Conrad (1985) notes that "compliance" is a medical term referring to how and why patients follow medical orders. One assumption underlying much compliance research is that individuals, when sick, should be passive and unquestioning recipients of medical care. A related assumption is that they do not have the capacity (both because of their ill health and because of their lack of training) to make informed, rational decisions about appropriate medication, therapy, or other kinds of treatment. Conrad points out that individuals who are patients do not view their responses to medical advice in terms of compliance/noncompliance at all. Rather, the issue is how to get on with their everyday lives, to assert control over their situation despite medical problems. From the perspective of someone who has had a stroke, the issue is how to reestablish "normal" everyday routines and negotiate one's identity during a period of profound uncertainty. The decision of whether to follow specific medical advice at any stage of the illness career is based on (1) the extent to which caregivers' rehabilitation goals "fit" patients' notions of recovery and (2) patients' priorities at the time the stroke occurred. Patients' decisions of when and why to "comply" with medical advice reflect their interpretation of the particular intervention.

Mrs. Smith shared the values of perseverance and work in therapy with her health care team, and she shared their ultimate rehabilitation goal of working toward functional independence. Yet she would not yield to the suggestions of the orthopedic surgeon because, at that moment in her illness career, his advice threatened her sense of self and purpose. Mrs. Jones did not share the underlying values of her caregivers, nor did she always cooperate with them. Her health care team assumed that if they could successfully monitor all her chronic conditions, alter her "negative" behaviors (such as smoking, resisting therapy, "disobeying" the proprietor), and prevent her from drinking, then all dimensions of her life would fall into place (i.e., her condition would be "stabilized.") Their approach, which encompassed so many dimensions of Mrs. Jones's life, assumed that practitioners know what is best for the patient and that patients can make profound behavioral changes quickly and easily (Zola, 1972).

Expanding Frameworks of Medical Care

Social scientists studying medicine in American society have recently described two contradictory, yet coexisting, interpretative frameworks to describe modern health care. The first framework, the "biopsychosocial" approach (Engel, 1977, 1981; Lock, 1982), posits that the patient's psychological, behavioral, and interpersonal attributes (as well as physiological and biochemical attributes) influence the course of an illness and are directly relevant for his or her medical care. This approach provides a conceptual framework that enables health care practitioners to comprehend and act upon the nonbiological aspects of patient care. It has come to represent a more humane medicine than the traditional, biomedical approach (Engel, 1977), which excludes psychological or behavioral dimensions of a health problem and addresses only measurable biological variables. The biopsychosocial approach has been advocated by social scientists, consumer advocates, and practitioners in a variety of medical fields.

The second interpretive framework, "medicalization," refers to a process whereby problems and behaviors are viewed as "disease," so that a mandate is given the medical profession to "treat" them (Arluke & Peterson, 1981; Zola, 1972). Classic examples of medicalization include alcoholism and drug addiction. More recent examples include pregnancy (Merkin, 1976) and menopause (Lock, 1982). These latter two represent the reinterpretation of normal, life-course processes, so that they become events requiring medical intervention. Social scientists have viewed this as a negative phenomenon.

The coexistence of the two interpretive frameworks presents an ironic situation regarding the practice of medicine and delivery of health services: the biopsychosocial approach to health care—by incorporating a range of dimensions of a person's life—appears to advocate intervention in so many aspects of a person's behavior (Lock, 1982). In recent years, the "consumer movement" (Berliner & Salmon, 1980) in health care has educated individuals to seek and demand medical treatment relevant to their lives within a sociocultural context. Individuals are asking health professionals to view them broadly as "people" who have illnesses that emerge from and are intertwined with various dimensions of their lives, not narrowly as "diseases."

The consequences of a more than biomedical intervention (Marshall, 1981), however, have yet to be fully understood. The danger of a medicine that encompasses all of life is that individuals, when "complying" with medical authority, must surrender their sense of self and purpose to an expanding arena of medical dominance. The medicalization of behavior by the broad, biopsychosocial approach to treatment presents a profound dilemma in the delivery of health care today. In order for both patient and practitioner to be satisfied with the level and range of care delivered, both parties need to be aware of the dilemma and its potential ramifications in specific cases. It is ironic that attempts to humanize health care may lead to loss of individual autonomy in decision making.

Vulnerability of the Elderly

Elderly individuals are both more vulnerable and more responsive to goals and expectations of various medical specialties—and thus the implication of medicalization—than are younger people, for at least two reasons. First, old age in American society is typically considered a time of sickness, infirmity, and impending death (Arluke & Peterson, 1981; Clark, 1972, 1973; Sankar, 1984). Sankar (1984) notes:

> For Americans old age is seen as a kind of disease, a terminal illness that uniformly begins in the sixties. This stereotype persists despite data indicating the relatively low incidence of institutionalization among people 65 and older (p. 251).

For the most part, health care practitioners share this stereotype. With old age defined in a medical idiom, the elderly themselves expect, and they are expected by others, to turn to the health care system for treatment, guidance, and understanding of all facets of old age itself. This widespread cultural conviction encourages the management and ultimately the control of the elderly for "medical" reasons.

Second, the elderly have more chronic conditions and more hospitalizations than do younger people, and they thus require significant medical and social support services (Becker, Pardini, Newcomer & Lee, 1983). To meet the health care needs of a growing aging population, a plethora of services that did not exist twenty years ago is now available to the physician for elderly patient referral. Moreover, there are now more professionals and paraprofessionals, trained in an ever-growing number of occupations, who are ready to extend the reaches of medical ideology and practice far beyond its traditional boundary of disease located within the body. Their efforts are intended to prevent institutionalization and repeated hospitalizations and promote "independence" and "quality of life" (Arney & Bergen, 1984). Paradoxically, services are delivered to the elderly in an attempt to preserve their autonomy while, at the same time, old age itself is construed as a medical problem requiring intervention (Arluke & Peterson, 1981; Zola, 1983).

If practitioners and patients can come to an agreement on the goals of the stroke rehabilitation process, and if they can agree on how much of a person's life requires medical intervention, then they can work together toward effective treatment. Without agreement or, at the very least, compromise, it seems unlikely that either goal—rehabilitation or recovery—will be attained.

NOTES

1. The term *illness* is used here as analytically distinct from the term *disease*. This distinction has been elucidated by many researchers in medical anthropology (see especially Eisenberg, 1977; Fabrega, 1975; Kleinman, 1978, 1980). *Disease* refers to "objective," discrete abnormalities or dysfunctions among body parts that can be identified by those trained in biomedicine. *Illness* refers to the subjective response of an individual to feeling poorly.

2. These are pseudonyms.

3. According to the Barthel Index [Mahoney, F. I., & Barthel, D. W. (1965). Functional evaluation: The Barthel index. Maryland State Medical Journal, 14; 61–65], a widely used standard of functional independence, Mrs. Smith scored 90 out of a possible 100 one month after her stroke. She scored 100 three months later. Seventy research participants (out of 102) scored below 90 following the stroke; half of those scored below 50.

4. Of the 102 people in the study, five have experienced hip fractures within the year since their stroke. Several others have fallen and fractured arms, wrists, or ankles. Physical therapists remark that hip and other fractures are not uncommon after strokes: the patient is getting better and forgets that one side of the body is weaker than usual.

REFERENCES

Arluke, A., & Peterson, J. (1981). Accidental medicalization of old age and its social control implications. In C. Fry (Ed.), *Dimensions: Aging, culture and health* (pp. 271–284.) New York: Praeger.

Arney, W. W., & Bergen, B. J. (1984). *Medicine and the management of living.* Chicago: University of Chicago Press.

Becker, G., Pardini, A., Newcomer, R., & Lee, P. (1983). *The health of older people: A framework for public policy.* San Francisco: Aging Health Policy Center, UCSF.

Berliner, H., & Salmon, J. W. (1980). The holistic alternative to scientific medicine: History and analysis. *International Journal of Health Services, 10,* 133–147.

Clark, M. (1972). An anthropological approach to aging. In D. Cowgill & L. Holmes (Eds.), *Aging and Modernization* (pp. 263–274) New York: Appleton-Century-Crofts.

Clark, M. (1973). Contribution of cultural anthropology to the study of the aged. In L. Nadar & T. Maretzki (Eds.), *Culture, illness and health* (pp. 78–88). Washington, DC: American Anthropological Association.

Clark, M., & Anderson, B. (1967). *Culture and aging.* Springfield, IL: Charles C. Thomas.

Conrad, P. (1985). The meaning of medications: Another look at compliance. *Social Science and Medicine, 20,* 29–37.

Eisenberg, L. (1977). Disease and illness: Distinctions between professional and popular ideas of sickness. *Culture, Medicine and Psychiatry, 1,* 9–23.

Engel, G. (1977). The need for a new medical model: A challenge for biomedicine. *Science, 196,* 129–136.

Engel, G. (1981). The clinical application of the biopsychosocial model. *Journal of Medicine and Philosophy, 6,* 101–124.

Fabrega, H. (1975). The need for an ethnomedical science. *Science, 189,* 969–975.

Helman, C. G. (1985). Disease and pseudo-disease. In R. A. Hahn & A. D. Gaines (Eds.), *Physicians of western medicine* (pp. 293–331). Dordrecht; Holland: Reidel, 1985.

Hsu, F. L. K. (1972). American core value and national character. In F. L. K. Hsu (Ed.), *Psychological anthropology* (pp. 241–262). Cambridge, MA: Schenkman.

Kaufman, S. (1986). *The ageless self—sources of meaning in late life.* Madison, WI: University of Wisconsin Press.

Kaufman, S., & Becker, G. (1986). Stroke: Health care on the periphery. *Social Science and Medicine, 22,* 983–989.

Kleinman, A. (1978). Concepts and a model for the comparison of medical systems as cultural systems. *Social Science and Medicine, 12,* 85–93.

Kleinman, A. (1980). *Patients and healers in the context of culture.* Berkeley: University of California Press.

Lifton, R. (1967). *Death in life.* New York: Basic Books.

Lock, M. (1982). Models and practice in medicine: Menopause as syndrome or life transition? *Culture, Medicine and Psychiatry, 6,* 261–280.

Maretzki, T. (1985). Including the physician in healer-centered research: retrospect and prospect. In R. A. Hahn & A. D. Gaines (Eds.), *Physicians of western medicine* (pp. 23–47). Dordrecht, Holland: Reidel.

Marshall, V. (1981). Physician characteristics and relationships with older patients. In M. Haug (Ed.), *Elderly patients and their doctors.* (pp. 94–118). New York: Springer.

Merkin, D. H. (1976). *Pregnancy as a disease: The pill in society.* Port Washington, NY: Kennikot Press.

Myerhoff, B. (1979). *Number our days.* New York: Dutton.

Pfifferling, J. H. (1980). A cultural prescription for medicocentrism. In L. Eisenberg & A. Kleinman (Eds.), *The relevance of social science for medicine* (pp. 197–222). Dordrecht, Holland: Reidel.

Reif, L. (1973). Managing a life with chronic disease. *American Journal of Nursing, 73*, 262.

Sankar, A. (1984). It's just old age. In D., Kertzer & J. Keith (Eds.), *Age and anthropological theory* (pp. 250–280). Ithaca, NY: Cornell University Press.

Strauss, A., & Glaser, B. (1975). *Chronic illness and the quality of life.* St. Louis: C.V. Mosby.

Strauss, A., Schatzman, L., Bucher, R., Erlich, D., & Sabshin, M. (1981). *Psychiatric ideologies.* New Brunswick, NJ: Transaction Books.

Zola, I. (1972). Medicine as an institution of social control. *Sociological Review, 20*, 487–504.

Zola, I. (1983). The medicalizing of society. In *Socio-medical inquiries* (pp. 241–296). Philadephia: Temple University Press.

6

Respite Care and Pride in Caregiving: The Experience of Six Older Men Caring for Their Disabled Wives

Aluma K. Motenko

Respite care originated in the United States in the early 1970s in response to the needs of parents of developmentally disabled children and as part of the deinstitutionalization movement. Recently there has been some interest in the concept of respite care for the disabled elderly, but few programs have actually been put into operation. With the growth of the elderly population and the rising costs of institutional long-term care, policy makers, legislators, and program administrators are seeking some alternatives to institutions. Many hope that respite care will encourage family support of the frail elderly and avoid or postpone unnecessary institutionalization or overmedication. Unfortunately, very little research has been undertaken to examine this idea fully.

My interest in studying male spouse caregivers arose from reading studies indicating that spouses may have unique caregiving experiences. Research has shown consistently that married elders are most often cared for by their spouses (Townsend, 1957; Shanas, 1979). Spouse caregivers are thought to be the greatest at-risk group of caregivers because they are themselves elderly and therefore subject to negative health consequences (Johnson, 1979; Fengler & Goodrich, 1979; Shanas, 1979). Their need for outside help, whether formal or informal, is likely to increase with the duration of the caregiving relationship (Myllyluoma & Soldo, 1980), and they are more likely to provide constant care and 24-hour care than other groups of caregivers, such as children, other relatives, and nonrelatives (Tennstedt & McKinlay, 1985). Spouses make more sacrifices to continue providing care and are less willing to consider other options and to use formal services than other types of caregivers (Tennstedt & McKinlay, 1985). The closer the bond between the caregiver and the frail elder and the more intimate the care required, the greater the strain in caregiving (Cantor, 1983; Johnson, 1979). Caring for a severely functionally disabled spouse is physically, socially, and emotionally taxing. It is believed that relief from these burdens in the form of respite care can help the caregiver maintain his or her spouse at home rather than having to resort to institutionalization. Respite care may also relieve the physical and psychological pressures associated with the burdens of caring for impaired elderly (Motenko, 1983).

Throughout the United States, states and agencies have been experimenting with a variety of programs and services to provide respite care (The Foundation for Long Term Care, 1983; Meltzer, 1982; Upshur, 1982; Yocom, 1982). The options include in-home and short-term institutional care, and the services include companionship and skilled nursing care provided by volunteers, paraprofessionals, and/or paid professional staff. Overnight and weekend care is available in settings ranging from the home, to nursing homes, to specially staffed apartments run by hospitals. These innovations are being tried in order to meet needs; they are not based on research. When research has been done, it has focused on services provided by institutions (Spence & Miller, 1985/86; Scharlach & Frenzel, 1986) rather than delivered in the home.

Similarly, male spouse caregivers have been underrepresented in research on aging. Although several studies have noted that spouses are the primary sources of informal support to married elders of both sexes (Treas, 1977; Shanas, 1979; Seelbach, 1978; Smallegan, 1985), the role of men as caregivers has received little research attention. In a related study, Vinick (1984) investigated 25 widowers who had taken care of their wives, but husbands have not yet been studied *while* they were giving care.

The Massachusetts program discussed in this chapter was initiated in 1981 by an Area Agency on Aging and is operated by a home health agency. Statewide program experimentation was launched in 1982 when the Massachusetts Department of Elder Affairs awarded three demonstration grants to home care corporations for respite care programs. A year later the National Council on Aging circulated a manual to help states develop respite care programs, based in part on the Massachusetts experience. Two years after that, in April 1985, Massachusetts embarked on a statewide program through the network of home care corporations.

Since a few programs are now in place it is possible to examine the beliefs mentioned at the start of this chapter. The hopes that are being expressed motivated me to examine the effectiveness of respite care. Does it provide the kind of support needed by families to continue caring for the frail elderly? Does it delay institutionalization? How does respite care fit within the system of family care? How does the spouse use informal help when respite care is made available? Is the spouse the primary caregiver even when receiving respite care? What role do offspring take in assisting the ill parent and the caregiving parent? Is caregiving in older married couples associated with great stress? Is caregiving as stressful for husbands as it is reported to be for wives and other family caregivers (Adams, Caston, & Davis, 1979; Archbold, 1983; Brody, 1981; Cicirelli, 1981; Horowitz & Debrof, 1982)? What are the needs of husbands in this situation, and what can respite care provide to meet those needs? Finally, what does caregiving mean to elderly husbands of frail wives?

In order to provide a focus for these questions, my study is organized around five hypotheses and three questions. The hypotheses are stated below without using the conventional null hypothesis format, since my design is qualitative rather than statistical:

1. Husbands using respite care take primary responsibility for care of their disabled wives within the informal support system of other family and friends and the formal network of paid professionals.
2. Caregiving is associated with stress, and spouse caregiving is particularly stressful.
3. Respite care supports the caregiver by providing relief from physical, social, and emotional burdens.
4. Respite care prevents or delays institutionalization.
5. Formal agencies need to take on or share the responsibility of caring for the frail elderly.

The three questions are concerned with the interpretive aspect of respite care:

1. What is the meaning of spousal care to male caregivers?
2. What is the meaning of respite care to male spouse caregivers?
3. What is the need for and utilization of respite care by male spouse caregivers?

METHODS

A pilot, exploratory study is an appropriate first step in studying a topic that has received little research attention. I hoped both to examine these hypotheses and to develop additional hypotheses that could be tested using varied sample populations and research methods.

The methods I drew on stem from Charmaz (1983), Glaser and Strauss (1967), Lofland and Lofland (1971), and Reinharz (1984). I interviewed six men in-depth in their homes, asking them to elaborate on their ideas with direct questioning. I also observed their behavior.

I was able to gain access to these individuals because I am a social worker with 10 years experience in planning and monitoring community and home-based programs to prevent and delay institutionalization for the elderly. Specifically, I had been the director of the Area Agency on Aging at the time the respite progam was started and funded by the Area Agency. Because of this connection, I was able to gain the cooperation of the agency in contacting husbands who were using their respite care program. All husbands receiving services for their wives at the time of the study were interviewed, excluding one whose wife was hospitalized during the period of data collection—February through July, 1984. With this exception, the six men represent the total population of husbands served by the home health agency, which is located in an urban area in the northeastern United States.

The agency defined eligibility for respite care on the basis of (1) a need for personal care, (2) residence with a caregiver who would assume responsibility for the client in an emergency and when the aide could not come to work, and (3) a need for relief. The first two criteria were the critical ones, because need for relief was not sufficient to merit eligibility in the program. Nevertheless, the agency was not able to develop its program on the basis of a uniform definition of respite care because none exists (Meltzer, 1982; Upshur, 1982).

The respite program was targeted to severely disabled older persons who required substantial assistance with activities of daily living such as toileting and bathing. The severe nature of their functional disability required the assistance of a skilled homemaker/home health aide with nursing backup. This is the frailest segment of the elderly population outside of institutions. Were it not for the assistance of their family, they would be unable to care for themselves and would be institutionalized.

Because of my extensive experience in this field, including home visits, I was very comfortable in my role as interviewer and observer. I enjoy speaking with older people. Their knowledge and experiences accumulated throughout their lifetimes fascinate me. In addition, the opportunity to hear these men speak lovingly about their wives, and my ability to observe their willingness to care for them, no matter how mentally or physically disabled, became a very positive experience for me.

Although I had wanted to interview and observe the husbands without the presence of their wives, this amount of privacy was difficult to come by. In some situations, the wife was preoccupied, resting, or mentally incapacitated, affording me privacy with the husband. In other cases, the wife was either a partner in the interview or was present during part of the interview. In these cases the presence of the wife was both a benefit and a hindrance. The wife presented her impressions, sometimes differing with her husband, giving me additional information about the family. In addition, this involvement allowed me to glimpse the marital dynamics of the couple. On the other hand, it is possible that when the wife participated, she inhibited the husband from complete disclosure or from expressing negative feelings or thoughts. In most cases I tried to allow time for the wife to join us for part of the interview but conducted the major part of the interview with the husband alone in a separate room of their home.

On the basis of these tape-recorded interviews and observations, 90 pages of field notes were assembled. Transcripts were made of illustrative segments of each interview and included in the field notes. After each interview I immediately made notes about the conversation. Then I listened to the tape, transcribed it, and typed my field notes.

In the analytic phase, I examined the transcripts of the interviews, paying close attention to interviewees' use of language. After completion of my study, I reported my results to the staff of the respite care program, thus repaying them in part for assisting me in locating these men. It is my hope that further research into respite care will enable us to develop a common understanding of what respite care is and should be.

THE SIX HUSBANDS

The men are white, first-generation individuals born in the United States to immigrant parents. They live in the working-class neighborhoods of a small city and its surrounding towns. All are retired except for Mr. Havighurst, a 61-year-old factory worker who works the night shift, making rubber gaskets, so that he can care for his 64-year-old wife during the day.[1] The highest level of education attained by the men is high school. The husbands range in age from 61 to 88 years, with a mean age of 73. Half of the couples are Medicaid-eligible and half are just slightly over-income for Medicaid benefits. They pay privately for their respite care. The physical health of the men can be categorized as mildly impaired in that their illnesses or disabilities (heart disease, high blood pressure, injured knee, back problems) require minimal medical treatment and minimally limit their functional capacity and independent living.

Mr. Black is a robust 88-year-old Catholic mason who has been retired for 20 years. His hardness of hearing and "weary" eyes do not stop him from socializing with his friends at the corner bar every day, listening to sports on the radio in the basement, and reading the newspaper with a magnifying glass. He appears to be in good health and is able to do all the cooking, laundry, and gardening, as well as monitoring his wife's medical condition and giving her her pills every day. She is 70 years old and has had a collapsed lung. For the past five years she has spent most of the day attached to a portable tank that supplies oxygen. Two married daughters and a son live nearby; they are devoted visitors and helpful with such things as taking Mr. and Mrs. Black to the doctor and seeing to household needs such as the purchasing of new curtains for Mrs. Black's room.

Mr. Wekstein is a 72-year-old Jewish butcher who sold his business 16 years ago to care for his wife, who had advanced Parkinson's disease. She can no longer feed herself, speak articulately, hold her head up, or keep her eyes open. Her movements are largely involuntary. Mr. Wekstein has heart disease and back problems. He can no longer lift his wife and maintain the household on his own, as he did until four years ago. He cooks for his wife, chops her food, and feeds her all her meals. He goes out every day to do his errands and to shop for food and medical supplies for his wife. Their two daughters live nearby. One visits, the other doesn't. Neither provides a significant amount of help. Mr. and Mrs. Wekstein moved to Oak Bluff when he retired and now live in public housing.

Mr. Oliver is an 80-year-old tool-and-dye maker who retired when he became allergic to the fumes in the plant. He uses a hearing aid and had prostate surgery one year ago. He moved into the "mother-in-law apartment" in his daughter's house six years ago when he required help with his wife, who has been diagnosed as having Alzheimer's disease. He does all the cooking, household chores, errands, and caregiving for his wife. He does not get along well with his daughter, whom he considers a "nervous wreck" and unhelpful. His other daughter lives farther away and is uninvolved.

Mr. Havighurst, a 61-year-old night-shift worker, is in good health. He complains about his knee, which was previously operated on for a bone chip. His daughter lives in the downstairs apartment of his two-family house and is available at night to care for Mrs. Havighurst when

Mr. Havighurst is at work. Mr. Havighurst does all the cooking, food shopping, laundry, cleaning, and caring for his wife. Their three daughters and grandchildren visit frequently and are an important source of companionship and joy for Mr. Havighurst and for Mrs. Havighurst, who has been bedridden for fourteen years with multiple sclerosis.

Mr. Evans is a 78-year-old machinist who has high blood pressure that is controlled with medication. He also had prostate surgery last year. His wife has been bedridden for the past three years, since a stroke left her paralyzed and unable to speak. She also has a long history of diabetes. Mr. Evans does all the cleaning, laundry, food shopping, cooking, and caring for his wife. He enjoys sitting down in the basement and doing the yard work. His only daughter and her children and grandchildren live too far away to visit regularly. The Evanses are extremely disappointed not to have the company of family at this crucial time.

Mr. Miller, a retired factory engineer, has mild diabetes and arthritis, which does not limit his activities. He drives a car to do the errands, completes the housework in the morning and enjoys sitting outside in his garden in the afternoon. His wife has had emphysema for 14 years. Her bone deterioration, a result of long-term drug therapy, requires her to use a wheelchair and a walker for short distances. She has trouble breathing and is attached to an oxygen tank, with tubes through her nostrils. The Millers' only son is married and lives next door. He helps with the lawn mowing and snow shoveling and other "odd jobs."

The couples' relationships with their children cover a broad range—from very active positive involvement; to active, but primarily negative; to not active, minimally positive; and finally to minimal, negative involvement.

Only Mrs. Oliver, the Alzheimer's disease victim, is able to go out of the house on a regular basis. Her husband takes her out every day to do their errands. All the other wives are homebound, although half are bedfast and half can ambulate short distances in the house. The husbands have been caring for their wives for either 14 to 16 years or three to six years.

THE MEANING OF CAREGIVING

To understand the meaning of respite care, one must understand what caregiving itself means to these men. How is it defined and experienced? In essence, I discovered that caring for their wives is a labor of love for these husbands. In the words of Mr. Oliver, who cares for his wife with Alzheimer's disease, "in order to take care of a patient, to start with, one of these patients, regardless of who they are, the first thing they must have for the patient is love. If they don't have that, forget it. Because husband and wife, they don't get along, they're not going to tolerate each other, for one thing. They'd be abusing the patient which is typical 'cause if you don't at least love a person forget it" (field notes and interview with Mr. Oliver).[2]

The husbands' desire to devote their later years to caring for their wives is motivated in large part by an appreciation of the care and support their wives provided them. In Mr. Oliver's words, "I'm giving her all I can. As I said, she's well worth it." This man expresses pride in his wife's past homemaking abilities. "She was very precise on everything. I'd say, work around the house she was one of the best there ever was. Taking care of the house, taking care of the food, taking care of me, she did a beautiful job."

When his wife needs special attention, he remembers the special things she used to do just for him. "This morning she was still in bed when I had my own breakfast. She was still asleep. So I just leave her there, sleeping, figuring all the years that she got up at 5 o'clock . . . what she did . . . the day shift. I'd leave the house at 6 o'clock to go to work. The many moons she did that for me. So I just look at her and say, go ahead, sleep." His desire to let her enjoy a few more minutes sleep is connected to his memories and appreciation of the hard work and loving attention she gave him when he had to leave the house very early in the morning. Now it is his turn to recriprocate. Mr. Oliver's present caregiving relationship with his wife is rooted in the relationship they had together in the past. In this way the past is part of the present and infuses meaning into caregiving. Caregiving is more than feeding his wife, making sure she takes her pills, cooking, cleaning, shopping, and the numerous other daily tasks that this entails. It is an expression of his appreciation and love for her. It is a desire to reciprocate loving care and perpetuate a relationship that continues to hold valuable meaning for him.

The guiding principles of love and commitment form the basis of the husbands' decision to pursue a lifestyle of caregiving. Mr. Wekstein says, "I want her to be with me. We have been married for 51 years. Why should I throw her out now, because she's sick? We were very close." He enjoys his wife's company even though she is bedridden and cannot communicate with him due to advanced Parkinson's disease. He has memories of the life they used to share, and he values the opportunity to continue to provide round-the-clock care to her as an expression of his love and commitment. What may seem like an irrational way of life to those who would recommend, and have recommended, institutionalization for Mrs. Wekstein, is very rational in his life-view. To put his wife in an institution now would go against the principles he has lived by all his life. He could not do that with a clear conscience.

The men realize that institutionalization is an option, yet they have chosen to care for their wives at home. Mr. Miller says, "I want to do it as long as I can." His wife is frustrated and angry at her disabilities stemming from emphysema and bone deterioration. She says, "I feel myself going downhill every day. I used to be very active. Now I can't go out with my husband or do nothing." Despite his wife's difficult physical and emotional state, Mr. Miller struggles emotionally and financially to keep her at home and to continue their life together. In the words of Mr. Havighurst, whose wife is bedridden with multiple sclerosis, "Put her in a rest home, hell no. I've been taking care of her all these years, I'm going to take care of her now."

Caring for their wives now provides the husbands with feelings of affection, approval, esteem, and a sense of security and belonging. They have a role in society. They are needed by their wives, and no one can replace them. No one can do what they are doing, because no one has the special relationship they have with their wives. In the words of Mr. Oliver, "No one can do what I do for my wife. When I go, they'll [the children] put her in a nursing home so fast." The relationship that developed over a lifetime of marriage can never be replaced. It continues to be an important part of their identity. The husband's basic social needs are gratified through the interaction of caregiving.

Mr. Oliver refers to caregiving as a job. "When you got a job to do, you got a job to do and that's it. If you can't do it . . . then you have to give it up. When they take laxatives they don't know what they're doing. Now that's a mess I have to clean up. It's part of my job if I want to stay on duty." Mr. Oliver's job has its pleasant and unpleasant duties. He feels that commitment to caring for his wife includes the responsibility for all the aspects that caregiving entails.

Caregiving is a job the husbands have chosen to do in repayment for past care their wives gave others. In the words of Mr. Black, whose wife has a collapsed lung, "She brought the kids up good, you have to give her credit for that. They all turned out good so I'm thankful for that." Mr. Black believes that his wife did her job well. Now she needs him and he wants to care for her, to do this job, with as much love and energy as she displayed in the past. The husbands put out a high level of energy and commit all their resources to caregiving. They derive pride in a job well done.

The overall experience of caregiving is not associated with stress by the husbands. It is associated with pride and responsibility—not resentment or burden. Indeed, the husbands derive self-esteem and security from maintaining continued close relationships with their wives and caring for them lovingly and attentively. However, the husbands do identify some negative aspects of caregiving. In the words of Mr. Evans, "It's the same thing every day. It gets on my nerves." Mr. Wekstein states, "There's not stress, just monotony, you get discouraged. After all nobody goes by here, just the people who live in this building." Strain is associated with the loss of their ability to socialize as they used to before their wives were sick and the loss of the ability to engage in varied interactions during the course of the day. The monotony of their daily routines is experienced in a way analogous to sensory deprivation. These findings allow us to differentiate between negative and positive aspects of caregiving. The unpleasant duties of caregiving are accepted by the husbands as being as much a part of the job as the pleasant. Loving commitment to one's wife make the caregiving experience a positive one overall, even though there are negative aspects to it.

THE MEANING OF RESPITE CARE

Given this definition of care, how do husbands using respite care view it? All the husbands consider themselves the primary caregivers for their wives. This means that they maintain responsibility for all areas of care. In the words of Mr. Oliver, "I do everything for her that she would do for herself." This includes personal care, such as toileting, bathing, dressing, lifting her into and out of the car, shaving facial hair, clipping toe and finger nails, and taking her to the hairdresser every two weeks; preparing the food she likes to eat and making sure that she eats properly; taking her to the dentist every six months for a cleaning; administering medications and laxatives when necessary; and providing the proper exercise. Mr. Oliver receives respite care once per week for two hours for bathing his wife. This allows him to rest and have a qualified worker perform an arduous task for a short period. Otherwise, his whole day is consumed with household and caregiving tasks. The brief time to rest each week enables him to avoid burnout and to maintain his high level of caregiving involvement. This corroborates Scharlach and Frenzel's (1986) finding that the vast majority of wives using nursing home–based respite care cited emotional and physical rest as its primary benefit. This brief respite allows husbands to provide more care for their wives, not less.

In addition to personal care, medical supervision, and overall responsibility, husbands do all the laundry, cooking, shopping, and maintenance of the house and grounds, including mowing the lawn, trimming the hedges, and gardening. In the words of Mr. Black, "Well, there ain't much to it when you come down to it. Easier to keep it clean, keep up with it, than to let it pile up. It's kind of an easy house to keep clean anyway. The only thing I don't like is dusting. Have to do it every day for the wife" (due to her lung condition). Mr. Black's house is immaculately neat and clean. He lives in the home that his father built and in which he grew up. Mr. Black's respite care consists of a home health aide for two hours two days per week for a bed bath, personal care, and some cooking. A homemaker comes three days for two hours from another agency to dust and clean the house. Mr. Black does not drive. The homemaker takes him shopping and helps him run errands. Mr. Black does all the laundry and gardening and the majority of cooking. When the home health aide comes, Mr. Black goes about his own business. He goes to the bar, reads his newspaper, or listens to the radio. Respite care allows him the free time to maintain his interests and activities.

Mr. Miller does all the shopping, cooking, cleaning, and laundry. He says, "There's really nothing to it." Before his wife became unable to do the housekeeping, he regularly did all the laundry, dishes and washing of the floors. He likes to go out in the morning to do the errands but doesn't like to leave his wife alone for a long time. When asked if he needs help with the work he replied, "I want to do it as long as I can." He receives a home health aide five days per week for one hour for bathing and personal care. He relaxes at home when the aide comes. The Millers also receive meals-on-wheels, which they pay for privately.

Housework is not difficult for Mr. Miller, Mr. Black, and the other husbands. Rather, they are accustomed to doing some housework and performing personal care, and they want to continue as long as they can. They do not want anyone else to take the responsibility for any of these tasks. Their day's work reflects a sense of competence if it is done well. Caregiving allows the husbands to have this psychological reward every day.

Amazingly, with their time-consuming workloads, the husbands not only attempt to provide what is necessary but also that which is pleasing to their wives. Mr. Evans, a small, robust man, has been caring for his wife, who is bedridden and unable to talk comprehensibly due to a stroke, for the past three years in their own home. "My wife likes to have a boiled egg, English muffin with jam (I have to be careful not to give her too much jam on account of her diabetes) and milk. She used to love coffee but now she only drinks milk. I drink coffee. This is what she likes for breakfast, so I eat it too." He grinds his wife's food so that she can swallow it, because she does not want to wear her dentures. He will go out of his way to prepare the foods she enjoys. He receives meals-on-wheels for himself and his wife five days per week. If the meal includes something his wife doesn't like, Mr. Evans will substitute a food that she enjoys. His respite care consists of a home health aide three days per week for two hours each day for bathing, a range of motion exercises, changing the bed and Mrs. Evans's clothes, and transferring her into the wheelchair so that she can sit out on the porch for a while. When the aide comes, Mr. Evans goes out shopping. In the afternoon, when Mrs. Evans takes her nap, her husband goes outside to mow the lawn and trim the hedges. He comes in every 15 minutes to check up on her. By attending to these details of caring, the husbands have the opportunity to exercise control, mastery, and competence in their lives.

A respite worker typically comes for a few hours. Viewed in light of the husbands' total responsibility, respite care takes on an ancillary position to the care they themselves provide. The free time allows the men to rest, go out to do errands, or pursue social and recreational activities. It does not release them from responsibility, but rather allows them to act on their responsibilities to themselves, to rest emotionally and physically to keep up their strength, and to maintain necessary personal activities, such as doctors' appointments and hair cuts. It also allows them to act on their responsibilities as primary caregivers by getting out to do the errands and shopping. The husbands provide the vast majority of care their wives require, which is considerable. This corroborates the basic theoretical premise of respite care—that respite care clients require a high level of care and are dependent on family supports (Howells, 1980; Meltzer, 1982; Yocom, 1982).

Because the men are proud of what they do and consider themselves knowledgeable and experienced in the care of their disabled wives, they require that respite workers be skilled and dependable. Mr. Havighurst, who has been caring for his wife for 14 years, since she became bedridden with multiple sclerosis, explained to me why a worker was not competent. "I had to show her how to change her position and how to put the pad underneath her. I do it all the time and get it right every time—no trouble. But when I had to show her, wouldn't ya know it, I had trouble getting it just right." The worker was not able to complete the tasks required with skill—that is, as well as Mr. Havighurst could. He considered this care inadequate. Respite care gives the husband another caregiving individual with whom to compare himself—to his advantage. This reinforces his sense of personal competence and control.

All the husbands spoke of workers who were not dependable in terms of cancelling visits, moving on to other jobs, and coming late. In the words of Mrs. Havighurst, "Tell them [the home health aides] not to come here anymore. I couldn't stand them anyway. They would go in the next room and make phone calls. Sometimes they didn't come or they would come later in the morning." Her husband added, "By the time they got here I had her all cleaned up anyway." The Havighursts receive respite care twice a week for two hours for a bed bath, cathetor care, and a range of motion exercises. Mr. Havighurst is proud of the high quality care he gives his wife. "Everyone is amazed that she has no bedsores." The doctor has told him how well Mrs. Havighurst is cared for. The doctor's praise reinforces the husband's sense of mastery and competence derived from caregiving.

It is Mr. Havighurst's responsibility to maintain acceptable standards of care. He exercises this responsibility by monitoring the care provided by the workers, deciding to dismiss unreliable or unprofessional workers and ceasing to use an agency if their workers are continually inadequate.

The men, who have devoted their later years to the care of their wives, pride themselves on maintaining high standards of grooming, cleanliness, and necessary medical monitoring. They do not relinquish care to respite workers with relief, but only entrust the temporary care of their wives to those who can meet these standards. In the words of Mr. Wekstein, "She [the home health aide] is a lovely person, likes my wife, and needs the money so it works out well. She gives her a bath in bed, gets her dressed, takes care of her catheter and dressings. She looks her over very thoroughly, and if anything is wrong she calls the office right away. This is her job." Mr. Wekstein's confidence in the worker gives him the comfort and peace of mind to leave the house to do an errand, knowing that his wife will be well taken care of in his absence. In this case the respite worker's good performance reflects the standards the husband sets.

ADULT CHILDREN'S CAREGIVING INVOLVEMENT

Do husbands maintain primary responsibility for caregiving when adult children and extended family are available to assist them? What is the nature of the husbands' relationships with their families vis-à-vis caring for their wives? Vinick (1984) states that widowers mentioned support from paid professionals but did not mention help from other family members in caring for their ill wives. Do men fail to perceive the support of others, or is such support not forthcoming? What kinds of services do men perceive as most wanted and needed from their families?

The husbands continue to maintain control of caregiving tasks when family is involved. They are vigilant in holding family members to their standards of care. Mr. Oliver must help his wife dress. "Putting on her pajamas over her head and taking them off is a problem. Sally [his daughter] says to let her sleep in her clothes. I'm not crazy, I wouldn't let her do that. I know that's not right." Mr. Oliver does not have confidence in his daughter's advice and consequently in her ability to care adequately for his wife in his absence. He hesitates to leave his wife with Sally. The men are equally as careful in monitoring the care another family member provides as they are in evaluating paid workers. Family members are part of the caregiving team, which is headed by the husband. The husband is thus able to continue to be master of all caring activities.

The help provided by children is considered supplementary to the load of the husbands. Mr. Miller's son, who lives next door, "does odd jobs." "I have a wonderful daughter-in-law. She brought over two slices of cake this weekend when she made a cake." The daughter-in-law does not bring over meals, she brings over cake. The son does not do the weekly shopping; he does occasional tasks. The children do not help out with the basic necessities of life. The Millers are managing adequately on their own and have a good relationship with their children. The companionship their children provide is greatly appreciated. Knowing that they are available when needed is a great comfort. This assistance supplements rather than supplants the care provided by Mr. Miller. Housework, personal care, and other caregiving activities are tasks that the husbands, themselves, want to continue doing as long as they can. It is a responsibility that they want to maintain primary concern for and one that they are coping with well.

Families such as the Havighursts, Blacks, and Millers rely on their children for companionship and "odd jobs." Others such as the Olivers and Weksteins regard their children's help as largely inappropriate. In the words of Mr. Wekstein, "I have no desire to go out. My children holler at me, 'Why don't you go out?' Last night my daughter called while I was eating my dinner. 'I want to come over and make shrimp scampi for you.' But I'm in the middle of eating my dinner. 'Put it away.'" She came over and made him the meal. When they were finished they wanted to take him out to the movies. He had no desire to go out. It was raining outside and unpleasant. "I want to stay home with Ma; after all, I can watch shows on TV. I don't need to go to the movies."

When asked if his children should help him more, Mr. Wekstein replied, "My daughter in Bridgeton, what can she do? She has a lot of trouble with her children. She can come down to see her mother and visit. My daughter in Shirley, what can I expect from her? A few times she has fed her mother. But to do anything, (pause) once in a great while." He does not expect his children to provide any substantial routine help.

It is Mr. Wekstein's responsibility, not his children's, to maintain his standards of care for his wife. Neither his children nor the professionals share in the responsibility for caring for Mrs. Wekstein. This responsibility is evident in each and every husband's view of caregiving. The husbands remain the most knowledgeable and experienced persons concerning their wives' care and take pride in their efforts. Their children's help is frequently inappropriate, rarely generous, sometimes rejected. At best, it supplements the care that the husbands themselves provide.

UTILIZATION OF RESPITE CARE FOR VACATIONS, HOSPITALIZATIONS, AND TEMPORARY INSTITUTIONALIZATION

The literature documents the use of respite care services by wives and adult children for vacations (Crossman, London, & Barry, 1981; Fengler & Goodrich, 1979). Husbands in this study, however, do not use respite care for vacations, because their identity is embedded entirely in their caregiving activities.

Three years ago Mr. Black's daughter was planning a trip and bought him a plane ticket to come along. "I would've liked to take the trip in a way, and then again, I didn't feel I could. I wouldn't leave her alone the way things are. I can take care of her better and so forth. If I was free or something like that, it probably would be different." Mr. Black would feel guilty taking a vacation even if his children would be around to care for his wife. He believes his wife would not get the quality of care that he can and does give. Nor would he properly fulfill his responsibility to his wife if he left her to enjoy himself.

Would Mr. Wekstein use respite care to take a vacation? "No, where would I go? I wouldn't enjoy myself. Honestly, she wouldn't know the difference. But I wouldn't enjoy myself, we were always very close." In addition, Mr. Wekstein would miss his wife. His place right now is with her, and that is where he wants to be. Husbands have legitimate reasons for not taking vacations, going out more, or enjoying themselves. Because caring professionals and family members may not understand these reasons, it is important to make an effort to gain a fuller understanding of a situation that appears irrational on the surface.

While overnight care for vacations is not desired, it is greatly needed for emergencies such as hospitalization of the husband. Such unexpected situations are a great worry to the husbands. In the words of Mr. Evans, "I want to take care of her as long as I can, but who will take care of her if something happens to me or if I have to go to the hospital again? When I had my prostate surgery last year, I had to make so many calls to find people to come and take care of her for 24 hours, and it cost so much. I told the doctor, 'I can't stay here [the hospital] I have to get home.'" It is extremely difficult to find 24-hour care and prohibitively expensive for the husbands when they do find it.

Experience with temporary nursing home placement was equally unsatisfactory for Mr. Oliver: "If you put a patient in a nursing home, many of them are in there, they can't get the care they get here. They call the nursing home the death sentence. They can't get the care. And if they don't eat, not being able to feed themselves, nobody's going to feed them. No one's going to cater to them. I put her in for a week. Went up to the nursing home to get her out. She was in the wheelchair, her pants is loaded. I raised hell. 'Your daughter didn't leave enough pants down here . . .' 'You take care of her right away or I'll take her into the bathroom right here myself.' They lost half of her stuff. The only way she'll really go into a nursing home is if something really happens to me. Because there's nobody here to take care of her. It's a 24-hour job, 24 hours a day." The nursing home didn't meet Mr. Oliver's standards for attending to Mrs. Oliver's toileting needs. The nursing home cannot "cater" to Mrs. Oliver in the same patient, attentive manner that he can.

The husbands' unsatisfactory experience with temporary nursing home placement and their lack of desire to get away from their wives to enjoy themselves are further testimony to their commitment to these women. They want neither relief from the caregiving responsibility nor the opportunity to get away from it. What is desired is ongoing backup support so that they can continue acting on their responsibility.

DEFINITION OF RESPITE CARE

On the basis of this research we can suggest a definition of respite care grounded in the experiences of males caring for their disabled elderly spouses rather than relying on a definition derived from the care of retarded children. First, we should recognize that the caregiver views respite care not as a relief from caregiving but rather as the opportunity to share the physical and emotional care of his wife so that he can maintain his role and his personal and caregiving responsibilities. Caregiving perpetuates meaningful marital relationships, which are a source of self-esteem. Caregiving provides a meaningful identity to the husbands. It allows the caregiver to exercise mastery in his daily life and to feel the psychological rewards of competence as a caregiver every day. Finally, respite care is part of a package of formal and informal supports that allows the caregiver to maintain the elder at home.

Good respite care is teamwork that meets the husband's standards. The husbands continue to maintain primary responsibility for their wives even when the worker is on duty. Respite care allows the husbands to rest, and to get out to take care of personal and household needs, to maintain quality care in their temporary absence, and to continue their role as principal caregivers. Even bad respite care serves to reinforce positive feelings by allowing the husbands to compare themselves favorably to the respite worker.

Important components of a uniform definition of elder respite care are suggested by these findings. Respite care should be defined in terms of providing essential support to the primary caregiver to avoid deterioration of the caregiver and premature institutionalization of the client. Psychosocial and medical assessment of the caregiver's functional ability to provide the care is equally as important as the assessment of the "disabled" older person's need for assistance. Defining respite care simply as relief from caregiving (Meltzer, 1982) is insufficient. Rather, it should acknowledge the caregiver's need for maintaining mastery and control in his role as the principal caregiver. This can be accomplished by striving for a teamwork approach that considers the husband's preferences and standards. If respite care is truly to provide emotional and physical rest for the caregiver, he must be assured that quality care will be maintained in his temporary absence. Such a respite service must meet the need of caregivers to maintain their standards of worker dependability, skill in the tasks and in the emotional requirements of caring for disabled elders. Finally, respite care is not temporary or intermittent service (as commonly defined, for example, by the Massachusetts Executive Office of Elder Affairs, 1985). Rather, it is ongoing support for caregivers available on a weekly or overnight basis in order to provide help in a manner that maintains family confidence in the worker, in the agency, and in themselves as long-term caregivers.

CONCLUSION

The findings of this study support the first hypothesis explored; i.e., husbands take primary responsibility for caregiving for their wives and managing the other family and paid sources of help. This corroborates Horowitz and Debrof's (1982) documentation of the primary role of the spouse in maintaining principal responsibility for caregiving tasks, household chores, and medical supervision of the older person. Other members of the informal and formal network are secondary and ancillary to the responsibility of the spouse. While other studies have documented the importance of children as the major source of support for the elderly (Frankfather, Smith, & Caro, 1981; Morris & Sherwood, 1984), this study indicates that their help is *supplementary* to that provided by the husbands. Retired husbands are the major caregivers both in providing to their frail spouses more varied types of help and more hours of help than other individuals. The help provided by children must conform to the husbands' standards of caregiving and homemaking, as well as to their personal needs and desires. Children who do not meet or understand these personal desires and standards are considered by the husbands to be inappropriate caregivers. Husbands in this study think of themselves as knowledgeable and experienced in providing the best possible care for their wives and want to continue doing so as long as they can.

The second hypothesis—that caregiving is associated with stress and that spouse caregiving is particularly stressful—was not supported in this study. The husbands associate caregiving with pride and responsibility, not with stress. They do not resent the caregiving role. True, they are disappointed that their retirement years are not what they had expected. Nevertheless, caregiving gives them an outlet for activity and emotion. It allows them to express their love for their wives, their commitment to them, and their appreciation of them in the past. Caregiving gives a positive meaning to their present lives by perpetuating their identity as husbands. What stress there is, is associated with loss, for example, the inability to socialize as they did before their wives were sick and the monotony of their daily routines, rather than with responsibility. The activity and commitment of caregiving may also serve to allay stress. The love, self-esteem, identity, and pride help to heal the husband and to maintain the existence of his world. Where there is love, spouse caregiving is experienced as pride in a job well done and the perpetuation of close and meaningful marital relationships—not as stress.

The third hypothesis concerned the effects of respite care. Does respite care support the caregiver by providing relief from physical, social and emotional burdens? I found that respite care does support the caregiver, but not as a relief or as a release from responsibility. Rather it is an aid to acting on responsibility. Respite care is not used as a vehicle for disengaging from caregiving tasks, because these tasks are not considered a burden by the husbands. Respite care is used instead to maintain responsibility as the primary caregiver and to allow the spouse to perform his role. It affords the caregiver the opportunity to share the physical and emotional care of his wife with a qualified person for short periods so that errands, needed rest, chores, and personal needs can be attended to. It allows the caregiver to be hospitalized for medical purposes and yet be able to return home to continue caring for his wife.

The fourth hypothesis concerned institutionalization. Does respite care prevent or delay institutionalization? It is clear that the husbands have considered institutionalizing their spouses. One husband briefly placed his wife in a nursing home and was dissatisfied. Another has been told by professionals that his wife belongs in a nursing home and was denied home care services by the agency for this reason. Nonetheless, it is important for him to continue caring for his wife at home. He will continue to do so despite the efforts of professionals to the contrary. Others resist institutionalization for fear of financial devastation. The husbands are deliberately trying to delay institutionalization. As noted by Vinick (1984), husbands want to continue to care for their wives until their own health fails and they are no longer able to do so. Respite care provides them with the cushion of support they need to maintain their responsibility as primary caregivers and to keep their wives out of nursing homes.

With regard to the fifth hypothesis, respite care by paid professionals does not supplant the care provided by families. It supplements that care. Formal agencies do not take over, nor even share, the responsibility of caring for the frail elder when the elder is at home. Husbands retain primary responsibility for their wives even when they are out of the house for short periods. By giving husbands the time and "peace of mind" to take care of necessary tasks, agencies supplement the care husbands provide. Respite care workers function under the direction of the husbands and must maintain the husbands' standards of care. At no time do respite workers take over responsibility from husbands.

The husbands in this study are white, semi-skilled, low-income, male retirees who could be assumed to have particular ways of using and defining respite care. The positive caregiving experience of these husbands may be a result of traditional marital bonds not found in all groups. On the other hand, loving marital relationships rather than traditional definitions of marital responsibility may be the key factor in defining respite care. Respite care may not be beneficial to abusive families, nor to those whose marital commitment and relationship are weak. It may also not be effective in families that desire privacy and isolation.

Socioeconomic status may be an additional influence on the utilization of respite care. Working-class, older husbands may have a life history of involvement in household chores and instrumental support to their wives, as a result of both partners' having worked outside the home throughout their married life. Husbands who never "helped out" at home, either because their wives did everything or because they had hired help, may not be able to use respite care. In addition, all of the men save one were retired, thus limiting their obligations elsewhere and allowing them to devote full time to their wives and home. Middle-class husbands may wish to continue part-time employment and/or commitments to community or other activities that are important sources of identity for them. They may not want to devote all their attention to the care of their wives and may therefore need different types of respite or paid caregiving support. Finally, respite care was chosen by these men. The husbands are independent and self-sufficient. Perhaps this is a critical personality factor behind their search for and utilization of respite care. It is evident that we need research to determine the factors influencing the utilization of respite care, as well as comparative studies of men and women as caregivers and respite care users. In addition, understanding the effects of socioeconomic status, varied types of marriages, retirement and employment and gender differences would improve our understanding of the meaning of caregiving and respite care.

Why do husbands experience caring for their wives as pride in a job well done and the perpetuation of close and meaningful marital relationships? In channeling their energies and activities into caring for their wives, the husbands maintain continuity in their habits and preferences. Continuity theory in gerontology explains the behavior of older persons as the continuation of habits, commitments, preferences, and dispositions of lifelong experiences (Atchley, 1972). Caregiving, then, gives older men continuity in their status as husbands. It allows them to continue to express their love and commitment to their wives and to maintain a home and life together. It maintains the integrity of the husband's self, family, and home.

Lowenthal and Haven (1968) have shown that intimate relationships may serve as mediating, palliative, or alleviating factors in the face of social losses. They maintain that intimacy through the maintenance of closeness with another is the center of existence up to the very end of life. In stubbornly and fiercely maintaining control over their role as caregivers, the husbands are expressing their closeness and intimacy with their wives and prolonging its existence as long as possible. Intimacy serves to allay the stresses of the loss of healthy, active retirement years with their wives, as well as the loss of stimulation in the husbands' environment.

Why is women's care of husbands found to be stressful while men's care of wives is not? Gilligan (1982) suggests that men have a dramatically different psychological make-up from women. Men are motivated by individual achievement. Women, however, strive for a more interdependent self through caring and nurturance. The husbands in this study derive a sense of personal achievement in the day-to-day concerns of being good caregivers for their wives. They have a great sense of pride and fulfillment in a job well done. Their sense of achievement is the core of their self-esteem and well-being. This sense of control, mastery, and self-efficacy may be the critical factor in the positive mental health of men at this stage in the life cycle.

Application of these theories to the husbands enables us to understand their behavior. What appears to be a stoic commitment to devoting their later years and energies to caring for their wives at home, no matter how ill their wives are, can now be seen in a new light. What we may view as the husbands' fierce independence to maintain control as the principal caregivers amidst informal and formal support is seen now as an expression of interdependence—of maintaining continuity in their home and family life and a meaningful role in retirement. If the husbands let others perform the bulk of caregiving tasks, what will they do? What will be their role in their later years? In contrast to viewing the husbands' caring as obsessive, we now see it as the fulfillment of intimacy with their wives. If they lose the opportunity for meeting these important needs through caregiving, how will they cope with their stress and maintain their sense of well-being?

This study suggests that helping husbands maintain their wives at home is essential to their psychological and physical well-being, as well as to the well-being of their wives. For these men, caregiving signifies the meaningful aspects of their lives. Without caregiving they would suffer additional, even more devastating losses. The positive benefits of caregiving compel mental health providers and policy analysts to strengthen and support spouses in their efforts to preserve an optimum quality of life for themselves and their chronically impaired family members.

In order for respite care to be effective it need not provide many hours of services to a couple. These findings support Horowitz and Debrof's (1982) conclusion that the *quantity* of service support is less important than the *presence* of service support if it is perceived as adequate to meet the needs of the family. This respite service was perceived as adequate in providing ongoing backup for needed rest and household and personal maintenance, with the exception of not providing in-home overnight emergency care. This is an important need that respite care should fulfill. Minimal respite service should not be equated with providing minimal benefit. The common assumption of policy makers and administrators that respite care dramatically increases health care costs may be unfounded. This study suggests that minimal respite services meet the caregivers' needs to maintain responsibility for their wives and to maintain themselves and their households.

More important than the *quantity* of service is the *quality* of service. A respite care service must meet professional standards of expertise and dependability before it is worthwhile for caregivers to consider. Husbands would not utilize a service in which they did not have confidence.

In addition, respite care must be seen as a team effort, with the elderly caregiver as an important team member and client. The goal of respite care should be to help husbands retain their roles as caregivers; that is, to help them act on their responsibility rather than to supplant that responsibility.

This study demonstrates the salutary benefits of caregiving in promoting the optimum quality of life for elderly men married to chronically ill wives. Respite care allows men to meet social, emotional, personal, and household needs that are likely to be neglected as a result of the relentless demands of caregiving. It allows men to continue their desired role as primary caregivers for their wives. It preserves loving marital ties and allows for the fulfillment of individual achievement, both of which are sources of well-being for elderly men. Respite care has the potential for strengthening and supporting elderly caregivers in their pursuit of satisfying and meaningful lives and avoiding the breakdown of the family caregiving capacity.

NOTES

1. Names and places have been changed to maintain the confidentiality of the study participants.

2. All quotations are taken from interview transcripts and field notes collected in this project.

REFERENCES

Adams, M., Caston, M. A., & Davis, B., (1979, November). *A neglected dimension in home care of elderly disabled persons: Effect on responsible family members.* Paper presented at the annual meeting of the Gerontological Society, Washington, DC.

Archbold, P. (1983). Impact of parent caring on women. *Family Relations, 32,* 39–45.

Atchley, R. (1972). *The social forces in later life: An introduction to social gerontology.* Belmont, CA: Wadsworth Publishing Company.

Brody, E. (1981). Women in the middle and family help to old people. *The Gerontologist, 21*(5), 471–480.

Cantor, M. (1983). Strain among caregivers: A study of experience in the United States. *The Gerontologist, 23,* 597–604.

Charmaz, K. (1983). The grounded theory method: An explication and interpretation. In R. Emerson (Ed.), *Contemporary field research* (pp. 109–126). Boston: Little, Brown and Company.

Cicirelli, V. (1981). *Helping elderly parents: The role of adult children.* Boston: Auburn House.

Crossman, L., London, C. & Barry, C. (1981). Older women caring for disabled spouses: A model for supportive services. *The Gerontologist, 21,* 464–470.

Fengler, A.P., & Goodrich, N. (1979). Wives of elderly disabled men: The hidden patients. *The Gerontologist, 19,* 175–183.

The Foundation for Long Term Care. (1983). *Respite care for the frail elderly, a demonstration project. A summary report on institutional respite research.* 194 Washington Avenue, Albany, New York, 12210.

Frankfather, D., Smith, M., & Caro, F. (1981). *Family care of the elderly.* Lexington, MA: Lexington Books.

Gilligan, C. (1982). *In a different voice: Psychological theory and women's development.* Cambridge, MA: Harvard University Press.

Glaser, B. G., & Strauss, A. L. (1976). *The discovery of grounded theory: Strategies for qualitative research.* New York: Aldine.

Horowitz, A., & Debrof, R. (1982).*The role of families in providing long term care to the frail and chronically ill elderly living in the community* (Methodological Report). Health Care Financing Administration. Washington, DC: U.S. Government Printing Office.

Howells, D. (1980, November). *Reallocating institutional resources: Respite care as a supplement to family care of the elderly.* Paper presented at the annual meeting of the Gerontological Society, San Diego, CA.

Johnson, C. (1979, November) *Impediments to family supports to dependent elderly: An analysis of primary caregivers.* Paper presented at the annual meeting of the Gerontological Society, Washington, DC.

Lofland, J., & Lofland, L. (1971). *Analyzing social settings: A guide to qualitative observation and analysis.* Belmont, CA: Wadsworth.

Lowenthal, M. F., & Haven, C. (1968). Interaction and adaptation: Intimacy as a critical variable. In B. L. Neugarten (Ed.), *Middle age and aging: A reader in social psychology* (pp. 390–400). Chicago: University of Chicago Press.

Massachusetts Executive Office of Elder Affairs Program Instruction for the Expansion of Home Care Services Through the Addition of Respite Care. (1985). Boston, Author.

Meltzer, J. (1982). *Respite care: An emerging family support service.* The Center for the Study of Social Policy, 236 Massachusetts Avenue, N. E., Suite 405, Washington, D.C., 20002.

Morris, J., & Sherwood, S. (1984). Informal support resources for vulnerable elderly persons: Can they be counted on, why do they work? *International Journal of Aging and Human Development, 18*(2), 81–98.

Motenko, A. (1983, November). *Respite care: Support for families caring for their parents.* Paper presented at the annual Scientific Meeting of the Gerontological Society of America, San Francisco, CA.

Myllyluoma, J., & Soldo, B. (1980, November). *Family caregivers to the elderly: Who are they?* Paper presented at the annual meeting of the Gerontological Society, San Diego CA.

Parmelee, P. (1981). *Spouse vs. other family caregivers: Psychological impact on impaired aged.* Cleveland, OH: The Benjamin Rose Institute.

Reinharz, S. (1984). *On becoming a social scientist: From survey research and participant observation to experiential analysis.* New Brunswick, NJ: Transaction Books.

Scharlach, A., & Frenzel, C. (1986). An evaluation of institution based respite care. *The Gerontologist, 26,* 77–82.

Seelbach, W. C. (1978). Correlates of aged parents' filial responsibility, expectations and realizations. *Family Coordinator, 27,* 341–349.

Shanas, E. (1979). The family as social support system in old age. *The Gerontologist, 19,* 169–174.

Smallegan, M. (1985). There was nothing else to do: Needs for care before nursing home admission. *The Gerontologist, 25*(4), 364–369.

Spence, D., & Miller, D. (1985/1986). Family respite for the elderly Alzheimer's patient. *Journal of Gerontological Social Work, 9*(2), 101–108.

Tennstedt, S., & McKinlay, J. (1985). *Social networks and the care of frail elders.* Boston: Boston University.

Townsend, P. (1957). *The family life of old people: An inquiry in east London.* London: Routledge & Kegan Paul.

Treas, J. (1977). Family support systems for the aged: Some social and demographic considerations. *The Gerontologist, 17,* 486–491.

Upshur, C. C. (1982). An evaluation of home-based respite care. *Mental Retardation, 20,* 58–62.

Vinick, B. (1984). Elderly men as caretakers of wives. *Journal of Geriatric Psychiatry, 17*(1), 61–68.

Yocom, B. (1982). *Respite care options for families caring for the frail elderly.* Pacific Northwest Long-Term Care Center, University of Washington, Seattle, WA 98195.

7

Stories Told:
In-Depth Interviewing and
the Structure of Its Insights

Robert L. Rubinstein

In this chapter I consider the usefulness of two sorts of qualitative methods in gerontological research that are variants of in-depth interviewing. I also consider some of the insights about our informants (or subjects) available to us through these methods. Two specific research projects with the elderly offer evidence of the utility of these methods.[1]

Qualitative interviews are research interviews that range from the inclusion of a few semistructured or open-ended questions nested in primarily structured research interviews to fully open-ended conversations on wide-ranging topics. Typically, the qualitative interview has a range or agenda of topics that forms the focus of inquiry. My interest here is with the topically oriented qualitative or in-depth interview. The topically oriented, open-ended, in-depth interview is related in form to the ethnographic interview described by Spradley (1979) and to the biographic interview described by Levinson (1978, p. 15), who noted that the biographical interview "combines aspects of a research interview, a clinical interview, and a conversation between friends." For purposes of gerontological research, the topically oriented, in-depth interview may be undertaken as a one-time event or as part of a sequence of interviews. It may be focused narrowly on a specific topic or broadly on general areas. In addition, questions may be sharply focused or more general.

In qualitative interviews, statements made as asides, as introductory remarks by the informants, as commentary, as stories told to accompany some point, constitute a very important source of data. The informed researcher does not tune out such "extraneous" comments, because they are important in several ways. They show the informant's awareness of the interview situation as a social interaction. Comments about the interview interaction represent a running analysis of the situation by the informant. The kinds of statements made by the informant may be especially revealing, not only of her personality and orientation, but also of specific events in the individual's life that would not be revealed in any other context. The comments may exhibit a series of associations that indicate what sorts of ideas "belong together" from the point of view of an informant's organizing scheme. And, perhaps most important for gerontological research, such comments and asides often represent important statements that older informants make about themselves. From the qualitative perspective, it is good scientific method to note and include "outside" responses.

One point often missed about in-depth interviewing in the social sciences is that it can represent a specific focus within a larger overall research framework. In-depth interviewing may be viewed as a phase in the participant-observation or field work process, although it may, of course, take place without the umbrella of participant-observation or field work *per se*.

How can this be? Keith (1980) has suggested that the methodology of participant-observation (a major component of field work) consists of three stages, which move from the greatest degree of "outsideness" for the investigator to the greatest degree of "insideness" over time. Keith's Stage 1 has as its goal initial participation in as many activities as possible so as to permit the participant-observer to gain a generalized knowledge of a community and its residents. In Stage 2, research activities become more focused as generalized activities give way to commitment to specific areas of research interest. In addition, recording data becomes more specialized. In Keith's scheme, Stage 3 represents a period of hypothesis testing, involving measurement and use of diverse research instruments, and comparison of data collected with that of other studies.

I believe it is possible to view in-depth interviewing within this framework, but only if we modify Keith's Stage 3. That is, the experience of field workers would follow Keith's scheme with the exception that, instead of specific hypothesis testing in Stage 3, this last stage would represent the most focused form of data gathering for those researchers whose primary interest is in "subjective culture" or subjective aspects of experience. Certainly, in-depth interviewing would be a key component of the collection of such data. This redefinition of Keith's Stage 3 occurs for two reasons. First, in cross-cultural research

situations, language competence is often delayed and temporally corresponds to this last period. Second, and more important, personal
associations have now had some time to evolve, and the degree of trust
necessary for the conveyance of private or difficult material would
most likely have been achieved in this period.

In-depth interviewing *can* take place either as part of a larger fieldwork experience, and therefore as part of an overall participant-observation enterprise, or independently, as part of an in-depth interviewing
strategy that is not part of a larger overall project. Where in-depth
interviewing is associated with field work, it might take place as part of
Keith's Stage 2. Most certainly it will take place as part of Stage 3.

In-depth interviewing that takes place independently of large research projects may be viewed as isomorphic in structure to Keith's
three stages of participant-observation. In viewing in-depth interviewing from this perspective, Stage 1 drops out, especially if research is
being undertaken in the researcher's own culture, since a lot of background investigation may not be necessary. We already have information about the meaning of important concepts, since we share these
with our informants. A course of in-depth interviews follows from the
knowledge of general background information and general subcultural
(ethnic, occupational) information, to the most focused, topical interviewing as trust and rapport are gained over time. Thus in-depth
interviewing, occurring independently of a larger research project such
as field work, can be viewed as analogous to parts of Stages 2 and 3 in
Keith's scheme.

One other difference between in-depth interviewing as part of or as
independent of participant-observation should be mentioned. If in-depth
interviewing is carried out in the field work context, the interviewer will
be enmeshed in the community she or he is studying. She or he will know
not only the informant but also the informant's friends, neighbors, and
family. The fact that the interviewer is known by these persons may
inhibit or affect the interview process in some way. For in-depth interviewing independent of participant-observation, such as the gerontological research I am describing here, the interviewer is usually not known by
the social circle of the informant and is therefore socially neutral and an
outsider. This neutrality may aid in the interviewer's task.

IN-DEPTH INTERVIEWING AS AN INTERACTION SETTING

As a data-gathering procedure, the in-depth interview is much more
than the actual content of the questions asked, the number or frequency of the interviews in the series, and the vagueness or the sharp-

ness of the questions. There are several important additional aspects to the in-depth interview. First, it is an environment or setting for the production of statements. It is a form of social interaction between two persons. In contrast to the social setting in which a close-ended or structured interview is used and in which the subject is dissuaded from making extraneous comments, the in-depth interview invites statements of all sorts, not just specific answers to specific questions. The goal of managing interview demand characteristics in in-depth interviewing is to create a supportive and encouraging environment for the informant to say whatever he or she wants to about the issue at hand. Qualitative researchers generally acknowledge extraneous comments in the interview situation but do not write about them. This may be because qualitative researchers themselves may be constrained by a consciousness of the quantitative model, may have no positive qualitative framework in mind, or may be swamped by the combination of data and impressions. Yet it is my feeling that acknowledging the real nature of this interaction can only lead to deeper understanding and that such interaction should be included in reports of qualitative research.

If attention is paid to all remarks made by an informant, the researcher is likely to find important material about an informant's identity and self-concept. It is my view that the base of all in-depth interviewing of older people (and, indeed, other people as well) is a concern for the *identity* of the informant. That is, statements made by an informant in this social setting for the production of statements are colored by a particular core sense of who he or she is and how events throughout life have contributed to making that core sense as it now exists. Essentially, an in-depth interview asks our informants for summative statements about their identities and biographies. People do not usually carry such summative or programmatic statements around, but they are constructed during the interview process (Frank, 1979). Ultimately, whatever its topical orientation and degree of specificity, in-depth interviewing is concerned with the core sense that individuals have of themselves. Many of us who have done in-depth interviewing with older people have had the experience of hearing two sorts of statements, often as asides, from our informants. I will call these identity statements. The first type is one in the following vein, "I am the kind of person who likes to do X or who must do X or who is very X" or, "I was always very X or I always enjoyed doing X" (Rubinstein, 1986), in these cases referring to some personally meaningful characteristic. These are statements of personal identity that are produced as part of the in-depth interview as social setting for the production of statements. The second kind of statements are statements of identity based on culturally central notions, such as family, love, duty, sacrifice, spouse, and

children. An example here is, "Doing my duty has always been important in my life." In an important paper, Sharon Kaufman (1981) has
identified *themes*, or "cognitive areas of meaning," that older people use
to structure and organize their biographies. Identity statements may be
akin to such themes.

In-depth interviews should be understood as operating on two epistemological levels. The first is the dialogue of question and answer,
probe and response. This is what the interview is all about. The second
is a metalevel, which itself has two components. The first represents
the informant's (and the interviewer's) comments and asides about the
interview and about the material raised during the exchange. For example, in interviews I have done, I have seen a rather simple question
asked at the beginning of a general interview about a person's marital
status (e.g., "What is your marital status?") trigger lengthy responses
about the history of the informant's marriage. Such questions may lead
independently to other topics. This is more than the information
needed to answer the particular question, yet the response constitutes
important data in the sense that we have learned about what happened,
about what a person thinks is important to her, and about the way
material is ordered. The second component, and the more difficult one,
deals with the transference and countertransference that goes on in the
interview arena. By this I mean the psychodynamic reactions we as
interviewers have to people we interview, derived from our reactions
to and feelings toward important individuals in our private lives. This
reaction holds for our informants' reactions to us as well. Those of us
who are younger than our informants may experience the interview as
a child experiencing the parent or grandparent. This perspective shapes
the way we ask our questions, how we select our questions, and how
we present ourselves.

In the in-depth interview we meet our informants as individuals, and
this puts a special responsibility on us. For example, when I interviewed
older men, I was the first person some had really talked to about their
wives' deaths. Even if I had not been interested in this material (which I
was), I would still have had a responsibility to listen to it, since these
men needed to present or discuss it. The need to talk, triggered by the
interview-as-social-interaction, should be respected, both as a way we
can be of use to our informants and as "good science" that provides us
with information an informant deems important.

The element of time plays a very important role in in-depth interviewing. While one may conduct an in-depth interview in one session
(particularly with a cooperative informant about a relatively focused
and public topic), frequently in-depth interviewing in gerontological
research requires multiple sessions. In this chapter I discuss a short-

term series of interviews with a fixed number of sessions and contrast these with a long-term series of sessions with a somewhat open termination point ("we'll see how it goes"). By short term I mean two to 10 interview sessions, while long term means 10 or more sessions. From the point of view of data gathering, differences in the length of an interview series have implications for the type of informant/interviewer relationship established, for the degree that material of interest to the interviewer is fully covered, for the interviewer's ability to ascertain ongoing events in the life of an elderly informant, and, indeed, for an assessment of the accuracy of responses.

What follows are two examples of the use of topically oriented, in-depth interviews in the study of aspects of the lives of the elderly. The first is an example of a short-term series of interviews with a fixed number of sessions. What is noteworthy in terms of the dynamics of in-depth interviewing mentioned above is that the interview sequence provided the opportunity for informants to revise statements they had initially made. Changes were made either in response to a growing understanding of what was required of them or to a growing sense of relaxation with the interviewer. The second is an example of an extended series of interviews that permitted the investigator to see and discuss, over a significantly long period of time, distinctive changes in the relationship of an elderly informant to her home environment.

THE SHORT SERIES OF INTERVIEWS WITH A FIXED NUMBER OF SESSIONS

In 1981, the Department of Behavioral Research at the Philadelphia Geriatric Center began a project to gather data about community-dwelling older men and to examine the quality of their lives on the basis of differing marital statuses and living arrangements. Funding was acquired for an anthropologist to interview older men *living alone* about their lives, their daily and preferred activities, and their social relations and affective states. The research, designed by M. Powell Lawton, called for a series of five two-hour interviews with each of the men in the sample, half of whom were associated with senior centers and senior-only housing units, and half of whom were not so associated. The men were interviewed in sessions that occurred once a week for five or six weeks.

Forty-seven older men were interviewed (30 widowers, 11 who had never married, and six who were separated or divorced). All but one of these men lived alone at the time of the interviews. Most of the men were interviewed from nine to 15 hours each. The average age of the sample was about 78. Slightly more than half were affiliated with a senior center or senior-only housing unit. There was great diversity of background, income, ethnicity, health status, and educational level.

One particular problem addressed by the research was the paucity of data about older men who had never married. These men were known primarily through reports on specialized environments, such as single room occupancy hotels (SROs) in which such men live at a higher frequency than does the general population. For example, 22% of Eckert's (1980) SRO sample were never-married men, as opposed to about 5% in the general population (U. S. Senate, 1982). Little has been reported on never-married older men in nonspecialized communities in the U. S. The existing literature (Gubrium, 1974, 1975) suggests that loneliness is not a problem for these individuals. Since the occurrence and experience of loneliness was one topic of interest to us in the interviews, we dealt with it specifically in a series of questions in the first or second interview. Most men were asked, "Are you ever lonely?" and, "If so, how often?" Some attempt was made to ascertain who the informant missed if this remained unspecified. Our sequence of five interviews had a structure. The initial interview dealt with a general set of topics, and each of the remaining interviews covered a review of the previous day's activities as well as detailed questions on specific topics, such as important life events, relations with family, favorite activities, and feelings about old age.

Initial responses to the question about the occurrence of loneliness revealed that six men were often lonely, 19 sometimes lonely, and 17 rarely or never lonely. Because the interviews generally extended over five or six weeks, we were able to follow-up the initial answers and representations of loneliness. The opportunity to follow-up enabled us to rate loneliness on the basis of three additional factors: (1) an "admitted" change in the level of loneliness noted during the initial assessment, (2) statements that showed loneliness to be a problem despite continued insistence, in reply to a direct question, that it was not, and (3) other indicators that the person was lonely. In this second or composite rating of loneliness, 11 men were judged to be lonely often, 22 men sometimes, and 10 men rarely or never.

The fact that the amount of loneliness came to be revised upwards in a number of cases was the result of continued contact beyond the first interview. I will describe two instances in which the amount of loneliness was revised upwards through the course of the interviews with two never-married elderly men.

Mr. Kooper

Aged 82 at the time of the interviews, Mr. Kooper[2] lived alone in a two-story row house in a predominantly white, lower-middle-class neighborhood of Philadelphia. He had lived in or near this neighborhood all his life. Mr. Kooper never married. His closest relatives were two nephews, sons of a sister, who lived in nearby suburban counties and whom he saw or spoke to irregularly. Mr. Kooper had not seen his brother, aged 86, for three years; his brother lived in the Midwest. Mr. Kooper said that he did not know if this brother was still living. Six sisters had all passed away.

During our second interview, Mr. Kooper described himself as not too lonely, although he noted that living alone was "bad," especially with regard to the possibility of illness. Earlier in the year he had been hospitalized, and the unpleasantness of this experience had been magnified by the fact that he had had to face it alone, without family. In fact, it was a social worker at a senior center who had arranged for his hospitalization.

Our first interviews were difficult. My attempts to ask questions about current activities and life-history events were met by Mr. Kooper's own agenda, which included discussion of his religious background; security problems at home; the difficulty he had in gaining part-time jobs, which had been his mainstay throughout his working life; and his difficulty in relating to people. My impression of him during our first three interviews was as someone who either did not seem to understand what was required of him during the interview, or as someone who did not wish to answer many of the questions I asked. He was someone who really needed to do it his way. At a short first meeting, prior to beginning the interviews, I explained the nature and purpose of the research. He was, I believe, fully aware of this, as well as his rights to refuse to answer questions or drop out at any time. Yet, for whatever reason, he continued through the five interviews. During the last three interviews he became more comfortable.

In the third interview, we discussed loneliness again. He noted, "I do get lonely, yes." He said that he was lonely frequently. I asked him what he did when he got lonely, how he managed to deal with it, and he answered that he reacted to loneliness by reading the paper or taking a walk. He noted, "I wish I had somebody sensible to talk to," and added that although there was a man whom he liked, a man from a local chapter of a religious sect, "all that man talks about is Jesus." The fact that Mr. Kooper did not marry was still a problem for him. "Women just want and want . . . I almost got married when I was younger but two things stood in my way . . . the difficulty in making a living and the difficulty I might have in getting along with any wife." Yet at times he talked about marriage as if it were still a possibility. Another object of loneliness was his mother. At times, she played a central role in his loneliness: "At times I sit on the front porch and cry, because I miss my mother."

To a certain extent his daily participation at a senior center helped him assuage his sense of loneliness, which he now began to talk about more openly. There were certain activities he especially liked, but his pleasure at the center was compromised by a few people he did not like at all. He noted that he did not really feel close to any of the people who attended the center, although he especially liked some of the staff. It was clear, however, that his participation in the center during the previous two years had opened him up to a variety of new experiences and people.

Mr. Kooper began the fourth interview with a statement about the young vandals whom he believed had broken his cellar window. In order to fill in a list of his places of residence during his life, I asked him about his residence in a particular neighborhood. This elicited a discussion of ethnic changes and ethnic groups and led to a discussion of his family and to some very frank statements about how his nephews *really* felt about him. My attempt to return the interview to a discussion of residence led to a recounting of disputes among his family members that had flared over the disposition of his parents' house. The profound sense of loneliness this man experienced came out further in this interview. Later on I asked him about his outlook for the future. He stated, "I always wanted to be a lawyer. I was the second smartest person in my class. I never accomplished this, however. I could always speak in front of my class . . . What am I now? I wind up in a center! I didn't even want to go, but its better than staying home."

A final interview covered some preplanned topics, but it also left room for Mr. Kooper to talk. He covered several areas but also returned to the theme of trouble with relations. He noted at one point, independent of any specific question I had asked him, "I can't figure life out . . . I suppose it would have been better to be married." He began to assess a number of younger widows that he knew and, toward the end of the interview, began asking for advice on how to approach a certain woman who lived on his street.

Emerging Insights

The interviews with Mr. Kooper moved from an initial portrait he presented of himself as relatively untroubled, to a point at which he described himself as subject to numerous conflicts in various areas of his life and as an individual who experienced loneliness. Initial representation of his social relations as somewhat satisfying gave way to a new image in which social relations were difficult. Real loneliness became part of the picture.

Mr. January

From the start, it was clear that Mr. January was lonely and that this loneliness was part of a larger, profound depression related, among other things, to his health status: he had emphysema. At some level he knew he was dying, although at times he tried to present himself as living rather normally. In fact, from the time I first met him, he had less than a year to live. In his late seventies at the time of the interviews, Mr. Janury had smoked several packs of cigarettes a day for many years earlier in his life and had worked in some of the textile mills that formerly made up a good deal of Philadelphia's industrial infrastructure, in both instances exposing himself to the possibility of respiratory disorders.

A small and fragile-looking man when I met him, Mr. January had withered from the more robust person in photographs he showed me of him and his family. His attitude toward life was stoic. When I asked him initially if he was lonely, he just shrugged. In thinking about his response, retrospectively, after I got to know him better, I decided that the shrug indicated that loneliness was not something that pertained to him because his life had moved beyond the realm of the ordinary evaluation of human emotions into an existence in which many emotions were luxuries and therefore could not matter too much. Here was a man conditioned by canons of "male inexpressiveness" (Balswick, 1982), with no close relatives and few social relations of any kind, who was terminally ill.

The first three of our five interview sessions were quite tense. Mr. January resisted attempts to discuss topics he considered too personal. Since the first three interviews with Mr. January were taped, I quote from the transcripts:

RLR: You mentioned your niece. Do you feel pretty close to your niece?

AJ: Yeah.

RLR: You talk to her at least once a week?

AJ: Oh, yeah.

RLR: You said that she called you up "to see if [you] were still alive." Does that mean that . . .

AJ: (Interrupts) Well, I call her up. I report to her every week.

RLR: If you are feeling depressed or anxious or lonely, do you talk to her?

AJ: No, I'm not that close with anybody.

RLR: If you do get anxious or depressed, what do you do? How do you handle it?

AJ: Just get over it.

RLR: Do you have any particular way of handling it? Do you pick up something (to do) to get it off your mind?

AJ: I can't say I do, no.

RLR: It just passes in time?

AJ: Yeah, sure.

RLR: Do you think a lot about the past?

AJ: I guess I do. At my age, everybody does.

RLR: Is there any period in particular you think about?

AJ: No, I don't know what to tell you . . .

RLR: Do you think about your parents?

AJ: Yeah.

RLR: Growing up?

AJ: (No response) . . . (long pause) . . . One thing that makes me depressed is not being able to get out like I used to.

Deflections away from the painful past were common, and this is one of many instances where discussions of the past were limited.

The first three interview sessions were held at Mr. January's kitchen table. He lived on the ground floor of a row house that had been converted into two apartments. The house was poorly maintained by the realtor. In addition, Mr. January's own apartment was incredibly filthy and messy. He did not clean because he was unable to do much physical work and, in addition, was too depressed. He had to muster his limited energy for projects that were more vital, such as shopping or washing his clothes. The apartment had three rooms, the living room in front, the kitchen/dining room in the middle, and the bedroom behind. Most of the living room furniture was covered with a thick coat of dust and was used by Mr. January primarily for storage. Beside the broken and dusty furniture, major features of the room were several hundred books (he was an avid reader) and a large, nonfunctioning refrigerator (he had damaged this beyond repair when he tried to defrost the freezer using an awl and had punctured the freezer lining).

Emerging insights

After the third session, because things were not going too well and because I feared I was putting too much pressure on Mr. January to talk when he did not want to, I gave up use of the tape-recorder and relied on written notes. In fact, I often avoided writing during the interviews, making notes in my car from memory after the sessions were over. For the fourth and fifth interviews we sat and talked, no longer facing each other, on Mr. January's enclosed porch, which overlooked a major Philadelphia thoroughfare. I included more conversation in the interview. Mr. January's mood brightened; it could be that he was feeling better, or that he felt more comfortable with me, or that he was happy to have the tape-recorder turned off, or that the weather had improved and he was happy because he could get out more. He even made a joke. A mother with a young child passed by; the child had a bottle. Mr. January said, "The kid has a bottle . . . just like his old man." Mr. January had frequently observed the father and his drinking companions.

He began to open up. He talked more about his family; his parents' separation at the height of the Depression; how he resided with his father until the 1960s, when his father died from liver disease related to his drinking; and how his sister went to live with their mother after their parents' separation and continued to live with the mother even after her own marriage. A more coherent picture began to emerge of his loneliness for his parents, his bitterness over their separation, and the sadness he felt over the ensuing turmoil and over his own missed opportunities. He frequently asked me whether I knew any "wealthy widows." While this was stated in jest, I believed it belied a sense of continuing conflict over his solitary status, a conflict that also emerged in other statements.

Initially I interpreted Mr. January's shrugged response to my question as a statement that he was lonely only sometimes. But it became clear over time that loneliness was a frequent component of his daily life and was profound and complex, involving feelings about parents and others.

About a year after the interviews were completed, I learned from his neighbor that Mr. January had died. The neighbor knew it, he told me, because he had seen Mr. January's niece putting most of his belongings on the curb for the trashmen to take away. Hearing this story forced into view for me a sense of the tremendous ambiguity that we have as interviewers. We are privileged to hear intimate details of people's lives and at some level may become close to our informants. However, our own lives go on and ultimately, despite our knowledge, we remain distant. Future contact with our informants may pull us in two directions, toward and away.

In both of these cases, the short-term, fixed series of topically oriented, in-depth interviews proved a useful method to look, in some detail, behind first responses. It facilitated gathering many responses to simple questions, as well as rich, contextualized data about informants' feelings and experiences and the ways in which these are organized.

A LONG-TERM SERIES OF IN-DEPTH INTERVIEWS

In late 1982, I began a three-year research project entitled "The Meaning and Function of Home for the Elderly," designed to describe and assess some of the sense of attachment that older people have for their homes. The research was designed to be carried out in three phases, a short, preliminary phase in which young, middle-aged, and older persons were interviewed about the concept of and their attachment to home; a one-year period of in-depth interviewing of a small number of older persons about their lives and homes; and, finally, a follow-up structured interview with 100 older persons about their homes. Here, I discuss the in-depth phase of the interviewing.

The period of in-depth interviewing with the small sample of older individuals was designed to take place over the course of a year and to include three four-month periods of in-depth interviewing. That is, over the initial four months I would see each of three or four informants once a week for a morning or afternoon, thus making for a total of about 16 lengthy interviews for the entire four-month research period for each informant. In fact, what has happened is that I have remained in touch with many of these informants beyond the four-month period, so that I have been able to follow ongoing events for almost two years in some instances.

This period of in-depth interviewing had three goals: (1) to come to know the individuals and their lives and daily routines well enough to gain some knowledge of what "home" meant to them; (2) to establish some knowledge of how these informants organized their identities thematically (Kaufman, 1981) and how these identity themes related to concerns and feelings about the home environment; and (3) to gain some knowledge of the "lived world" and "everyday life" of each informant so as to better understand the role of the home in the maintenance of these entities.

Selection of informants was dictated by interviewer perception of informant articulateness and reflectiveness. Seven informants, four women and three men, form the core of the informant base. Material gathered from these seven individuals forms the descriptive basis of a work on aging and the environment (Rubinstein, in preparation).

In the remainder of this section, I will describe some of the effects of a long-term series of in-depth interviews on ability to gather data on changes in an elderly individual's relationship with her home environment.

Mrs. Quinn

As of this writing I have known Mrs. Quinn for two years. During a period of four months, I saw her once a week for our "visits." Since our "official" interviews stopped, I have visited her about once every three months. Mrs. Quinn is a short, thin woman, who was almost 80 at the time of our first interview. She lives in a two-story row house in a middle-class neighborhood in Philadelphia.

At our first meeting, when we were introduced, Mrs. Quinn impressed me as a strong-willed person. At this initial meeting, when we hardly knew each other, I was again witness to the telling of important stories. My explanation of the research project and of my desire to visit her on a weekly basis was accepted and agreed to. In addition, my presence triggered a number of stories that, as I was to recognize later, hinged on a number of rather fixed thematic foci, particularly the need to struggle against great odds. The central story she told me concerned events surrounding her beloved husband's death in the 1940s, her family's poverty after his death, the shame she felt when some of her children had to turn their earnings over to her for support of the family, and her resolve, despite her considerable misgivings about her abilities and strength, to secure employment and keep her family together. Somewhat later on, she told me she had managed to attain one thing in her life that she had never really thought possible, ownership of a home.

In the early interviews with Mrs. Quinn, as with the other informants, my strategy was to steer away from direct discussion of the meaning of home in hope of ascertaining how much this topic was of concern to the informants independent of my research interests. I also wanted to establish a picture of each informant's life as she herself described it. The first interview with Mrs. Quinn covered general topics and some life-history information. We discussed her birth, her health problems, significant dates in her life, her seven children (six living), her numerous grandchildren, her contact with her children and grandchildren, her income, and some of the places she had lived. In the second interview, I asked her about "best" and "worst" things in her life right now and the things she did "yesterday." This latter question was enough to induce lengthy discussion and narrative (the interviews generally took about three hours). In the last two months of the four-month period, I began to introduce questions about her home and its significance. But throughout the course of the interviews, I was careful to pay attention to remarks Mrs. Quinn made about her home and to observe her behaviors in her home.

Emerging Insights

It eventually became clear that one of Mrs. Quinn's major concerns was her ability to remain in her home, given the various physical declines she was experiencing. Much of what she talked about independently reflected or referred to this struggle. In order to describe the process of this discovery, I will use the term *saturation* or *pattern saturation*. I have borrowed this term from Bertaux and Bertaux-Wiame (1981), who used it to describe the process by which an investigator learns that particular, long-term behavioral patterns are typical of a group of people (in their case, the events described in the life-history narratives he took from persons sharing a particular occupational niche in France). Eventually, when one hears enough similar narratives, one's knowledge of these events is saturated by the pattern and therefore complete. In the sense I am using the concept here, it refers to the recognition on the part of the investigator that the structure or content of the informant's narrative or statements returns again and again to specific foci. After a time, I began to see that the stories about her past Mrs. Quinn told me at our first meeting (when I was a stranger, but a person assigned to the particular role of interviewer) were significantly related to her present-day conflicts. Initially, the death of her husband left her to be supported by children until she got herself moving and "took the bull by the horns." Her current conflicts continue this theme, relating to her ability to continue in her home, her own physical decline, conflicts over support from children, and (unrealistic) expectations about herself and her abilities to "take charge" of the situation given the physical decline she was experiencing.

After the four-month interview period had been completed, I visited Mrs. Quinn periodically. While I would call her on occasion, she would also call me, sometimes in a panic, claiming that "everything was falling apart," that she did not know what was happening to her, and that she was concerned about the continuing effects of her physical decline. At times there was a sense of terror, which was new. I would talk to her on the phone and arrange to go to her home to talk some more about her concerns.

What emerged from all the interactions was a picture of a woman whose relationship to her environment was changing. Initially, during the four-month interview period, she was experiencing physical decline—decreased stamina, strength, energy, and endurance—and had been experiencing this for some time. Nevertheless, the *rate* of decline was usually manageable. Although Mrs. Quinn was aware of the decline and, certainly, at some level, of the conflicts it engendered within her, these were usually manageable. They were manageable in the sense that her physical abilities had declined rather gradually and over a lengthy period of time and that her sense of self had evolved with these physical changes. In response to this gradual decline she had constructed a daily and weekly routine, characterized by a degree of regularity. Her daily routine was constructed to absorb the gradual changes in her physical state. Health conditions and difficulties in managing her environment (vacuuming, cleaning, moving furniture, climbing the step ladder, and other chores) were known, predictable, calculated, and built into her daily routine. Change was not sudden. Thus, given the fixed, gradual rate in the decline of her physical abilities, a lot of these problems could for the most part be tuned out in her day-to-day routine.

Sometime after the four-month period of interviewing had elapsed but during the first year in which I knew her, the pace of Mrs. Quinn's physical decline increased. Previously, consciousness of decline had emerged as something to notice (to direct consciousness to) once a week or more infrequently. Now difficulties were noticed more frequently and they impinged increasingly upon her normal routine.

As the rate of decline increased, Mrs. Quinn hoped her decline would stabilize and things would return to the way they had been. Her discussion with me began to focus around the key theme of, "How do I maintain myself in a situation of decline?" In my observations of how Mrs. Quinn reacted to the changes going on in her life, four constructs emerged.

First, she evidenced increasing environmental microsensitivity. Lawton and Nahemow (1973; Lawton, 1980) have suggested that as an individual's overall competence or competence in selected domains decreases, environmental press, or environmental constraint on behavior, increases. Over the period of time I visited Mrs. Quinn, she became increasingly sensitive not only to environmental barriers (e.g., stairs, folds in the carpet, furniture in corridors) but to such environmental factors as the way her body was positioned and the need for handholds.

Second, physical changes put increased pressure on identity maintenance, that is, on maintaining the core feeling of who she was and what was "correct" for her. In our most recent contacts, explanatory narrative has become more sharply focused on the central issue of how to maintain herself despite decline. Formerly separate issues, such as her relationship with her children, now figure more prominently in this dominant concern.

Third, what may be called environmental trade-offs occurred. The goal of such trade-offs is to give up certain activities (thus defining them as peripheral to the central project of maintaining oneself) in order to rescue as much energy as possible for this central project. The goal or central project is to retain as much as possible of what constitutes normal, routine behavior. Thus, over time, five days a week at the senior center become four, then three; a daily highlight (Rubinstein, 1986), which may consist of four elements (going to three stores and then to evening mass), now consists of three, then two elements. A cleaning day that once included vacuuming, laundry, kitchen jobs, and cleaning the bathroom now includes just the laundry. There is simply no energy for the others.

Clearly there are some choices in how to work this. For example, Mrs. Quinn could give up *all* cleaning and *all* other activities, contenting herself solely with attending the senior center five days a week. Yet she has chosen to try to retain activities from as many different domains as possible, cutting back some of each to retain elements of all. The apparent goal of this is to retain "the week" as the major experiential unit, as the unit of time and activity that seems natural, unquestioned, and uninterrupted, in which, for her, threats to the self seem manageable. A fallback position is to give up the week as the unit and to "live one day at a time." At my last meeting with Mrs. Quinn, about a month before writing this chapter, it became clear that she was losing control of her weeks and more and more had to see "how it was going" each day before she could get on to those things she wanted to do.

Finally, I was able to observe another change over time. The spatial analog of the temporal construct of trade-off is something I call environmental centralization. In the process of environmental centralization, peripheral areas of the home become increasingly secondary to the maintenance of "the day" or "the week" and thus of personal identity. In the case of Mrs. Quinn, centralization means giving up the use of areas of her home, such as the second bedroom, most of the basement, and the backyard, and restricting most of her living to a central corridor in her home. Even in those rooms she has continued to inhabit, peripheral areas have developed. The central core of her dining room (her most used room), for example, includes the TV, telephone, an eating table, and a sideboard where she keeps her keys, checkbook, and bills. In this room, the corners and side areas, formerly kept clean and free of clutter, have now become repositories for her shopping cart, vacuum cleaner, and other items as the sides of her dining room more and more become storage areas as her basement used to be.

The long-term strategy of topically oriented, in-depth interviewing, a strategy that acknowledges and includes asides, comments, and stories as an integral part of the interview process, has permitted the observation and investigation of significant changes in elderly individuals' central identity, processes affecting these changes, and the relationship of individuals to their environments over time.

CONCLUSION

This chapter has discussed two types of topically oriented, in-depth interviewing, a short-term series with a fixed number of interviews and the more long-term type. In many ways, our understanding of the types and contexts of research methods and strategies, with the elderly or with others, is in a nascent phase. The two sorts of interview strategies described here both have ramifications for the types of data gathered, as do such other strategies as community-based participant-observation and one-time surveys. Investigators should be able to choose from a palette of methods, combining them when necessary, rather than going through an endless "blue period." The interview strategies described here are well suited for gerontological and other behavioral science research. As the use of such interview strategies increases, it is important that we analyze their use to enhance our understanding.

NOTES

1. Data reported in this paper were gathered in two research projects supported by two different sources. The project on older men living alone was supported by the Frederick and Amelia Schimper Foundation; the project entitled "The Meaning and Function of Home for the Elderly" was supported by the National Institute on Aging (Grant Number AG03509). I wish to express my gratitude here to both these organizations. Some of the material presented in this chapter appeared initially in a paper entitled "The Experience of Loneliness: Older Men Living Alone," presented at the annual meeting of the American Anthropological Association in 1982. In addition, I wish to acknowledge the support of M. Powell Lawton, Ph.D., and Miriam Moss, M.A., of the Behavioral Research Department of the Philadelphia Geriatric Center, as well as the supportive environment for research at the center. I wish to thank Allen Glicksman and Miriam Moss of the center and the editors of this volume, who read an earlier draft of this chapter and whose comments greatly helped to improve it.

2. For all the cases discussed below, all names are pseudonyms and some situations have been disguised.

REFERENCES

Balswick, J. O. (1982). Male inexpressiveness. In K. Soloman & N. B. Levy (Eds.), *Men in transition: Theory and therapy* (pp. 131–150) New York: Plenum Press.

Bertaux, D., & Bertaux-Wiame, I. (1981). Life stories in the bakers' trade. In D. Bertaux (Ed.), *Biography and society: The life history approach in the social sciences*. Beverly Hills, CA: Sage.

Eckert, J. K. (1980). *The unseen elderly: A study of marginally subsistent hotel dwellers*. San Diego, CA: The Campanile Press.

Frank, G. (1979). Finding the common denominator: A phenomenological critique of life-history method. *Ethos, 7*, 68–94.

Gubrium, J. (1974). Marital desolation and the evaluation of everyday life in old age. *Journal of Marriage and the Family, 36*, 106–113.

Gubrium, J. (1975). Being single in old age. *International Journal of Aging and Human Development, 6*, 29–41.

Kaufman, S. (1981). Cultural components of identity in old age: A case study. *Ethos, 9*, 51–87.

Keith, J. (1980). Participant observation. In C. L. Fry & J. Keith (Eds.), *New methods for old age research: Anthropological alternatives* (pp. 8–26). Chicago: Center for Urban Policy, Loyola University of Chicago.

Lawton, M. P. (1980). *Environment and aging*. Monterey, CA: Brooks/Cole.

Lawton, M. P., & Nahemow, L. (1973). Ecology and the aging process. In C. Eisdorfer & M. P. Lawton (Eds.), *The psychology of adult development and aging* (pp. 619–674). Washington, DC: American Psychological Association.

Levenson, D. J. (1978). *The season's of a man's life*. New York: Knopf.

Rubinstein, R. L. (1986). *Singular paths: Old men living alone*. New York: Columbia University Press.

Rubinstein, R. L. (1986). The construction of a day by elderly widowers. *International Journal of Aging and Human Development. 23*, 161–173.

Rubinstein, R. L. (in preparation). *The meaning and function of home for the elderly*.

Spradley, J. P. (1979). *Participant observation*. New York: Holt, Rinehart & Winston.

U. S. Senate, Special Committee on Aging. (1982). *Developments in aging: 1981*. Washington, DC: U. S. Government Printing Office.

8

The Transition to Self-Care: A Field Study of Support Groups for the Elderly and Their Caregivers

Mary Ann Wilner

This study is about coping. Specifically, it is about how some elderly people have begun to use the self-help movement to grapple with the difficulties of growing older and being stigmatized in a youth-oriented society, and how families of the cognitively impaired elderly have turned to each other for support and sustenance.

I used data collected from field observations in two self-help support groups to answer three broad questions. Why do some people turn to the self-help movement for support? What do they receive from the groups? What changes do they experience as a result of their participation in these groups?

One self-help group, in Georgetown[1], was sponsored by a regional mental health agency and held at the Council on Aging office of a small older city in the eastern United States. The second group, sponsored by a metropolitan mental health center, was held biweekly at a local public library of a small city within the confines of a major eastern metropolitan area. Both groups were facilitated by licensed social workers from

---

[1]The names of the locations and participants of the groups have been changed to preserve confidentiality.

the sponsoring agency and held sessions that lasted for an hour and a half.

Members of the Georgetown group were aged 55 and over. Their concern was coping with their own aging and the accompanying problems in a society where youth is valued more than advancing age. Members of the second group were primary caregivers of relatives with Alzheimer's disease. They were experiencing the wrenching process of caring for and separating from relatives suffering from this degenerative, chronic, and terminal illness whose most devastating manifestation is loss of cognitive functioning.

Two different philosophies of group facilitation were evident in the groups. The social worker of the Georgetown group followed a packaged curriculum oriented toward older people. Issues such as personality, self-esteem, assertiveness, change, and limitations were among the topics of discussion. The facilitator of the Alzheimer's group took a more passive role. Although she was an attentive listener, she did not set an agenda. Typically, a participant would simply start talking and venting about a recent experience or feeling.

The groups also differed in their life tenure. The Georgetown group had 10 meetings. Theoretically, members were to attend only this 10-week session, but because of their expressed interest and demand, participants rejoined subsequent sessions. Although 12 people were enrolled during the session I observed, only 10 attended any given meeting. The Alzheimer's caregiver group met consistently throughout the year. New members could join at any time, at the invitation of the facilitator. During the meetings I observed, attendance of the six members was almost 100 percent each week. Only failure to obtain a respite caregiver for their afflicted relative prevented them from attending.

Using the method of grounded theory discovery developed by Glaser and Strauss (1967), I entered the field and began observations without the development of prior hypotheses.

My interest in the question developed over time. My own familial experience with Alzheimer's disease made me acutely aware of the difficulties experienced by caregivers. My professional and academic experience in long-term care and with a variety of self-help situations among older individuals increased my curiosity about the efficacy of self-help groups. Some initial reading about the topic also helped me formulate questions about the role of self-help groups for the elderly and their caregivers. However, as much as possible, I refrained from developing hypotheses in the early stages of the research. Other than writing a short prospectus about the topic of study to gain admission to the sites, I acted solely as an observer in the initial stages of the study.

I was introduced to the groups by the social workers and invited to bring a chair to the discussion table, but I did not join in the discussions. At the last meeting I observed in each group, I asked several questions developed from themes that had emerged from earlier observations. This direct approach to collecting data changed the nature of the group dynamics and seemed to hamper the participants' ease of conversational exchange. Consequently, the findings presented in this chapter derive almost exclusively from my observations, not from the few questions posed directly to the groups.

Following each session I typed, in copious detail, field notes of each of the conversations and interactions from the session. The notes were then studied for emerging themes. Analytic memoranda were subsequently developed to explore further the themes and to substantiate thematic links within each session and between the sessions. The findings described below evolved from the field notes and analytic memoranda. Quotations are taken directly from the field notes.

The research was time limited, completed within the confines of a four-month graduate course in qualitative methodology at Brandeis University. From a total of 15 hours of observations, similar themes emerged from both groups.

This description of the research is separated into two parts: first, an annotated description of the findings from the field observations; second, a review and integration with relevant literature.

MAJOR THEME

The most prevalent theme in both groups was the use of the group by its members to transcend their position of being neglected and rejected by societal institutions. Members become more masterful at negotiating with representatives of these formal and informal institutions. Underlying this overall theme were three subthemes—dissatisfaction with family, friends, and professionals. Specifically, members of both groups repeatedly mentioned their neglect by and dissatisfaction with their families and friends, as well as the professional service, medical, and business establishments with which they interacted. Notable from the group discussions was the members' increasing ability to interact with individuals in these institutions in a more assertive manner, leading to enhanced life satisfaction, strengthening of coping abilities, and ultimately self-care.

GEORGETOWN AGING SELF-HELP GROUP'S SUB-THEMES

Family Losses

The most acute loss of family members felt by the Georgetown self-help group participants was the loss of their spouses. Eight of the 10 women were widows, and both men were widowers. Although most had children, they expressed disappointment that their children did not phone or visit more often. Ida made excuses, claiming that "younger people today are so busy . . . they don't have time to come visit. . . . Even those who are middle-aged are . . . trying to give their children a college education." Alice disagreed and did not see this as a valid excuse. She thought her generation had not been firm enough with their children in instilling the values and morals of taking responsibility for their parents.

Some of the women experienced disapproval from their children. Mary talked about having friends of different ages, saying that her son never understands her friendship with a woman who is his age. She gets criticism from him, yet this woman calls her all the time and worries if she can't reach her. Lucy asked, "How can we cope with people who want us to be like they are?" The facilitator responded by noting the difference between receiving advice and making decisions. Alice said that she has to be "flexible and changing with her family or else they will leave her behind and [she] does not want that."

These comments suggest uneasy ties between the group members and their children; relationships could not be taken for granted. The women had to work to maintain the ties, for they were no longer the family matriarchs.

Loss of Friends and the Ability to Make Friends

This theme was introduced by the facilitator, who verbalized that as one's spouse and friends die, there is a loss of friends as well as a loss of opportunity for making new ones. He asked if the theory was true that older people are not as likely to strike out and make friends. The group agreed, although most of the members were active in the community. Nevertheless, these people complained of not having close friends and of having difficulties making new acquaintances.

Neglect by Professionals

Feelings of abandonment by the professional and business worlds were mentioned often. Ingrid noted an episode where she was "put on hold" by an insurance company. When the woman returned to the phone, Ingrid said, "I am not a machine but a human being and you did not ask me if it was convenient to wait." She mentioned at another time that before joining the group she was quite intimidated by and afraid of doctors. "Now that is much easier . . . although [she] is afraid of professionals." Janet said she would feel more comfortable going to the mental health center if she had to. "That would not be as scary, intimidating, or distasteful now."

As can be seen from these brief examples, members of this group had experienced intimidation and rejection by many of the institutions with which they had to do business. Participation in the group seemed to have helped them become more assertive and satisified with their responses from representatives of these various institutions.

ALZHEIMER'S GROUP SUB-THEMES

Family Relationships

Members of the Alzheimer's group had experienced similar failures in receptivity by, and service from, societal institutions. Their most acute and painful rejection, however, was from their families. Most members of the group were the primary caregivers of the Alzheimer's victim. They were the ones who lived daily with the person, noted the changes, acknowledged the disease, and gradually gave over more of their own lives to taking care of the person. These people also took responsibility for making the decision to place their loved one in an institution.

Members of this group spoke of their anger, disappointment, and exhaustion from the lack of support from other family members. They experienced lack of empathy, distancing, and denial from their families. Ruth lived on the second floor of a duplex. Her sister-in-law, who lived downstairs, offered very little help and had little knowledge of the status of Ruth's husband. She watched him one day for 20 minutes and realized that he did not respond, yet she had heard Ruth talking to him all the time. She could not understand this discrepancy and did not seek to become more involved in providing emotional support or assisting with physical caregiving.

Ruth, who was over 65, had great physical difficulty giving her husband a shower. She was afraid they would both fall. For years her son could not accept the existence of the disease and offered no help. It was an important day when the son called and offered to come over and bathe his father. Afterwards, the father turned to his son and thanked him. This was a remarkable breakthrough for the son, who had denied the father's illness, and for Ruth, who was now able to receive help from her family.

Paula had been experiencing marital difficulties because of her care-taking responsibilities for her mother. She said, "Family members who are not with the person all the time or who are not acknowledging what is happening are of no use, only the group members can really be of support." She said that, in the beginning, her brother and husband thought she "was a little nuts and making it all up." She said if only "she had had some phone calls from family and friends during the day asking how [she] was doing, that would have helped [her] so much and helped [her] mother because [she] would have had more energy and strength to offer better care to [her] mother."

Paula said how awful it was when no one else in the family acknowl-edged her mother's condition. She felt vindicated when "last week [her] brother picked up their mother from the nursing home and called [her] five times in an hour because the mother was so anxious and dis-tressed." He brought her over to Paula's house and asked Paula to feed her since his wife was not at home. Paula later said to him, "You never see it, but now you do, that is what is going on and what has been driving me nuts."

Loss of Friends

These caregivers were also experiencing a lack of contact with and support from their friends. Their isolation and lack of time due to caregiving responsibilities, as well as withdrawal by friends, contrib-uted to the loss of this important support. Few members mentioned visiting friends, having friends come by the house, or talking with friends on the phone. Paula is the only one who said that the only thing that got her through was being able to phone a different friend once each day and cry on the telephone.

Neglect by Medical, Service, and Business Worlds

These people also experienced neglect by the business and professional worlds. They had difficulty finding and purchasing clothes and bedding materials that were appropriate for their Alzheimer's relative. Before the formal start of one session, Ruth shared with Paula and Mrs. Samuels, another group member, information about a "dignity pant" that she had found in a mailorder catalogue. The price was less than from any other store, and the product was exemplary for her purposes:

changing with ease and frequency the wet pants of her incontinent husband.

Of most significance was neglect and misuse by the medical and service establishments. Group members' worst frustration was their doctors' inability to make an accurate diagnosis of Alzheimer's disease. I asked a question about experiences with doctors. Paula rolled her eyes. She said she "has a young local family doctor. He will never say it is Alzheimer's, only senile dementia. He thinks it's a good idea that [Paula] goes to the group, but he won't say or write down that [her] mother has Alzheimer's. [She] thinks he does not want that on her record because the label would hurt her chances of getting accepted to a nursing home."

Marge talked about her mother's previous doctor, who would say of her Alzheimer's-afflicted sister, "She's old, what do you expect?" That infuriated Marge and her mother. Although Alzheimer's can only be accurately diagnosed through an autopsy of the brain, most of the group members reached the diagnosis of Alzheimer's through their own reading and discussions. They had little information or support from their physicians, but instead often supplied information and suggested readings to their doctors.

Mrs. Samuels, a doctor's wife, had experienced her own difficulties with physicians. As the group was leaving after one meeting, she noted that she had just fired her lifelong family doctor because she discovered that he was not, in fact, visiting her husband in the nursing home. Everyone congratulated her for having taken that action, which they knew was difficult.

Group members complained that even when the medical profession was reaching out to families with Alzheimer's disease–afflicted relatives, they were not doing an adequate job. For example, Paula commented that the language at the hospital's community session on Alzheimer's was too medical for her.

Group members were also experiencing neglect from the service system. Those members still caring for their Alzheimer's-afflicted relative at home needed respite care, a service not adequately provided. Ruth filled many sessions talking about her problems with respite care workers. On one occasion, a conversation developed about who made an appropriate respite worker. It was agreed that an 18-year-old girl cannot be a good one. Ruth found that "the younger girls are afraid of [her] husband and one does not want to take him to the bathroom, that one came and while he slept she just curled on the couch and slept." Another respite care worker stole a bag of her groceries.

WHAT HAPPENS IN THE GROUPS THAT PROMOTES CHANGES AND SELF-CARE?

Emotional Support

In contrast to the loss and rejection members experienced from families, friends, and professionals, group participants served as a source of caring, support, and modeling for each other. The groups served a function that neither family nor friends performed. Edith mentioned several times that she had learned she was not alone in her experience as a widow wanting to retain closeness with her children. She found great comfort in knowing others shared the same situation.

Group members actively affirmed each other's activities and responses to new situations. Such validation served to bolster feelings of self-esteem and accomplishment. For example, one of the Georgetown men was repeatedly complimented for his excellent leadership skills when the group went to the flower show. They were so thankful that no one became lost. In another meeting Janet, who was an avid library patron, recounted that earlier in the day the librarian had asked her to speak at the town budget hearings in support of the library. She was afraid to speak at a large gathering. Everyone in the group congratulated her on what an honor it was to be asked to speak. They offered suggestions on how to speak publicly. The most useful and caring piece of advice was offered with humor: Sam told her to stand at the back of the hearing room with the microphone and no one would see her.

Group members spoke often about how their peers in the group were so different from friends and family. They experienced mixed feelings about their families. They loved and treasured them, and they did not want to burden them with their problems and concerns. Most wanted never to live with their children, and they enjoyed the freedom from full responsibility for their grandchildren. They did not want to be criticized or ordered around by their children. They wanted children and grandchildren in their lives, but they did not feel free to be themselves in their presence. With group members they "could let their hair down," as one woman commented. In the group they could say anything and be understood. They knew others were listening attentively in a nonjudgmental way.

Members of the Alzheimer's group exhibited similar expressions of caring, listening, and concern. There was an empathic and supportive aura underlying the verbal exchanges. Each session began with members asking each other about their Alzheimer's relative. When Paula said that her brother and sister-in-law had begun to help her, the group was ecstatic.

Paula said that, "In the group . . . people know your situation, and they don't criticize you for what you've done, or tell you you're wrong, or your behavior or diagnosis is wrong, because they know exactly what you are talking about." She also learned from others. She said she came to her first meeting and "cried for one and a half solid hours before complete strangers but [she] did come back and each week has been wonderful."

Marge said that her doctor ordered her to continue coming to the group. She "guesses it just helps to come and unload and get rid of all the terrible tension, and cry a little, that it is really very helpful. Where else could [she] come cry except in the group?"

The group was also a place to laugh and experience comic relief from the intensity and tragedy of their lives. "Laughter might be called a gift to help our sanity in the face of trouble" (Mace & Rabins, 1981). The participants howled at Ruth's story about her fear that the neighbors would think she takes in laundry for money because she always has so many clothes out drying. Her husband is incontinent, and she is constantly washing because she "can't stand dirty laundry around."

The members were very attentive listeners. They shared a respect for each other and an acceptance of people as they are, rather than because of any particular achievement. Ruth always brought her husband along because she has no one to leave him with. Mrs. Samuels commented that "she was lucky she could still bring him, and she should continue to do that as long as she could." When he started to move and utter sounds one day, Micky and Mrs. Samuels quickly riveted their attention on him. They seemed to know that the Alzheimer's victim can often grasp the outer world and can respond to attention and care.

The facilitator told the group that she was impressed with their ability to find each other at a larger community meeting held at a local hospital. She told me that the group is effective because the members are homogeneous. "The group is much more together now. At the beginning there were two women whose husbands were already in a nursing home, and the others were barely at the stage of acknowledging the disease, much less talking about a nursing home. This discrepancy caused a lot of pain and friction because the members with spouses in the nursing home were hearing over again about the experiences of those at the early stages of the disease and that was painful to them, and the others were hearing about the nature of the disease and the prospect of institutionalization and that was painful to them. . . . It did not work well at first."

Subsequently, the facilitator discouraged other people who had relatives already institutionalized from entering the group. This suggests that some of the efficacy of the group process may be due to selection of participants who share quite similar experiences. The actual homogeneity of the group members could not be verifed because data about members' characteristics or the admission process were not collected, since the focus of the study was exclusively on their participation in the group.

Exchange of Information

Besides empathic and supportive emotional exchange, members of this group provided each other with specifics about management of their relatives. Mrs. Samuels's husband was the only member's relative who was institutionalized because of Alzheimer's, and she was the most knowledgeable about the disease. She offered many suggestions about management of the relatives, a contribution that grounded the others in information about the disease. This helped them to see the symptoms as a disease, not a chosen behavior. Marge asked about "the crying, [she] finds that hardest of all to take. . . . [She] wondered if it was depression." Ruth said her husband went through a period of that. Marge asked Mrs. Samuels if that was the nature of the disease and how long would it last. Mrs. Samuels said it does end. "They go through a period of depression, but then they work it out."

Mrs. Samuels offered practical suggestions, such as telling Paula to put her mother's name on the waiting list of the local nursing home so she could have access to that facility. She also asked Ruth if a safety net would help keep her husband in his chair. Later she suggested that Marge ask her sister's doctor for liquid medicine so she could give her sister the medicine in juice. Here she was offering a new way to use the medical profession. Ask them for what you need, instead of waiting to get help that often is not forthcoming.

Mrs. Samuels also offered suggestions to the caretakers for their own self-care. Many times she told Ruth that she needed time for herself. When Paula told the story of leaving her mother with her sister-in-law for the first time, and not feeling guilty about not leaving a phone number where she could be reached, Mrs. Samuels supported her wholeheartedly and encouraged her to increase the frequency of such actions.

The facilitator also offered medical information and suggestions about management of the Alzheimer's relative. People "wondered at the number of people with Alzheimer's that we never knew about and why don't we know about them?" The question of shame came up. Marge especially, but also everyone else, could not understand what was embarrassing or shameful about having the disease. The facilitator talked about the difference between what is seen as physical and mental illness. She said people will talk all day about the symptoms and problems of someone with a physical illness in the family, but they will not talk about a mental illness.

CHANGES DERIVED FROM GROUP PARTICIPATION

The most notable changes among the Georgetown group members were their enhanced self-esteem and ability to be assertive in the familial and professional worlds. This meant an increased ability to care for themselves. Pamela "had learned to be assertive and not let the kids take over." Anne's kids were "far away and [her] husband is dead, and [she] had to know how to do things for [herself] and speak up." Ingrid said "the group had helped [her] be lighter and laugh more and enjoy life more . . . " She thought coping with aging had been her problem, but she "realized the difficulty was coping with life." Many mentioned that they now listen better to others. Edith learned "that there are many people in [her] same position and [she] is not alone, and that has helped [her] a great deal."

These women had learned how to take better care of themselves. One mentioned she would go to the local mental health center if she felt the need. Another found it easier to go to a physician. Anne learned that she felt much better from getting out and being active. Despite the barriers of inadequate transportation and cold New England weather, she felt better being active out of the house.

These people also felt better about themselves. They felt more self-assured and better able to cope with life—whether that meant business-people, children, the loss of a spouse, or increasing physical limitations.

One of the ways members of the Alzheimer's group learned to take better care of themselves was by arranging for time away from their ill relative. Paula was successful at ensuring that her brother assumed more responsibility so that she could get away for a few hours. She also noted that "this group is what led [her] to get into counseling and that has been wonderful and enormously helpful." She began seeing a professional therapist with her husband, which helped reduce many of the misunderstandings and tensions in her family. Marge, whose sister had Alzheimer's, rotated caretaking responsibility with other siblings and nieces. She felt that her sister's husband was suffering the most because he never left his wife's room. He was enormously stressed and was never able to give himself even an hour's respite.

Participants seemed to learn to listen more carefully to others, and that helped them take better care of themselves. For months, Mrs. Samuels had offered numerous suggestions to Ruth, who did not seem to hear or reply to them. Later Ruth was able to hear a Veterans Administration doctor caution her to get help for herself. The group facilitator noted that several months earlier she would not have heard or heeded the doctor's advice.

Changes were subtle in the Alzheimer's group. Mere attendance at the meetings, implying an acknowledgment of the presence of the disease, reflected substantial change. Being able to make plans for moving the relative, when necessary, to a more appropriate caregiving environment was enormously significant. Paula had spent her first several months in the group just determining if her mother had Alzheimer's disease. In less than six months, not only had she placed her mother in a rest home, but she talked about the realization "that [her] mother will not live the rest of her life in a rest home either, but will have to be moved again to a more intensive care facility."

The use of the Alzheimer's group seems to have prevented the premature placement of a relative in an institution. The discussions suggest that group members learned to make appropriate use of doctors, institutions, and social workers because they learned to use the group for the more basic information about the nature and management of the disease, and for necessary tension release and mutual support.

INTEGRATION WITH THE LITERATURE

Themes that emerged from field observations of these two support groups complemented findings from the literature regarding self-help groups and management of Alzheimer's disease. Many of the earlier writings show that people who join these groups need assistance in coping, defined by Donald Warren (1981, p. 11) as "a process of mobilizing and utilizing supports, skills, and assistance available in a person's 'social network' for dealing with and solving problems." Examples in the first section of this chapter illustrate that members of both groups learned to use each other and their lifelong informal supports, as well as formal providers, in ways that were more helpful to them.

In their classic work on self-help groups, Katz and Bender (1976) schematically described what they termed essential conditions for self-help groups: (1) a source of dissatisfaction with daily living patterns;

(2) sharing of discontents instead of internalizing them as private agendas; (3) an element of deprivation inherent in the dissatisfaction; and (4) an individual's perception that some possessed quality (status, social acceptance, etc.) has been withheld when it is due. The Georgetown women, who complained of rejection and impotence in their interactions with the business community, and the Alzheimer's caregivers, who felt stigmatized due to the nature of their loved one's disease and shunned by the medical community, slip easily into this framework.

Hess (1976) and Hochschild (1973) characterize old age as a period of "decreasing involvement in family, neighborhood and work networks, whether voluntary or not" (Hess, 1976, p. 55). Consequently, older people often "devise spontaneous helping patterns which frequently mirror those of extended families" (Hess, 1976, p. 59). Hochschild describes these ties as "'backup relations,' social insurance policies for the times when the complementary bonds of parent and child, husband and wife, . . . fail, falter, or normally change" (Hochschild, 1973, p. 96). In *The Unexpected Community* (1973) Hochschild observes residents of Merrill Court, a housing project for older, lower-income people. She finds that the women treasured their children and loved to visit and talk with and about them, but they did not want to live with them or to have them visit for long periods of time. These are the same concerns expressed repeatedly by members of each of the observed groups.

Groups offer to their members a "kith and kin" support that provides continuing guidance and direction as well as self-validation. The joiners are on a "quest for community," a place where they can depend on others in intimate relationships for psychic and material support and for "sharing and shaping interpretations of the world" (Hess, 1976, p. 55).

Caplan (1981, p. 419) explains how high levels of social support, as exemplified in a mutual aid group, can "protect individuals against increased vulnerability to illness . . . associated with high stress." According to Caplan, participation in the group enables members to develop "mastery" skills, which mobilize their internal and external resources to develop capabilities to change their environment or relation to it, as well as reduce feelings of emotional arousal. This is analogous to the psychic and material support described by Hess (1976). The group members provide each other with concrete help and skill training, enabling them to operate more effectively in frustrating or confusing situations. Data from the Georgetown and Alzheimer's groups repeatedly reveal exchanges of concrete information. The Alzheimer's caregivers were constantly sharing with each other ways to manage different behavioral manifestations of the disease.

Caplan (1981, p. 417) notes that especially in grief work, which characterizes both these groups, long-term support is best offered by a "nonprofessional mutual help organization of other bereaved persons. These people have the motivation to persevere in this way because they identify personally with those they are helping and because they themselves receive reinforcement of their mastery of their own loss each time they offer help to a fellow sufferer." Here Caplan offers further explanation of the manner in which these groups work. His thesis of mastery of social support, leading to a "recovery of a sense of well-being" as well as a modification of the environmental situation, is strikingly similar to the themes derived from this study's data: that support group participation teaches the development of coping abilities, leading to enhanced self-care.

Research on support groups specifically for caregivers of Alzheimer's patients is recent and rather sparse. Barnes, Raskind, Scott, and Murphy (1981) note a need for controlled evaluation of the efficacy of these support groups. However, there are serious ethical problems in imposing a controlled evaluation on this population. Caregivers of Alzheimer's patients find it difficult to follow directives of a group leader or even to listen to an informal talk about Alzheimer's. Imposing structured questionnaires, validated tests, and controlled interviewing would be disrespectful to these caregivers, and many of them would find it very difficult to respond.

Another methodological problem has been the small numbers inherent in the nature of the support group structure. It is encouraging that findings from this research and a few other qualitative studies have replicated each other. Together these studies add up to a larger population. Their many similar findings contribute to the accumulating body of knowledge and add new information specific to the support group process and its effectiveness.

A variety of qualitative studies and personal accounts have already revealed the enormous benefits gained by participating members. Significant changes—such as acknowledging the presence of the disease, being able to make plans for eventual institutionalization of the relative, and learning to incorporate other family members in offering emotional support and caregiving—are mentioned in each of the studies (Zarit, Reever, & Bach-Peterson, 1980; Aronson, Levin, & Lipkowitz, 1984; Heston & White, 1983; Mace & Rabins, 1981; Clark et al., 1984; Roach, 1985). The groups are important in strengthening the morale, emotional well-being, and treatment skills of care-providing families. Such factors are critical in attaining optimal health and functioning of the Alzheimer's victim (Barnes et al., 1981). Roach (1985) poignantly describes her realization that, if placed in a nursing home, her mother would receive not only good care, but stimulation and perhaps the skills to become less helpless.

The members of the Alzheimer's group in this study and in earlier research mentioned similar concerns, fears, and angers. They were distrustful of physicians who tended to withdraw once the diagnosis was made, "communicating a sense of hopelessness, and leaving the family without a source of information about how to care for the patient" (Barnes et al., 1981, p. 81). In the midst of their enormous caregiving responsibilities spouses often neglected their own personal needs and interests. Families felt isolated and unsupported by friends and the community at large. They found day care facilities reluctant to care for the cognitively impaired, and respite workers inadequately trained for the work.

Earlier studies report that the group served as a new support system as well as a social outlet. Meetings gave members "an opportunity to share concerns, clarify problems and roles, develop skills for . . . coping" and to learn about the nature of the disease and available community resources (Hudis, 1977, cited in Zarit, Reever, & Bach-Peterson, 1980, and in Mace & Rabins, 1981). The groups offered friendship and an outlet for emotional tension: "sharing these feelings can be comforting and can give you the strength you need to continue to care for a declining person." Grief "is eased somewhat when it is shared with other people who are also living with [this] unique tragedy" (Mace & Rabins, 1981, p. 164).

A friend with a brain-damaged son wrote to Marion Roach, who had a mother with Alzheimer's disease: "When I finally stopped [crying] and went to the bookstore, I found almost nothing. I was looking for a book on how to cope, just cope. I wasn't even looking for a cure. I just wanted to know how to live with this" (Roach, 1985, p. 172). What has emerged from my study is that through participation in self-help groups, people learn how to cope.

Although the focal issues of the two groups studied here varied, members who joined with feelings of impotence in dealing with their worlds learned to see the similarity in their experiences, to share valuable information, and to practice skills necessary for taking care of themselves and enhancing their life satisfaction.

REFERENCES

Aronson, M. K., Levin, G., & Lipkowitz, R. (1984). A community-based family/patient group program for Alzheimer's disease. *The Gerontologist, 24,* 339–342.

Barnes, R. F., Raskind, M. A., Scott, M., & Murphy, C. (1981). Problems of families caring for Alzheimer patients: Use of a support group. *Journal of the American Geriatric Society, 29*, 80–85.

Caplan, G., (1981). Mastery of stress: Psychosocial aspects. *The American Journal of Psychiatry, 138*, 413–420.

Clark, M., Gosnell, M., Witherspoon, D., Huck, J., Hager, M., Junkin, D., King, P., Wallace, A., & Robinson, T. L. (1984, December 3). A slow death of the mind. *Newsweek*.

Glaser, B. G., & Strauss, A. L. (1967). *The discovery of grounded theory: Strategies for qualitative research*. New York: Aldine.

Hess, B. (1976). Self-help among the aged. *Social Policy, 7*, 55–62.

Heston, L. L., & White, J. A. (1983). *Dementia: A practical guide to Alzheimer's disease and related illnesses*. New York: W. H. Freeman.

Hochschild, A. R. (1973). *The unexpected community: Portrait of an old age subculture*. Berkeley, CA: University of California Press.

Katz, A. H., & Bender, E. L. (Eds.). (1976). *The strength in US: Self-help groups in the modern world*. New York: New Viewpoints.

Mace, N. L., & Rabins, P. V. (1981). *The 36-hour day: A family guide to caring for persons with Alzheimer's disease, related dementing illnesses, and memory loss in later life*. Baltimore: The Johns Hopkins University Press.

Roach, M. (1985). *Another name for madness*. Boston: Houghton Mifflin.

Warren, D. I. (1981). *Helping networks: How people cope with problems in the urban community*. Notre Dame, IN: University of Notre Dame Press.

Zarit, S. H., Reever, K. E., & Bach-Peterson, J. (1980). Relatives of the impaired elderly: Correlates of feelings of burden. *The Gerontologist, 20*, 649–655.

9

Empowering Nursing Home Residents: A Case Study of "Living Is For the Elderly," an Activist Nursing Home Organization

Kathleen Kautzer

This chapter presents a field study of Living Is For the Elderly (LIFE), a Boston-based nursing home rights organization that promotes self-help and political activism for nursing home residents. LIFE activates nursing home residents by devising strategies to bolster their self-esteem, expand their social networks, and provide them with dignified and challenging social roles.

At first glance one might consider an activist organization to be ill suited to the needs and capacities of nursing home residents. After all, policy makers in the long-term care field have consistently assumed that nursing home residents are incapable of asserting their own rights or monitoring the quality of care they receive.

For example, in his highly acclaimed account, *Unloving Care*, Vladeck concludes that upgrading nursing home services requires primarily increased professional monitoring of service delivery because, in his words, "the need for government regulation arises from the weakness of consumers" (Vladeck, 1980, p. 155). In the same vein, Callahan and Wallack's goals for long-term care, which are shared by most policy

163

makers in the field, are concerned exclusively with the rights and responsibilities of care providers; they provide no right for clients to participate in the design of their own service plan or the policies of the institution where they reside (Callahan & Wallack, 1977). Mendelson (1974) is considerably more explicit and emphatic in her rejection of client empowerment. Since she defines powerlessness as "the essence of the patient's condition," she concludes that "no patient organization, no guarantee of legal rights is going to change the realities of the nursing home patient's plight" (p. 240). Finally, even those policy makers who place priority on increasing the autonomy of long-term care clients limit their reform proposals to new methods of financing services, rather than methods of involving clients in the design and administration of services (Farrow, Joe, Meltzer, & Richman, 1981).

Policy makers' negative assessments regarding the activist potential of nursing home residents are shared by advocacy organizations representing both elderly and disabled persons. Generally speaking, organizations representing both the elderly and disabled have neither actively recruited nursing home residents as members nor vigorously promoted their political interests. Rather, both types of organizations have devoted their advocacy efforts to legislative reform aimed at enabling their members to avoid institutionalization by expanding community services for the disabled.

For example, the Independent Living Movement has focused its lobbying efforts on legislation aimed at opening up new educational and employment opportunities for the disabled and making public buildings, housing, and highways barrier-free (DeJong, 1979). Similarly, the 1972 White House Conference on Aging, which included a large number of advocacy organizations for the elderly, issued recommendations that made only token reference to the institutionalized elderly but expressed strong support for increased public funding of in-home services for the disabled.

Although political activism to date has remained confined primarily to noninstitutionalized persons, the emergence and growth of the LIFE organization suggests that nursing home residents can engage effectively in self-organization and political advocacy. I chose LIFE as the setting for my research because I was interested in ascertaining the impact of activism on the well-being of nursing home residents. LIFE represented a unique opportunity to observe the effects of activism because it is one of only three nursing home rights organizations in the U.S. that is composed primarily of nursing home residents,[1] and its members enjoy a wider range of activities than are available to most nursing home residents.

RESEARCH METHODS

The research was conducted over a two-month period (March 8–May 4, 1983). The study included 20 hours of observation of four separate LIFE events and 12 interviews (with four LIFE staff persons, seven LIFE members, and one activities director for a LIFE-affiliated nursing home). In addition, data were acquired by examining literature published by or about the LIFE organization between January 1980 and June 1983.

Upon entering the field, my own prior research and personal beliefs had led me to suspect that activism would have positive benefits for nursing home residents. Nonetheless, I entered the field with no prior knowledge about what types of activities were possible for nursing home residents or what the exact nature of benefits would or could be.

I encountered no difficulty in gaining access to this research setting—LIFE officers readily approved my research plan and actively encouraged staff members and residents to cooperate with my requests to attend LIFE events and conduct interviews. LIFE officers also placed no restrictions on my access to data or my right to quote them by name in published research reports. In addition, all interviewees consented to my quoting them by name. Far from fearing violations of confidentiality, LIFE staff and resident activists were eager to counter the anonymity that typifies institutionalized persons.

THE LIFE ORGANIZATION

The LIFE organization was founded in 1972 by two male social workers who were employed at the Veterans Administration Hospital in Bedford, Massachusetts. As a result of their experience in placing veterans in nursing homes, they became concerned about the lack of recreational and advocacy activities available to nursing home residents. Lacking both funding and official sanction, the two men began holding meetings in several nursing homes in the Bedford area.

Over the past 13 years the LIFE program has expanded to include over 100 nursing homes in five geographic regions within the Greater Boston Area and has enrolled approximately 1,000 nursing home residents as members.[2] LIFE's growth has been facilitated by a series of public and private foundation grants that enabled the organization to gradually expand its paid staff. In 1985 LIFE had a paid staff of eight persons and an annual budget of $100,000, most of which was received from the federal Department of Health and Human Services under Title III of the Older Americans Act. LIFE is governed by a 15-member board of directors, composed of three nursing home residents and 12 community volunteers.

Nursing homes are selected for membership in LIFE on the basis of location. When LIFE receives funding to provide services within a given geographic region, it invites all homes within the area to participate. LIFE conducts in-house meetings to introduce the program to residents, and residents become members simply by paying a $5 membership fee.

From its inception, founder Ed Alessi envisioned a political role for LIFE, since he recognized that nursing home residents lacked any form of political organization and consequently were not consulted in the legislative process that determines public funding and regulation of nursing home services. One might label this problem "regulation without representation." LIFE's political activities have taken the form of joining or forming coalitions to lobby at the Massachusetts State House for legislation to upgrade the rights and living conditions of nursing home residents. LIFE members mobilize support for LIFE-sponsored legislation by participating in demonstrations at the State House, conducting phone-calling and letter-writing campaigns to legislators, and testifying at legislative hearings.

Beyond its political activities, LIFE also offers a variety of social and recreational events that are designed as a stimulating alternative to the mindless, lowest-common-denominator programs (such as bingo games and birthday parties) that are standard fare in most American nursing homes. For example, LIFE sponsors fall foliage tours, outdoor concerts, boat rides in Boston Harbor, and the annual LIFE Olympics (an all-day event featuring athletic contests specifically designed for frail and disabled participants).

HOW LIFE ACTIVATES NURSING HOME RESIDENTS

LIFE succeeds in activating nursing home residents by designing organizational strategies that accommodate both the frail and/or disabled status of residents and the institutional constraints of nursing homes.

To begin with, LIFE staff carefully nurture prospective activists by lavishing a great deal of personal attention on interested members.

Several members whom I interviewed reported that they decided to run for leadership positions after receiving persistent encouragement from a LIFE staff person.[3] Most activists whom I interviewed described their friendships with LIFE staff persons as one of the highlights of their association with the organization. Given that nursing home residents tend to be socially isolated, the personal attention they receive from LIFE staff is a strong motivating factor for becoming involved in LIFE.

Second, LIFE's ability to recruit activists is facilitated by the patient and sympathetic attitudes exhibited by LIFE staff in their interaction with active members. LIFE staff recognize that many nursing home residents have difficulty assuming responsibility due to failing memory and/or the fact that they have been forced into a passive, dependent position and are no longer expected to be responsible for aspects of their lives. Both interviews and observations of LIFE staff confirmed that they readily forgive LIFE members when they occasionally fail to fulfill responsibilities they have assumed; for example, they may "forget" dates of meetings and be unavailable when a driver arrives to transport them to LIFE events, or they may fail to distribute newsletters, solicit new members, or collect dues.

Third, the assistance LIFE receives from nursing home staff is a critical factor in overcoming transportation and communication barriers faced by nursing home residents. Transportation is a major problem for LIFE, since nursing homes tend to be geographically isolated and many residents lack fare for taxis or mass transit, as well as contacts in the community on whom they can rely for rides. The most expensive and time-consuming transportation problems are posed by nonambulatory residents who cannot even attend in-house meetings without escorts and who require specially equipped vans or buses to attend events in the community. LIFE staff also encounter difficulty in communicating with residents by telephone, since the only phone available to most residents is a busy pay phone or a house phone located in a noisy lobby or corridor. Nursing home staff, particularly activities directors, help LIFE circumvent these obstacles by transporting and escorting nonambulatory residents to LIFE meetings, posting meeting notices, recruiting residents to attend LIFE meetings, and assisting residents in fund-raising and lobbying activities.

Fourth, far from shunning more disabled members, LIFE takes pride in the participation of handicapped members and assures them a visible role in LIFE events. LIFE operationalizes its self-help philosophy by selecting activities that are appropriate for the varying capacities of members and by cultivating respectful and supportive attitudes toward disabled participants. For example, LIFE staff welcome the attendance of all residents at in-house meetings, even those who appear disoriented, doze frequently, and/or require medication to be administered during meetings. Surprisingly, my observations of LIFE meetings indicated that the presence of disoriented residents did not disturb other residents, since the disoriented residents were a familiar presence and remained quiet and passive throughout the meeting.

Even more important, LIFE members create a comfortable, secure environment for disabled members by enthusiastically soliciting and rewarding their participation. The 1983 LIFE Conference featured speakers who were blind, epileptic, disfigured, and/or in wheelchairs. The 600 residents who attended the conference listened attentively during two hours of speeches, even to speakers who had poor diction. Many persons in the audience would nod frequently during speeches, as if to reassure the speaker, particularly if the speaker was stuttering or temporarily forgetting lines. All speakers received enthusiastic applause and numerous friendly pats and words of praise as they left the podium.

LIFE staff are also inventive in designing technical aids that bolster the confidence and opportunities for participation of disabled members. One resident informed me that she was persuaded to deliver testimony at a State House hearing, despite a recent cataract operation, by a member of the LIFE staff who prompted her speech with cue cards printed in enormous letters.

Fifth, in recognition of the low-income status of most nursing home residents (Butler & Newacheck, 1981), LIFE charges only nominal dues and fees for its events and frequently waives expenses for indigent members. LIFE members are also encouraged to cover their own expenses or those of indigent members from their own nursing homes with monies they collect during fund-raising events sponsored by LIFE, such as raffles, flea markets, and community suppers.

Sixth, LIFE's ability to activate residents is probably enhanced by the fact that it is quite literally "the only game in town," the only organization actively seeking the participation of nursing home residents.

A final advantage enjoyed by LIFE is the fact that members do not become targets of derision or retribution as a result of their political activism, particularly since staff in LIFE-affiliated nursing homes tend to support and encourage the participation of residents. In contrast, activists in many social movements have been forced to cope with various forms of harassment and retaliation from those who oppose and/or feel threatened by their reform proposals. For example, histories of the American labor, civil rights, and feminist movements (to name but a few) describe activists as frequently subjected to jeering, verbal insults and threats, loss of jobs and/or property, imprisonment, and even murder (Zinn, 1980).

IMPACT OF ACTIVISM ON NURSING HOME RESIDENTS

LIFE affects the well-being and life satisfaction of its members by socially constructing new identities and social roles for nursing home residents. The interpretation of these data assumes that human beings' sense of self, modes of thought, and choice of actions are shaped and limited by the social context in which they occur (Berger & Luckmann, 1966). My research findings indicate three major areas in which LIFE alters the social context of nursing home residents: (1) self-image, (2) social ties, and (3) empowerment.

Self-Image

LIFE literature emphasizes that LIFE activities are designed to improve the self-image of nursing home residents:

> LIFE helps nursing home residents to help themselves by putting the "I" back into their lives. The "I" stands for independence, initiative, involvement and image of one's self. The focus is on abilities rather than limitations (LIFE brochure).

The task of augmenting the self-esteem of nursing home residents is a formidable one, considering the dramatic loss of status encountered by persons upon becoming nursing home residents. Perhaps the most severe shock to the personal identity of residents occurs when they are first admitted to a nursing home. Virtually all residents whom I interviewed described themselves as depressed at the time of their admission. None wanted to enter a nursing home—it was a choice forced on them when they became disabled and/or required nursing care following hospitalization.

Newly admitted residents frequently must come to terms with irreversibly diminished physical and mental capacities. Persons whom I interviewed entered nursing homes after loss of voice, sight, or hearing capacities or paralysis of limbs. My interviews with residents also revealed that they are painfully aware of negative societal attitudes toward the disabled, particularly those in nursing homes. Listed below are responses I received to the question: "What do you think are society's attitudes toward nursing home residents?":

> They think we're all senile, tied up in chairs, don't do anything.

> They think we're all put out to pasture.

Some people think "Oh they can't do anything. What's the sense of bothering with 'em?"

In addition to loss of physical or mental capacities, residents usually must relinquish personal belongings such as homes, cars, and pets and leave behind familiar neighborhoods and social networks. Losses of this magnitude clearly have an impact on personal identity, since many persons view personal belongings as a measure of self-worth and rely on familiar social networks for recognition based on past achievements and contributions.

Not only do people enter nursing homes with diminished self-esteem, but also their sense of self-worth is likely to decline even further during institutionalization due to the dehumanizing treatment accorded many nursing home residents. One of the most disturbing forms of degradation experienced by residents is the treatment they receive from significant others, who often assume new attitudes toward the institutionalized person. Pat Johnson of the LIFE staff explains:

> It's hard for the public to understand that even their own mother is not a different person because she went into a nursing home. They say: "Oh, she's in a nursing home now. She can't do that."

A vivid demonstration of this phenomenon was related to me by LIFE's executive director, Margaret Cronin. She described an in-house meeting in which a resident's daughter publicly apologized to her father because she thought he was "crackers" when he initially told her he had testified at the State House on behalf of LIFE legislation.

It is also a well-documented fact of institutional life that staff tend to depersonalize residents under their care, since they do not have sufficient time or flexibility to respond to individual needs (Goffman, 1961). Although my interview subjects spoke highly of staff in their homes, several residents admitted that they were sometimes offended by "the way they speak to you." I personally heard staff use terms such as "sweetie" and "dearie" when addressing residents, even though these terms are considered demeaning by many persons because of their implication of false intimacy and their use with children.

Finally, the institutional regulations of nursing homes impose a dehumanizing regimentation of the daily lives of residents, who lose control over the most simple aspects of their lives, such as choice of food or room decor and scheduling of meals and activities. Loss of autonomy is particularly severe for those residents who require the assistance of staff to dress, eat, or perform toileting functions. Privacy is almost nonexistent for most nursing home residents, very few of whom can afford private rooms or personal phones (Vladeck, 1980). Most of the residents I interviewed had three roommates, and their "personal space" was limited to a bed and several square feet of floor space.

Given this bleak environment, what can an organization like LIFE do to reintroduce some measure of dignity and self-esteem into the lives of nursing home residents? To begin with, a primary objective of LIFE is to promote more positive attitudes toward residence in a nursing home and to challenge the notion that it should be viewed as shameful or morbid. LIFE's literature and public statements by LIFE staff repeatedly emphasize that residence in a nursing home is a sensible and desirable option for many disabled persons, since it provides security, services, and opportunities for socialization not available in the community. For example, one LIFE leaflet boldly asserts: "Entrance into a nursing home should not be considered the end of life, but the beginning of a new kind of life." Statements of this sort are not just platitudes—the entire LIFE organization is designed to create a "new kind of life" for residents by providing them with activities that are genuinely stimulating and self-enriching.

When I asked residents to describe the benefits of membership in LIFE, their answers suggested that LIFE had indeed restored their interest in a future existence. Consider the following typical responses: "LIFE gives you something to live for. You're not just sitting in a corner." "LIFE gives me something to look forward to." "LIFE makes you feel like living."

The self-help orientation of LIFE represents a major component of efforts to affirm and develop the self-esteem and competence of nursing home residents. The emphasis is not "taking care of" or "representing the interests of" residents, but rather providing them with encouragement and opportunities to advocate on their own behalf. LIFE staff demonstrate their respect for residents by assigning them visible roles of power and influence within the organization, including testifying at State House hearings, chairing LIFE functions, and representing LIFE at community forums and in television and radio interviews.

Clearly, public speaking is a prideful occasion for most persons, but these events take on special significance for nursing home residents. Nearly every resident whom I interviewed identified speaking at the State House as their favorite LIFE activity. Residents gave me detailed accounts of their testimony, even when it had been given several years previously (no memory problems here!).

Public speaking also affords residents the chance to publicly affirm their status as nursing home residents. For example, Roy Smith, a wiry paraplegic with an elfish grin, opened his speech to the 1983 LIFE

Conference by proclaiming: "I want to tell you all how much I enjoy being in a nursing home. I'm still happy, what more can I ask?" Another conference speaker, Margaret Carey, a witty and outspoken blind lady, confessed to the audience: "I was complaining a lot when I first came there. I didn't want to be in a nursing home. Now I've been there four years and I just love it." The remarks of these two speakers expressed the sentiments of other LIFE members, judging by the vigorous rounds of applause both speakers received after delivering these lines.

In addition to public speaking, LIFE provides ample opportunity for its members to receive awards and/or titles. Since every LIFE chapter elects three officers annually, there are leadership roles available to a large number of members. Several chapters also conduct elaborate "swearing in" ceremonies for newly elected officers, complete with wine and dancing. In the same vein, the two major annual LIFE events, the LIFE Conference and the LIFE Olympics, include numerous contests in which awards are conferred on the winner of each contest and, in some cases, even to the highest-scoring resident in each nursing home.

By all accounts, these formal symbols of recognition are meaningful to LIFE members. All award recipients at the LIFE Conference accepted their trophies with broad smiles and enthusiastic acceptance speeches. When I visited nursing homes, several interviewees proudly showed me their LIFE award certificates, which they had posted in their rooms or stored in their bedside tables.

Given the large number of awards and leadership roles allocated by LIFE and the relative ease with which they are acquired, some persons might view them cynically. Yet for LIFE members they appear to be highly valued. This may in part reflect the pressing need of residents for some form of recognition, but I think it also reflects the background of LIFE members. Since many nursing home residents are from low-income backgrounds, they may have had little opportunity to participate in formal organizations and acquire official titles. Also, this cohort of elders grew up during a period when formal awards and titles may have been even more highly valued than they are today.

My interviews with LIFE members confirmed that residents acknowledge and appreciate efforts to bolster their self-esteem. Specifically, all the residents whom I interviewed claimed that they were attracted to LIFE because it enabled them to maintain their dignity and enhance their self-image. The following lines recurred throughout resident interviews: "They [LIFE staff] treat you like a human being." "LIFE makes you feel better about yourself." "LIFE makes me feel like a person."

Social Ties

Contrary to what one might expect, residents within a nursing home frequently do not form close social bonds. LIFE's executive director, Margaret Cronin, confided to me her initial shock at the low levels of interaction:

> I've had meetings where people from the same nursing home sat next to each other and have never spoken to each other. It's unbelievable! And they eat together every day without speaking and don't even know each other's names.

Considering the depressed state of many nursing home residents and the unstimulating environment, it is not surprising that many residents exhibit antisocial behavior. LIFE activist Arthur MacGuire described to me his own isolationist tendencies when he first entered a nursing home, explaining:

> You gotta go. If not you're stuck. You get complacent. You get dumb. After that you don't want to do anything. You become a recluse.

Recognizing that loneliness and isolation are major problems for nursing home residents, LIFE activities are designed to enable residents to "broaden their social life beyond the confines of their home" and "to become an integral part of the community" (LIFE leaflet). Almost every resident I interviewed spoke of the social benefits of belonging to LIFE, especially that it enabled them to meet residents in other nursing homes. Commenting on the social stimulation members derive from LIFE events, Annette Caranchi, activities director at Wellington Manor, observed:

> And just to see them when they go out to these activities, how excited they get! They tell me: "Hey, we're going to see such-and-such a person today."

The nonambulatory residents whom I interviewed were particularly appreciative of the mobility acquired through participation in LIFE. Mary Dorlay probably expresses the sentiments of many nonambulatory residents in her "letter of appreciation," which appeared in the December 1982 LIFE newsletter:

> I would like to express my thanks and appreciation for your thoughtfulness in inviting me to the concert. Also, the Long Island picnic in Sep-

tember was most enjoyable. It was the first time I went on a public function on my own. Both were terrific!

LIFE meetings also provide members with opportunities for physical contact, which may be otherwise totally missing in their lives. Ballroom dancing, which requires physical contact, is a frequent form of entertainment. LIFE staff also tend to be very "physical" in their interaction with residents; they frequently kiss cheeks and shake hands. At the 1983 LIFE Conference, every resident who appeared on the speaker's platform was ceremoniously kissed and hugged by LIFE's chairman of the board, Ed Alessi.

In addition to the overt social benefits of participation, my research also uncovered a number of indirect methods whereby LIFE's socialization process enables residents to strengthen social ties. First, LIFE activists serve as role models for other residents by demonstrating the vitality and variety of experiences that are possible for nursing home residents. One activities director describes the influence of LIFE activist Phil Burns as follows:

> Phil is a good role model. He's out as much as he can be. He goes to plays downtown, dances, goes to mass, swims, visits the community center. Other residents see that and say: "Hey just 'cause I'm here doesn't mean I have to stop living."

Second, LIFE affirms the needs of residents to keep in touch with and express their emotions. Some nursing home residents may suppress emotions in an attempt to deny or control anger, fear, or loneliness. While this is a logical coping mechanism, it also robs them of the opportunity to experience pleasure, joy, and communion with others. LIFE constructs opportunities that enable members to express themselves without fear of retaliation, rejection, or ridicule. For example, Pat Johnson of the LIFE staff told me she advised one very angry and irritable resident:

> Hey, Mona, cool it! Don't take your anger out on staff. It's not their fault. Direct your anger at the legislature where it will do some good. They're the ones who give you only $40 a month.

According to Johnson, this woman became one of LIFE's most active and assertive members, and in the process became a more sociable and considerate person.

Mirroring the philosophy of Kübler-Ross (Kübler-Ross, 1969), LIFE affirms the right of members to grieve and acknowledge the reality of death. It used to be standard practice in nursing homes to not even inform residents when someone died and generally to deny the morbidity that is commonplace in nursing homes (Gubrium, 1975). In stark contrast to such policies, LIFE dedicates all of its major events to recently deceased members and offers support services to grieving members. For example, when LIFE activist Mona Thorton died recently, LIFE arranged transportation for residents to attend her funeral and even sponsored a memorial service for her at her nursing home.

LIFE also encourages its members to experience the more positive emotions of joy and affection. LIFE events are characterized by laughter and merrymaking. For example, the audience at the 1983 LIFE Conference laughed heartily at the humorous lines delivered by a variety of speakers. Judging by the volume of laughter, the most popular lines were delivered by Margaret Carey as she teasingly recalled how residents trick nurses to avoid taking medicine. She quipped: "Aides ask me how I am, and I say: 'Oh, pulling the devil by the tail!'"

I was genuinely amazed at the spontaneity and vitality exhibited by those who attended the 1983 LIFE Conference. This was clearly a music-loving crowd, singing along every time folk singers led songs from the podium. Some residents even stood in the aisles and danced; those in wheelchairs swayed their heads in tune with the music. Two of the most well-attended conference workshops were "Creative Movement" and "Fit as a Fiddle," in which scores of residents enthusiastically danced or performed exercises in unison. Perhaps vanities and inhibitions diminish for persons who are close to death and who have few opportunities for merrymaking. These people seem to be more considerate of one another than others in our society, perhaps as a result of their own personal experiences with failing health and the pain and stigma that accompany it.

The third method LIFE employs to strengthen the social ties of residents involves enabling residents to interact on the basis of reciprocity rather than dependence. Many social theorists contend that the strongest social bonds require some degree of exchange, since reciprocity contributes to mutual respect and control between partners (Gil, 1976). Consistent with this theory, LIFE provides its members with a number of opportunities to reward and provide for others. For example, residents vote for and confer awards upon both legislators and nursing home staff on the basis of their contributions to LIFE. For the same reason, LIFE periodically conducts fund-raising drives for the St. Jude Children's Hospital, and LIFE member Bessie Lindenbaum appeared on a TV telethon several years ago to donate $400 that LIFE had collected for this cause. LIFE also sponsors a series of intergenerational exchange programs in which residents meet with youngsters and share details about life when they were growing up. Several LIFE members serve as volunteers at a local day care center. Hence, LIFE not only extends the social networks accessible to nursing home residents, but also enhances their willingness and capacity to form social ties by providing them with role models, supportive environments in which to express their emotions, and resources that enable them to interact on the basis of reciprocity.

Favorable comments regarding the benefits of LIFE's socialization process were forthcoming not only from LIFE members, but also from family members and nursing home staff who interact with residents on a regular basis. According to LIFE staff, many family members and nursing home staff generously donate funds and volunteer services to LIFE after witnessing how participation in LIFE improves the morale and well-being of residents. For example, a son of a LIFE activist, who regularly serves as a volunteer chauffeur for LIFE, credits the LIFE organization with enabling his mother to forgive her children for their decision to place her in a nursing home. (Reportedly his mother was initially so outraged by this decision that she refused to speak to her children during the first year of her residence in a nursing home.) An equally favorable reaction to the LIFE program was expressed by a nursing home administrator:

> Ya, the LIFE program, oh, it's a pain in the neck . . . but you know the LIFE program is the best thing that ever happened to my nursing home. I used to have people whining in my office. Now I have people you can really talk to. It makes it a much nicer place to work for all of us.

These testimonials on behalf of the LIFE program support LIFE's contention that alternative socialization patterns can alleviate and even reverse the depressed and isolationist behavior exhibited by many nursing home residents following institutionalization. LIFE's contention is also supported by Blackman, Howe, and Pinkston (1976), who found that nursing home residents exhibited increased social interaction in response to increases in scheduled activities.

Empowerment

LIFE founder Ed Alessi describes the goals of the program in essentially political terms:

> The LIFE program centers itself on people who live in long-term care facilities. It works toward having them take control of their own lives, destroying damaging stereotypes and attitudes that plague, and expanding their role in our society.

Undeniably it is LIFE's political goals that pose the greatest challenge and frustrations for both staff and members of LIFE, but it is also LIFE's political achievements that represent the organization's greatest source of pride and its most tangible accomplishments.

The internal politics of the LIFE organization demonstrate the problems and contradictions involved in transforming the identities of severely oppressed persons. Although LIFE staff express strong commitment to self-help principles, they also candidly admit that, in Margaret Cronin's words:

> It's a very hard thing to get people to help themselves and not impose your own values, or where you want to go professionally. It's a hard job.

My ability to assess the degree of control exercised by members in the LIFE organization is limited, since I did not attend any policy-making meetings. On the one hand, Alessi insists that membership input determines all major policy decisions, particularly choice of legislative proposals, and my own interviews with residents confirmed their strong support for LIFE-sponsored legislation. Allocating public speaking roles to members also represents a form of power sharing, and LIFE staff apparently make no attempt to censor or manipulate speeches delivered by members. One speaker at the LIFE Conference told me that LIFE staff had advised him to speak on "any topic you like" and had not read his prepared text in advance of the conference.

On the other hand, my observations of LIFE meetings suggest that the leadership roles assigned to LIFE members tend to be symbolic rather than substantive. During the in-house meetings I attended, the role of the resident officers was primarily ceremonial, i.e., taking roll and calling the meeting to order. LIFE staff prepared and narrated the agenda for the meeting and recognized and replied to inquiries from the floor. In all probability the limited role assumed by resident officers resulted from practical rather than political constraints—many officers have impaired visual, speech, and hearing capacities, and the hectic schedule of LIFE staff probably prevents them from consulting individually with officers about agenda creation and narration. Nonetheless, there is no denying that LIFE staff must maintain a delicate balance in assigning responsibilities to residents in order to avoid condescension and paternalism at one extreme, and undue pressure and unrealistic expectations at the other.

LIFE's internal political constraints pale in comparison with the external political obstacles the organization encounters in its efforts to empower residents. The organization's ability to challenge the authority of nursing home administrators is severely undermined by the fact that access to residents is dependent on the cooperation and assistance of nursing home staff. Until recently, LIFE could gain legal access to residents in a given home only by obtaining the approval of the nursing home administrator. The very homes that refuse to participate in LIFE may be ones whose residents have the greatest need for a program like LIFE. These administrators, in many instances, may have something to hide (substandard or abusive care) or may have paternalistic attitudes regarding the rights of residents to join an organization like LIFE.

In order to counteract this problem, LIFE joined a coalition that recently won passage of the Ombudsman and Community Access Bill[4] granting Massachusetts nursing home residents the right to invite any organization of their choice to conduct in-house meetings without the approval of the nursing home administrator. Nonetheless, this bill may only marginally improve LIFE's access to residents, since uncooperative administrators could probably sabotage LIFE's entry into their home by instructing their staff to refuse to post meeting notices, escort nonambulatory residents, and/or penalize residents who become members.

Despite these far from ideal conditions for advocacy, LIFE does retain some ability to correct the power imbalance that exists between residents and administrators of nursing homes. Since LIFE staff frequently visit LIFE-affiliated nursing homes, they have some opportunity to observe conditions in the home and intervene on a resident's behalf. Pat Johnson of the LIFE staff informed me that she habitually consults with nursing home staff when she notices a marked deterioration in a resident.

LIFE empowers its members, in a very real sense, simply by its ability to enhance their self-esteem and provide social contacts within and beyond the confines of the nursing home. Those residents with a higher degree of self-confidence are less likely to be tolerant of abuse and mistreatment, particularly when they have outside contacts in the community to rely on for information and support. At the 1983 LIFE Conference, Margaret Carey served as a role model of an assertive resident when she advised her colleagues:

> If you have some difficulty, speak right up. There's nothing they can do to you . . . I don't have any problems but if I did I would surely tell you people.

LIFE members in the Martin Home in Dorchester presented compelling evidence that nursing home residents are indeed capable of engaging in assertive, collective action when they sent a delegation to confront neighborhood children who were throwing stones at residents and calling them names. This delegation not only convinced the children to cease their harassment, but also persuaded them to run errands for residents.

Beyond these indirect forms of empowerment, LIFE assists its members in forming in-house resident councils, which consist of elected resident delegates responsible for presenting grievances to the nursing home administrator. Furthermore, legal rights are a frequent topic of discussion at LIFE meetings, and information brochures on "The Legal Rights of Residents" are widely distributed among the membership.

Another political aspect of LIFE involves efforts to break down the isolation and societal stigmas surrounding nursing home residents by promoting interaction between nursing home residents and members of the communities in which they reside. According to Alessi, before the existence of LIFE, it never occurred to community organizations to include nursing home residents in their activities. LIFE staff seek to increase the visibility and accessibility of nursing home residents by soliciting invitations for LIFE members to participate in social events (such as local talent shows or baking contests) and to speak at community forums (such as "elderly speak-outs" and meetings with public officials). As a result, Alessi boasts: "Now whenever an organization wants a nursing home resident to talk about aging, they call LIFE." In addition, LIFE members have also gained access to some of the publicly funded services available to elders in the community—for example, the Senior Shuttles in various locales now provide transportation services to LIFE members.

Finally, it is the legislative arena that most clearly reveals the possibilities and limitations involved in realizing LIFE's political goals. As a small grassroots organization, LIFE lacks both the numbers and finances that enable conventional interest group lobbies to obtain attention and concessions from legislators (Lowi, 1969). Yet despite its limited resources, LIFE has achieved an impressive number of victories at the Massachusetts State House, including a series of increases in the Medicaid personal allowance[5] (which raised the allowance from $30 to $55/month over a 5-year period), the security bill (which guarantees each resident a locked space), and the telephone privacy bill (which requires a soundproof telephone booth or cubicle in every nursing home). My interviews with residents indicate that the most popular LIFE-sponsored bills are those increasing the Medicaid personal allowance. Although both the security bill and the telephone privacy bill have encountered implementation difficulties, LIFE staff report that a majority of LIFE-affiliated homes have complied with this legislation.

LIFE has achieved these political victories by forming coalitions with other groups (including church groups, advocacy organizations for the elderly, and service providers) and by appealing to the humanitarian values of legislators. When residents testify at State House hearings, they articulate the human costs and benefits of public policy decisions as they affect their own lives. The following account of LIFE members' testimony at a State House hearing demonstrates the clever and dignified manner in which residents command the attention and respect of legislators:

> One congressman said to Helen: "We used to give you people $48" [referring to the Medicaid personal allowance, which had been reduced from $48 to $40]. She said: "That's right, sir, we are only asking for $45, so you're saving $3, do you realize that?" Well, it brought the house down.
>
> So then I spoke on the access bill. I had not regained my sight fully, so I used cue cards with my speech printed in big letters. I said: "Speaker of the House, don't be alarmed, sirs. This isn't as bad as it looks" [referring to her cue cards]. Well, I got a chuckle out of him.

Several legislators have indicated strong support for the goals of LIFE by repeatedly sponsoring LIFE legislation and making guest appearances at LIFE's annual conference to accept honorary awards. Most notably, Senator Gerald D'Amico (Democrat, Worcester) demonstrated an understanding of the philosophy of LIFE in his remarks to the 1983 LIFE Conference. He commended residents for "taking control of your own lives, you haven't delegated the responsibility."

LIFE's political accomplishments are particularly impressive when one considers the low levels of political organization available to nursing home residents nationwide. According to LIFE staff, Massachusetts is one of only three states where nursing home residents testify at State House hearings and communicate on a regular basis with state legislators.

Despite their exceptional nature, however, LIFE's political victories reveal both the possibilities of and limitations to empowerment faced by a grassroots organization of disenfranchised persons. More specifically, LIFE's legislative victories are precisely the type of reforms most likely to survive the American legislative process; i.e., they are incremental reforms that require minimal public expenditures and/or only marginally infringe on the prerogatives of service providers. By their very nature, these reforms represent only slight improvements in the living conditions of Massachusetts nursing home residents, whose legal rights and discretionary income remain woefully inadequate.[6] Clearly, more complete and enduring forms of empowerment for nursing home residents would require more extensive and costly reforms, such as legislation that dramatically increased the Medicaid personal allowance and/or granted residents the right to participate in governance of the institutions where they reside.

It seems unlikely that LIFE wields the political leverage necessary to achieve reforms of this magnitude, which would no doubt meet with intense and concerted resistance from powerful lobbies representing taxpayers and nursing home owners and administrators. In summarizing the political constraints faced by poor people's movements, Piven and Cloward (1979, p. 3) state:

> In these major ways protest movements are shaped by institutional conditions, and not by purposive efforts of leaders and organizers. The limitations are large and unyielding. Yet within the boundaries created by these limitations, some latitude for purposive effort remains.

LIFE has acquired some degree of political influence by identifying and maximizing the "latitude for purposive effort" available to nursing home residents. The boundaries restricting LIFE's advocacy efforts will be revealed only if and when LIFE pursues more ambitious political objectives and/or political organization among nursing home residents becomes more widespread.

POLICY IMPLICATIONS OF RESEARCH FINDINGS

The LIFE organization presents vivid evidence that nursing home residents are not only capable of becoming more cognizant and assertive regarding their legal rights, but they also consider advocacy to be enjoyable and rewarding. LIFE also demonstrates that residents are not likely to become more assertive in isolation but require an organization like LIFE to provide them with collective strength, mobility, and a therapeutic environment in which to explore new social roles. At present one can only speculate about the extent to which increased empowerment of residents can reduce or eliminate abuse or substandard care. This would be a fruitful topic for future research and certainly should be a priority consideration of long-term care policy makers, particularly since many policy makers admit that regulation can only marginally improve service quality in nursing homes (Vladeck, 1980; Kane & Kane, 1981).

The success of the LIFE organization also challenges the now prevalent assumption of policy makers that expansion of in-home services for the disabled is the most promising policy option in the long-term care field (Butler, 1979; Callahan & Wallack, 1977). When I questioned LIFE staff about the deinstitutionalization issue, they consistently expressed concern that exclusive interest in this option could divert attention and resources away from nursing home residents. Their concerns appear well-founded when one considers the outcome of the movement to deinstitutionalize mental patients. This policy was justified on humanitarian grounds but utilized by cost-conscious public officials to reduce expenditures on mental patients.

LIFE staff also pointed out that many persons prefer residence in a nursing home; they cited several LIFE members who had been placed in community residences but returned to nursing homes because they felt lonely or insecure living alone.

LIFE activists present a compelling argument that it is possible to lead an enjoyable and rewarding life while residing in a nursing home, provided there is an organization available to mitigate the dehumanizing aspects of institutionalization and empower residents to pursue respected and challenging social roles.

NOTES

1. The two other nursing home rights organizations similar to LIFE are the Nursing Home Residents Advisory Council, Minneapolis, MN, and the Coalition of Institutionalized Aged and Disabled, New York, NY.

2. Most LIFE-affiliated nursing homes are classified as Level III by Massachusetts regulatory agencies. Massachusetts nursing homes are classified into four levels, based on the amount of nursing care provided. According to LIFE staff, residents of Level III homes benefit most from an organization like LIFE, since they are less incapacitated than residents of Level I and II homes but lack the independence and mobility available to residents of Level IV homes. It is not possible to assess whether LIFE members are "representative" of Level III residents or nursing home residents in general, since LIFE does not compile demographic data on members.

3. In the interest of brevity, I report research findings without identifying the specific interviews or field notes on which they are based. Extensive documentation is provided in Kautzer (1983). All quotations cited in this chapter are taken from transcripts of interviews conducted during the research project.

4. This legislation won the approval of the Massachusetts legislature under the Chapter 544 Acts of 1983 and is now contained in Massachusetts General Laws, Chapter 19A, Sections 27–35.

5. The Medicaid personal allowance is the only income available to Medicaid patients for all personal expenses, including transportation, entertainment, nonprescription drugs, cosmetics, telephone charges, clothes, snacks, and so forth.

6. The legal rights of Massachusetts nursing home residents are restricted to resident control over personal communication, finances, and medical treatment and protection against arbitrary discharge and transfer. Even these rights can be abrogated by orders from a physician. For the 80% of Massachusetts nursing home residents who are Medicaid patients, their *only* source of discretionary income is the Medicaid personal allowance.

REFERENCES

Berger, P. C., & Luckman, T. (1966). *The social construction of reality.* Garden City, NY: Doubleday & Co.

Blackman, D. K., Howe, M., & Pinkston, E. M. (1976). Increased participation in social interaction of the institutionalized elderly. *The Gerontologist, 16*(1), 69–76.

Butler, L., & Newacheck, P. (1981). Health and social factors relevant to long-term care policy. In J. Meltzer, F. Farrow, & H. Richman (Eds.), *Policy options in long-term care* (pp. 38–78). Chicago: University of Chicago Press.

Butler, P. A. (1979). Financing noninstitutional long-term care services for the elderly and chronically ill: Alternatives to nursing homes. *Clearinghouse Review, 13*(5), 335–442.

Callahan, J., & Wallack, S. (1977). *Reforming the long-term care system.* Lexington, MA: Lexington Books.

DeJong, G. (1979). *The movment for independent living: Origins, ideology, and implications for disability research* (Occasional Paper No. 2). East Lansing, MI: University Center for International Rehabilitation, Michigan State University.

Farrow, F., Joe, T., Meltzer, J., & Richman, H. (1981). The framework and directions for change. In J. Meltzer, F. Farrow, & H. Richman (Eds.), *Policy options in long-term care* (pp. 1–38). Chicago: University of Chicago Press.

Gil, D. (1976). *The challenge of social equality.* Cambridge, MA: Schenkman.

Goffman, E. (1961). *Asylums.* Garden City, NY: Doubleday.

Gubrium, J. F. (1975). *Living and dying at Murray Manor.* New York: St. Martin's Press.

Kane, R. L., & Kane, R. A. (1981). The extent and nature of public responsibility for long-term care. In J. Meltzer, F. Farrow, & H. Richman (Eds.), *Policy options in long-term care* (pp. 78–118). Chicago: University of Chicago Press.

Kautzer, K. (1983). Do not go gentle: A field study of the LIFE organization. Unpublished manuscript, Heller School, Brandeis University, Waltham, MA.

Kübler-Ross, E. (1969). *On death and dying.* New York: Macmillan.

Lowi, T. J. (1969). *The end of liberalism.* New York: W. W. Norton.

Mendelson, M. A. (1974). *Tender loving greed: How the incredibly lucrative nursing home industry is exploiting America's old people.* New York: Knopf.

Piven, F. F., & Cloward, R. A. (1979). *Poor people's movements.* New York: Random House.

Vladeck, B. (1980). *Unloving care.* New York: Basic Books.

Zinn, H. A. (1980). *A people's history of the United States.* New York: Harper & Row.

10

Dilemmas of Participant-Observation in a Menopause Collective

Kathleen I. MacPherson

The passage through menopause is a key physiological experience that marks the beginning of old age for women. A group of women experiencing menopause and attempting to formulate a *new* definition of this phenomenon—the Menopause Collective—was the subject of my research. The Menopause Collective was a social-change organization of controversy and confrontation trying to show how menopause is far more than a biological process. My study of the group focused on how the members of the Menopause Collective managed their work. Other purposes included creating a historical record of the organization and providing a blueprint for other groups working on conceptual change.

An unusual methodological feature of the study is that I carried it out while I was a member of the group. Because of issues of trust and intimacy, I believe that only a member could have carried out the study. On the other hand, obtaining permission to study my group did not lead me into a comfortable research relationship with the members. On the contrary, I was led into the series of disconcerting dilemmas to be discussed in this chapter.

The focus of the chapter is threefold. First, I present the ideology of the Menopause Collective. Second, I provide a detailed discussion of dilemmas encountered when attempting to study a political group of which one is a member. Finally, I conclude by tracing some implications for future gerontological research.

IDEOLOGY

The Menopause Collective was an open membership group that began in 1978 when two women affiliated with the Women's Community Health Center in Cambridge, Massachusetts, assembled graduates of menopause self-help groups that they had facilitated over the years. The graduates of their groups who were interested formed an *ongoing* collective. The members of the Menopause Collective were women in their thirties, forties, and fifties who worked together to offer menopause self-help groups for community women, conduct research, and write about menopause and other health concerns of older women. At the same time, as a basis for their praxis, they engaged in ongoing "internal self-help"—sharing feelings, observations, and new information about themselves with each other.

The Menopause Collective was a direct outgrowth of the women's health movement. Initially, the women's health movement and the self-help centers and groups focused primarily on reproductive issues of younger women, such as contraception, childbirth, and abortion (Frankfort, 1972; Dreifus, 1977). As early as 1973 at the San Francisco Women's Health Center and the Women's Community Health Center in Cambridge, Massachusetts, a few older women who had been working with younger women in feminist health centers started self-help groups for menopausal women. Older women's health issues became an interest of formerly young health activists who were aging and becoming interested in mid-life and older women's health care. This process is illustrated in the Boston Women's Health Book Collective, whose third edition of *Our Bodies, Ourselves* (1984) has an expanded section on menopause written by members of the Menopause Collective, as well as increased content on aging. There has also been an outpouring of feminist self-help books and newsletters that include menopause as one of their concerns (Reitz, 1977; Page, 1977; National Women's Health Network, 1980; Santa Fe Health Education Project, 1980; San Francisco Women's Health Center, 1980; Millette & Hawkins, 1983; Voda, 1984).

The new self-help ideology of aging that was developed by the Menopause Collective and these other groups is basically that menopause is a normal part of the aging process for women. This is in direct opposition to the medical ideology of menopause, which increasingly has medicalized this universal life experience of women. Medicine first defined menopause as a deficiency disease requiring estrogen replacement therapy (Wilson, 1963). Next, the medical definition of menopause expanded from a deficiency disease to a syndrome that added osteoporosis (a condition in which bones become thin and easily fracture) to the "symptoms" of hot flashes, night sweating, vaginal dryness, and sundry other psychological and physiological conditions (Speroff, 1983; Greenblatt, 1974). An attempt has been made by Notelovitz (1984), formerly of the Center for Climacteric Studies at the University of Gainesville, Florida, and others to medicalize the *entire* climacteric period. These physicians, primarily gynecologists, are claiming that the period of life between ages 35 and 65 is potentially dangerous for women and harbors other threats, such as sexual dysfunction, in addition to menopause and osteoporosis.

The medical response to this "danger" is to recommend that women be under the care of physicians who commonly prescribe hormone therapy. This therapeutic response to menopause consists either of estrogen alone or estrogen combined with progesterone. We already know that uterine cancer is linked to using estrogen alone (Weiss, Szekely, & Austin, 1976). Progesterone is not safe either. As we learned from users of the birth-control pill, progesterone is associated with an increased rate of stroke (Smith, Prentice, Thompson, & Hermann, 1975; Stern, Byron, Haskell, Farquar, Wherle, & Wood, 1976). Transnational pharmaceutical companies also play a role in promoting the use of hormones by mounting vast pro-hormone public relations campaigns to influence both women (through articles in womens' magazines) and physicians (through medical journal advertisement and research grants) (Dejanikus, 1985).

The Menopause Collective's ideology that menopause is normal and not a disease was developed by the members' careful examination of scientific literature and their own experience. Their methods of developing a definition hinged on discussion, reading, and self-help. For example, the spacing and amount of menstrual flow commonly becomes quite erratic in the premenopausal period (one or two years before periods stop). Not deferring to physicians, the collective members themselves decided whether this experience fell within the parameters of "normal" in the majority of cases or was something that was abnormal and should be controlled. By observing how the group interpreted their experience and gave advice to others, I concluded that their ideology of menopause consists of the following beliefs:

1. If women were to discuss menopause, they could learn from other women and eliminate the stigma and shame associated with aging. Menopausal women, not male physicians, are the true experts on the menopausal experience. Women can define the parameters of what is normal if they share their experiences.

2. If women would share their experiences of coping with the bothersome aspects of menopause, they could be more self-reliant and menopause would not be defined by "scientific research" alone. A small number of women with severely handicapping physical changes (such as insomnia caused by very frequent hot flashes), on the other hand, should seek evaluation by a health care provider and benefit from low-dose, short-term hormone therapy.

3. Women would be safer if they distrusted physicians, particularly gynecologists, and were skeptical about medications such as hormone replacement therapy and other untested "new drugs."

4. Menopause—with its freedom from menstrual periods and unwanted pregnancies—should be redefined as a positive experience.

This set of alternative beliefs emerged during a five-year period from 1978 to 1983. During that time the group was committed to building an alternative organizational form, that is, a collective structure and process. These are common features of new alternative groups and settings providing feminist health services (Gottlieb, 1980).

STUDYING MY OWN POLITICAL SETTING

Although this study was designed in part to "experiment" with some novel methodological issues, it nevertheless builds upon traditional qualitative methods, particularly ethnography and in-depth interviewing. My orientation was primarily descriptive. The goal was to seek patterns emerging from the data. Seeking out and identifying patterns in the data might be termed "ethnoanalysis" and follows in the sociological traditions of such classical works as Whyte (1943), Liebow (1967), and Stack (1974).

Dilemmas encountered in doing this work resulted from attempting to study a political group of which I was and am a member. The study caused me considerable discomfort as I focused on the difficulties and pain in the group. Instead of retreating from this conflict, I tried to analyze it. I learned that there were specific stages underlying the incredibly long time it took to develop a group consensus. By observing how the group worked toward consensus, I uncovered how internal conflict is managed among self-identified feminists. Major debates confronting the collective included whether the packet of information the menopause collective mailed to local and distant women should contain articles with divergent views (including those of male gynecologists); how best to cope with multiple external demands on our limited woman power; and whether it was important to practice internal self-help at collective meetings.

I also experimented in my participant-as-researcher role. Combining these roles could lead to both role confusion vis-à-vis group members and criticism about objectivity from methodologists. Yet from a feminist research perspective, I was in a unique position to have intimate access to an unusual organization, a menopause collective, of which I had been a member since its inception. Feminist sociologists are addressing the methodological issue of "feminist distrust" of male-dominated positivistic research methods (Kantor & Millman, 1975; Westkott, 1979; Reinharz, 1984a). From this perspective I am a member of the only demographic category that could be "trusted" to do this study—a menopausal feminist. I was actually experiencing hot flashes as I carried out the research.

Sometimes I felt caught in a dialectic between my membership and researcher roles. Initially, I was aware that researchers are cautioned to avoid too much involvement (Gold, 1958); to strive for neutrality (Gans, 1968); and to seek an attitude of empathy rather than sympathy (Douglas, 1976). On the other hand, some field workers have emphasized that subjective experience is not only a source of bias, but also a source of insight and understanding, both for those studied and for the researcher (Wolff, 1964; Zola, 1982; Reinharz, 1984b).

Certainly this dual role gave me access to the emotional life of the group in a way that would have been impossible for an observer. At the same time, it left me subject to all the emotional turmoil of a member as well as the strain of researching the group. The small social setting (usually seven to 10 members at meetings) made it impossible to "hide in the woodwork" when difficult collective decisions had to be made or social activism undertaken, particularly since I wanted to retain the trust of the other members. Sustaining their trust became one of the most difficult tasks I had to face.

My decision to study a group in which I was a member was based on my political values and my view of research as political work. I needed to do research that had meaning for me personally. Other sociologists have expressed the same concern for conducting unalienated research that has both personal meaning (Reinharz, 1984b) and larger social relevance (Mills, 1959). I wanted to capture the process of this collective's work as it happened, because too many times in our past this kind of organization has become lost to history. Many years later, a scholar might attempt to reconstruct the life of this group after the members were dead, as Schwarz (1982) did in *Radical Feminists of Heterodoxy*, when not able to be there with them. I believe in the need for feminists (and other groups) to write our history as we make it, to let the living voices of activists describe their work, to allow the researcher to observe and record social activism in progress. Part of this historical record will consist of the contradictions and conflicts that arise among members attempting to present a coherent ideology to the outside world.

Other sociologists have participated both as researchers and as members of the setting studied. These role models enhanced my understanding of the risks and benefits of playing this double role: Roth (1963) did field work while a patient in a tuberculosis hospital; Thorne (1983) studied draft resistance movements; Jules-Rosette (1975) did research on an African apostolic sect; Posner (1980) studied relationships in a Canadian home for the aged; Van Maanen (1983) did field work with the police; Zola (1982) reported an insider's view of being handicapped; and Krieger (1983) studied a lesbian community.

In contrast to these supportive examples, other methodologists warn of the potential pitfalls of the participant-as-researcher role. They suggest that it is difficult to capture the interaction in a setting that has already become familiar (Bogdan & Taylor, 1975). Distance and detachment are required in order to look at a group sociologically (Emerson, 1983). Pollner and Emerson (1983) call this problem "engulfment": "Involvement may be so comprehensive, preemptive or entangling that the researcher's capacity to observe is undermined or threatened. . . . Instead of being *at* a scene, the observer finds he is *in* the scene" (p. 252). Janes (1961) refers to this phenomenon as "going native." Thus the central methodological question of my study became: could I be *at* the collective and *in* the collective at the same time?

Interestingly, the balance between these two stances was forged by help I received from others. By reading, teaching research methods to my students, and interacting with colleagues, I was reminded continuously to keep some distance within the collective. In addition, the collective itself provided barriers to engulfment. My contact with the members occurred on a biweekly or monthly basis, so interaction was infrequent even when intense. I continued performing my usual roles as a collective member—writing articles for publication, engaging in public speaking, participating in internal self-help, co-facilitating menopause "open-house" presentations, and other work. From the point of view of the members I had simply added a new function similar to group historian.

Despite the fact that I had been involved in the collective's work during the previous three years, I felt reluctant to ask the members' permission to study our group. This timidity came from having observed other professionals use grassroots organizations for their own career advancement without giving something back in return. I was also aware that doing this research could jeopardize the collective in terms of exposing our vulnerabilities. My hesitation was overcome when I realized that I could contribute to the collective's political work as I studied it. Also, as conflict escalated in the collective, I believed my research might help us make sense out of what appeared to be senseless at the time. New members were leaving, and the remaining members were split over goals and how to achieve them. Members felt as though the organization kept "spinning its wheels." When I first presented my proposed research to the group at the September 1982 meeting, responses ranged from concern over losing me as a productive member to wariness about the focus of the study. Permission was granted as soon as it was realized that my research would coincide with the objectives of the group:

> SALLY: Will this be in any way a psychological study of members? (She smiled as she said these words very slowly, and emphasized the word psychological). I wouldn't like that! (general laughter)
>
> KATHLEEN: No, not at all. I plan to focus on how we create and disseminate a feminist perspective of menopause.

The group agreed unanimously to support my research (field notes, September 1982).

As in many other organizations, a small number of women, the central members, did most of the work, came to meetings regularly, and were invested in keeping the collective viable. When four of these central members decided that a fifth would have to go in order to "keep the collective alive" I had to decide if I would go along with this decision.

The woman who was to be asked to leave, Nina, was seen as "having a corporate attitude" in her approach to collective tasks. More seriously, she repeatedly and gratuitously attacked another woman, Vicky, at meetings. Although she worked very hard on the collective's tasks, she was chronically dissatisfied and had threatened to withdraw from the collective several times. In March 1983 she was joined by another member, Nancy, who was unhappy that there was no physical space available to facilitate menopause self-help groups for community women. Both my participant and researcher roles pushed me to try to keep both women in the organization as productive, albeit dissenting, members. To help keep them in the collective, I located space for offering menopause self-help groups to community women in the Women's Center in Cambridge, Massachusetts. This is one example of how I actively kept creating the field I was studying. At other times I played a "diplomatic" or "group-sustaining role" to keep Nina and Nancy from resigning. I believed this was appropriate methodologically and as a group member, since I was not studying what makes such a group survive but rather how it creates a feminist ideology of menopause. In spite of finding the space, however, Nancy resigned in August 1983, leaving Nina without her closest ally.

On November 3, 1983, Sally, another central member, telephoned to say that she and several other women planned to confront Nina at the November meeting:

> We have been talking to each other and to former members who have left the collective [due primarily to internal conflict] and we finally know what the problem is . . . it's very painful, but she [Nina] spoils our meetings by being so hostile . . . people feel uncomfortable (field notes Nov. 3, 1983).

At this point, I was ambivalent about confronting Nina, so I took advantage of my research role and decided to interview her and four other central members. These interviews were a planned part of my data collection, but I timed them to get a better understanding of the process that led to the decision to evict Nina. These interviews revealed that Nina's behavior was viewed as so problematic that unless she left, the collective would "die." During her interview, Nina did not seem aware of the anger felt toward her and of the decision to confront and expel her. I fought my inclination to tell her, for by now I had decided that I would support the decision of the other central members. My decision to not inform Nina was also abetted by my researcher role of maintaining distance and "not telling." Nevertheless, this was a controversial choice from a "feminist process perspective" (Wheeler & Chinn, 1984). Decision making by consensus had not been achieved by the collective, therefore differences in beliefs and values were not discussed or viewed as possibly contributing to group strength. In part this resulted from our being physically separated by considerable distances. For example, I lived a hundred miles from Cambridge and traveled even farther for two months each summer. As a result I was not present during the heated discussions that occurred during the summer preceding Nina's expulsion. From a feminist process perspective, I would be criticized for not insisting, when I returned from vacation, that we talk to Nina in an attempt to understand each other's differences. On the other hand, if I had made this request after the decision had been made, I believe that I would have lost my sociological researcher role as well as the trust of the other central members.

Miller (1952, p. 98) warned researchers "not to become a mere machine, but in situations involving overt and covert controversy, he [sic] should be wary of identifying himself [sic] symbolically and emotionally with a particular group." He advised asking, "At what point does closeness to the subjects limit the research role?" In this case, I felt I needed to ask, at what point does distance from the subjects terminate access or even destroy the organization? Miller implied that the subjects are a homogeneous group. However, researchers of small groups quickly learn that there are sides within groups and the researcher's task is to navigate the rough waters among them. In essence, I chose to distance myself from one member, Nina, in order to not distance myself from the other four central members. Because the group was small I could not do as Ruzek (1978) had done in her study of the women's health movement:

> My decision not to actively work with or join any particular group was influenced by concern that "joining" would force me to take sides in schisms and squabbles. By maintaining some distance, I could learn more about all sides of disputes and could maintain a critical stance—difficult when too closely associated with one group (p. xii).

I had no choice about siding. There was no neutral third side. The only other choice I could have made was to resign from the collective when I started doing research. But this would have weakened the group, thus undermining my own political goals, and also jeopardizing the research effort. Because I had assumed a researcher role while fully participating in the group under study, I was compelled to take sides in disagreements as they arose. Furthermore, I personally had reached the same conclusion—Nina's behavior would destroy the group. On the other hand, I liked her and felt I had betrayed her.

On November 16, 1983, there was an open Menopause Collective meeting at which five central members, including myself, painfully discussed with Nina the impact, past and present, of her attitudes and behavior in the group. She agreed to leave without appearing to have "taken in" much that had been said.

Complications soon followed on the heels of Nina's departure. Mary, a marginal member who had not attended meetings for over a year, wrote a draft letter to all Menopause Collective members who had not been present at the open November meeting. She asked for signatures of protest over the process used to ask Nina to leave. Mary is a close friend of Nina's and a member of the Boston Women's Health Book Collective. I began to see, more and more, that doing this kind of research as a full participant put me at risk for alienating collective members like Mary, to whom I no longer could have access. I began to understand that the participant-researcher dilemma takes on different dimensions when the research site is conflict-laden and likely to produce a demand that the researcher take sides.

Nina has since taken on the important task of creating a mid-life women's self-help book similar in format to *The New Our Bodies, Ourselves*. Since she asked me to write a section on osteoporosis, I feel we have maintained an ability to work together on a project requiring trust. However, the structure of this work arrangement and our ensuing social relationship is more businesslike than the shared vision of work in the collective.

In summary, by studying my own group I was led into a series of disconcerting dilemmas: increasing my workload because I retained my group roles as well as my participant-researcher role; being forced, against my natural inclination, to take sides in conflicts; feeling guilty about possibly exploiting the group for my own purposes; wondering if I was exposing my group's weaknesses. There were, however, some positive features. First, I learned how to combine participant and researcher roles. Second, I learned that the group felt less concerned about my research than I; they were supportive throughout the study. Third, I probably contributed to the group's survival by sharing my analysis of some of its more difficult problems. Finally, my research role compelled me to remain involved in the group while I conducted research that has great meaning for me personally.

IMPLICATIONS FOR GERONTOLOGICAL RESEARCH

As a result of this study I recommend that the method of participant-as-researcher be used in gerontological research. New insights and understanding can be gained if a member of a group, with the same concerns as the group under study, conducts the investigation. However, this approach promises not only benefits but also several dilemmas.

In this particular study I was a member and also shared demographic characteristics with other research participants. Instead of being a male or a younger female researcher, I was a menopausal woman studying an organization concerned with menopausal women. I knew the history of the group, the old and new members, and the kind of political work in which the group was engaged. I could feel, as well as analyze, the internal conflicts that inevitably arise in such groups and also be in touch with the painful experience of taking sides in these conflicts. Finally, I experienced the shared relief of conflict resolution and an increased sense of group identity.

My study focused on older women in the women's health movement who became increasingly political as they took on the task of redefining menopause—a major benchmark of aging. Other benchmarks, such as grandparenthood, retirement, and entering a senior citizen residence, could also be studied in this way, with findings compared with insights derived from other methods.

Qualitative methods such as participant-observation and open-ended interviewing allow researchers to understand older people's definitions of their current situation. When carried out in activist organizations such research helps to eliminate a monolithic view of older people's lives, which frequently stresses passivity and loneliness. Gerontological researchers should take risks by becoming involved in older people's groups they are studying and sharing what they learn about themselves as they do their research:

> In social science, I think, we must acknowledge the personal far more than we do. We need to find new ways to explore it. We need to link our statements about those we study with statements about ourselves, for in reality neither stands alone (Krieger, 1983, p. 324).

As a person who hopes to conduct qualitative gerontological research with older women in the future, I will draw on an important asset—I am rapidly becoming an older woman myself.

REFERENCES

Bogdan, R., & Taylor, S. (1975). *Introduction to qualitative research methods*. New York: John Wiley & Sons.

Boston Women's Health Book Collective. (1984). *The new our bodies, ourselves* (3rd Ed.) New York: Simon & Schuster.

Dejanikus, T. (1985, May/June). Major drug manufacturer funds osteoporosis public education campaign. *Network News*, pp. 1, 3, 8.

Douglas, J. (1976). *Investigative social research*. Beverly Hills, CA: Sage.

Dreifus, C. (1977). *Seizing our bodies*. New York: Vintage Books.

Emerson, R. (1983). *Contemporary field research*. Boston: Little, Brown and Company.

Frankfort, E. (1972). *Vaginal politics*. New York: Quadrangle Books.

Gans, H. (1968). The participant observer as a human being: Observations on the personal aspects of fieldwork. In H.S. Becker, B. Greer, D.R. Reisman, & R.S. Weiss (Eds.), *Institutions and the person* (pp. 300–317). Chicago: Aldine.

Gold, R.D. (1958). Roles in sociological field observation. *Social forces 36*, 217–223.

Gottlieb, N. (Ed.). (1980). *Alternative social services for women*. New York: Columbia University Press.

Greenblatt, R. (1974). *The menopause syndrome*. New York: Medcom Press.

Janes, R.W. (1961). A note on phases of the community role of the participant observer. *American Sociological Review, 26,* 446–450.

Jules-Rosette, B. (1975). *Vision and realities: Aspects of ritual and conversion in an African church.* Ithaca, NY: Cornell University Press.

Kantor, R., & Millman, M. (1975). *Another voice.* Garden City, NY: Anchor Press.

Krieger, S. (1983). *The mirror dance: Identity in a woman's community.* Philadelphia: Temple University Press.

Krieger, S. (1985). Beyond "subjectivity": The use of the self in social sciences. *Qualitative Sociology, 8,* 309–324.

Liebow, E. (1967). *Tally's Corner.* Boston: Little, Brown and Company.

Miller S. (1952). The participant observer and "over-rapport." *American Sociological Review, 17,* 97–99.

Millette, B., & Hawkins J. (1983). *The passage through menopause: Women's lives in transition.* Reston, VA: Reston Publishing Company.

Mills, C.W. (1959). *The sociological imagination.* New York: Grove Press.

National Women's Health Network. (1980). *Menopause resource guide 3.* Washington, DC: National Women's Health Network.

Notelovitz, M. (1984). The menopause and climacteric—Three decades of clinical need. *Midpoint, 1,* 3–9.

Page, J. (1977). *The other awkward age: Menopause.* Berkeley, CA: Ten Speed Press.

Pollner, M., & Emerson, R.M. (1983). The dynamics of inclusion and distance in fieldwork relations. In R.M. Emerson (Ed.), *Contemporary field research* (pp. 235–252). Boston: Little, Brown and Company.

Posner, J. (1980). Urban anthropology: Fieldwork in semifamiliar settings. In W.S. Shaffir, R. A. Stebbins, & A.T. Turowetz (Eds.), *Fieldwork experiences* (pp. 203–212). New York: St. Martin Press.

Reinharz, S. (1984a). Feminist distrust: Problems of context and content in sociological work: In N. Berg & K. K. Smith (Eds.), *Exploring clinical methods for social research* (pp. 153–172). Beverly Hills, CA: Sage.

Reinharz, S. (1984b). *On becoming a social scientist: From survey research and participant observation to experiential analysis.* New Brunswick, NJ: Transaction Books.

Reitz, R. (1977). *Menopause: A positive approach.* New York: Penguin Books.

Roth, J. (1963). Information and control of treatment in tuberculosis hospitals. In E. Freidson (Ed.), *The hospital in modern society.* (pp. 293–318). New York: The Free Press of Glencoe.

Ruzek, S.B. (1978). *The women's health movement.* New York: Praeger.

San Francisco Women's Health Center. (1980). *Menopause: A natural process.* San Francisco: Author.

Sante Fe Health Education Project. (1980). *Menopause: A self-help manual.* Santa Fe: Author.

Schwarz, J. (1982). *Radical feminists of heterodoxy: Greenwich Village, 1912–1940.* Lebanon, NH: New Victoria Publishers.

Smith, D.C., Prentice, R., Thompson, D.J., & Hermann, W.L. (1975). Association of exogenous estrogen and endometrial carcinoma. *New England Journal of Medicine, 293,* 1164–1167.

Speroff, L. (1983, October). *Menopause.* Paper presented at the District III meeting of the American College of Obstetricians and Gynecologists, Copenhagen, Denmark.

Stack, C. (1974). *All our kin.* New York: Harper & Row.

Stern, M.P., Byron, W.B., Haskell, W.L., Farquar, J.W., Wherle, C.L., & Wood, P.D. (1976). Cardiovascular risk and use of estrogen or estroprogestagen combinations. *Journal of the American Medical Association, 235,* 811–815.

Thorne, B. (1983). Political activist as participant observer: Conflicts of commitment in a study of the draft resistance movement of the 1960's. In R. M. Emerson (Ed.), *Contemporary field research* (pp. 216-234). Boston: Little, Brown and Company.

Van Maanen, J. (1983). The moral fix: On the ethics of fieldwork. In Robert M. Emerson (Eds.), *Contemporary field research* (pp. 269-287) Boston: Little, Brown and Company.

Voda, A. (1984). *Menopause, me and you: A personal handbook for women.* Salt Lake City: University of Utah.

Weiss, N., Szekely, D., & Austin, F. (1976). Increasing incidence of endometrial cancer in the U.S. *New England Journal of Medicine, 294,* 1259-1262.

Westkott, M. (1979). Feminist criticism of the social sciences. *Harvard Educational Review, 49,* 422-430.

Wheeler, C., & Chinn, P. (1984). *Peace & power: A handbook of feminist process.* Buffalo, NY: Margaretdaughters.

Whyte, W.F. (1943). *Street corner society: The social structure of an Italian slum.* Chicago: University of Chicago Press.

Wilson, R. (1963). *Feminine forever.* New York: M. Evans and Co.

Wolff, K. (1964). *Surrender and catch: Experiences and inquiry today.* Boston: Reidel.

Zola, I.K. (1982). *Missing pieces: A chronicle of living with a disability.* Philadelphia: Temple University Press.

11

Contextual Issues in Quantitative Studies of Institutional Settings for the Aged

Eva Kahana

Boaz Kahana

Kathryn P. Riley

Science is absolutely not a system for frustrating the exercise of intuition and imagination. Rather it is a set of procedures for making such ideas as fruitful and productive as human ingenuity allows (Hoover, 1984, p. 12).

Studies in institutional settings comprise a large segment of published social gerontological research. In the majority of such studies, the general institutional context is little noted and remains in the background as an unwelcome, extraneous, or confounding variable.

There may be a number of reasons for the lack of attention to the context within which institutional research is embedded. Mainstream behavioral and social science journals seldom publish accounts that focus on the complex environmental or situational factors within which the research was conducted. When investigators note dynamic interactions within the environment that may have influenced the presumed neat causal sequence relating study variables, publishers often respond by requesting that such intrusions be deleted or may consider the study flawed and not worthy of publication. In a specific instance where one of the authors of this chapter related lack of cooperativeness by staff as an important contextual factor in a study utilizing a quasi-experimental design in an institutional setting, the editor returned the manuscript with the suggestion that the results were exciting, but the study required replication in nursing homes where all staff are cooperative and interested in participating in the study. Does such a nursing home exist? Can these variables be controlled?

Gerontologists, along with other social scientists, have the desire to collect data that permit generalizations about behavior in late life. In the search for increased generalizability of gerontological research (George, 1984), the context within which observations occur is often viewed as an impediment that complicates our efforts. Mishler (1979) argues, on the other hand, that the all-important influences of context render any attempts at generalizations futile.

In this chapter we take a position midway between these two extremes and argue for the importance of recognizing, describing, and utilizing context to improve the feasibility, validity, and meaning of gerontological research in institutional settings. Serious attention to the researchers' own attitudes and views about the institution as a context and to the research enterprise as a separate but related context constitutes an important first step in this process. Lawton (1980) has advanced this position by suggesting that a major goal of gerontological research is to specify those person–environment conditions under which well-being of the elderly is maximized.

Our discussion of the role of context will focus on understanding contextual issues that are likely to affect the very success of undertaking and completing a research effort in an institutional setting. We will also consider contextual issues that influence the quality and type of information obtained. Subsequently we turn to contextual issues that affect the interpretation and meaning of data. In the second part of our chapter we will illustrate the impact of some of the contextual issues discussed in terms of our own research.

CONTEXTUAL ISSUES IN THE IMPLEMENTATION OF RESEARCH IN NURSING HOMES

Gaining and Maintaining Administrative Cooperation for Research

Nursing home research presents numerous paradoxes for investigators. Often research is undertaken in institutions for the very ease with which captive populations concentrated in an accessible facility may be studied. Yet research in institutional settings presents many challenges stemming from the diverse constituencies to which the researcher must relate, coupled with the vulnerability and environmental docility of the elderly who are the subjects of research.

When research is not sponsored or invited by administrators of an institution, obtaining cooperation of the facility represents the initial hurdle for investigators. Academic researchers in particular often encounter problems in gaining access to institutions. Reluctance to participate in the research results from a number of factors. First, administrators may be hesitant to permit outsiders a close-up view of their operation. They may be concerned with potential negative publicity, especially in view of the poor image of nursing homes presented in the media and held by the public. Second, there is often little information about any benefits to the facility from an investment of staff time and permission for access to residents. Finally, there may be genuine motivation to protect the residents' privacy and concern about the stress of participating in a research project. All of these factors are likely to affect residents' responses to questions and their behavior during observation.

In order to assure cooperation and success in carrying out the study, the initial contact with the nursing home owner or administrator is critical. Investigators must establish themselves as reputable and responsible professionals. It is important to build contacts within the administrator's network prior to soliciting participation for a specific project or to have someone known to the administrator make the initial contact. A letter of introduction that describes the investigator's experience, credentials, and intentions may prove valuable. Following these initial steps, a meeting among the administrator, key institutional staff, and the investigator(s) is critical.

Concrete benefits to administration may include researchers' commitment to work with the administration to help correct problems uncovered in the course of research or to help develop programmatic guidelines. For example, in our study, which identified marked differences between staff conceptions and self-conceptions of the institutionalized aged (Kahana & Coe, 1969), a simple intervention strategy was used to familiarize all staff with the most important aspects of residents' self-perceptions. Providing administrators with previous written reports by the investigator may be both helpful and impressive. Active rather than passive cooperation with researchers may be facilitated by inviting administrators to review detailed research plans and to make suggestions concerning the conduct of the project.

It is important that investigators assure the administration of the confidential nature of the study. Discussion of precautions taken to insure ethical conduct of the study and concern for minimizing demands on staff time and resident resources should be included in this meeting. It is also useful to consider seriously the perspectives of administration and offer something in return for their participation. Summarized data about residents of the facility may be made available to the administration. There may be questions of particular interest to the administration or staff that could be included in the survey. Thus, in fact, the institution would gain valuable information—e.g., residents' preference for different architectural features or eating times—in exchange for institutional cooperation.

Where long-term care institutions sponsor in-house research departments, special issues in the initiation and conduct of research arise. Gaining entry to such facilities is likely to involve explicit agreements about collaboration in funding, the conduct of the study, and publications arising from the research. Researchers are likely to gain useful insights about the nature and philosophy of the organization during the course of negotiations to insure cooperation of the facility.

Organizational problems and attitudes also directly affect the implementation of research projects in institutions. Staff turnover, problems with staffing, or conflicts among staff members are likely to be translated into unforeseen obstacles in carrying out day-to-day research routines. Researchers may be informed mid-project that their procedures must be changed to conform to new organizational structures. Although the research may not be brought to a halt, the validity of the research may be seriously affected. Research projects may actually be aborted when internal audits or changes in administration take place. It is very useful in this regard for researchers to build up networks of cooperation at different levels of management and staff in order to prevent or overcome such difficulties if they should arise. At the same time, changes in administration, policies, or management are important to note as integral issues in description and understanding the environmental context in which staff and residents function.

Issues in Working with Staff

After obtaining agreement to participate in a research project from the administration, investigators must focus on developing good relationships with staff members, including "front-line" nurse's aides and assistants, as well as nurses, social workers, activity therapists, and other professional staff. Prior to implementation of the project, it is useful for the research team to spend some time in the facility, familiarizing themselves with the staff and with the physical and social environment and becoming acceptable additions to the institutional setting. In one study of age-integrated wards in a state psychiatric facility, the work of the research project was hampered by staff resentment of an order from the administration to cooperate with the investigators (Kahana & Kahana, 1970). This order was viewed as another example of the staff's powerlessness, and their resentment was overcome only through repeated contact and reassurance from the researchers.

Continued maintenance of cooperation and good will of institutional staff often falters because of problems and latent or manifest conflicts in the daily execution of research projects. This is an area in which researchers must be particularly diligent and sensitive in considering and seeking information about staff attitudes, workloads, and involvement in the research. Since the actual implementation of research projects is often left to research assistants, the principal investigator may not be aware of problems until they have reached sizable proportions. Roth (1966) has described many of the difficulties inherent in large scale "hired-hand" research, suggesting that involvement of research assistants and field workers in the planning and decision-making stages of data collection can prevent breakdowns in the field research process. Intensive involvement of principal investigators in the data collection process will also help prevent or identify problems that might occur.

Requests made of staff to provide ratings of residents are often viewed as posing additional workloads. Casual requests by researchers to "fill out these forms during your break" are seldom popular with staff. It is very helpful to designate a time period during working hours when forms may be completed. Researchers must also honestly confront the fact that completion of research instruments is of little personal value to many staff members, who may already feel underpaid, overburdened, and unappreciated in their job (Vladeck, 1980; Kayser-Jones, 1981). Such attitudes may be improved if researchers indicate that they value the staff's professional input regarding their residents or patients and make every effort to reinforce staff regarding the value of their contributions.

There is evidence from both qualitative (Annandale, 1985) and quantitative studies (Kahana & Felton, 1977; Kahana & Coe, 1969) that health care providers from different disciplines, as well as families and significant others, often hold divergent views and definitions of elderly patients and their needs. Thus the background of the informant characterizing the institutionalized patient represents an important aspect of the institutional context. Researchers must be particularly attentive to the staff subcultures of different professionals, which comprise an important influence on resident experiences.

Practical Issues in Implementing Research

The simple task of finding a suitable place for conducting an interview often poses difficulties for researchers. Physical and psychological symptoms may worsen when respondents are interviewed in an uncomfortable setting, at an uncomfortable temperature, or in an unfamiliar environment. Ultimately these environmental factors play important roles in affecting the quality, meaning, and generalizability of the data obtained. The presence of a roommate may present a distraction and influence the information provided by a respondent. The physical and social settings where interviews take place are likely to have an impact on the data obtained. Resident statements or testimonials on satisfaction with institutional care given in the presence of a staff member or fellow resident should be received differently from those given in privacy. In fact, the impact of a roommate during interviewing would be a useful subject matter for research. Having two interviewers interview two roommates at the same time or providing the excluded roommate with an alternative activity may prove helpful in dealing with such problems.

On the other hand, observations of interactions among roommates might yield invaluable information about the social world of the resident. Because quantitative research approaches are concerned with isolating the respondent, they may result in incomplete or distorted data about the resident's life. A case in point occurred in interviewing a friendly, compliant, and apparently satisfied resident. As the interviewer thanked her for her time and proceeded to leave, the resident turned to her roommate, who was just entering the room, and said in her native tongue, "This one won't be any problem. I sure sold him a bill of goods about how great this dump is!" In this case consideration of interactions among roommates sheds new meaning on data obtained in interaction between a respondent and an interviewer. Contextual data were also provided here about the undercurrent of communication among residents (Goffman, 1961). This encounter revealed a bond of understanding among residents who shared a common language and culture that set them apart from staff.

Logistical problems are also presented in scheduling interviews, given the structure of mealtimes, bedtimes, and visiting hours in institutional facilities. It is very important for researchers studying the life of residents in institutions to consider variations in the milieu at different times of the day and week. Researchers are likely to obtain valuable data on the milieu in which residents live if they interview during times that are not considered optimal for interviewing.

Informed Consent and Ethical Considerations in Institutional Research

Obtaining informed consent from captive populations in general and from the vulnerable aged in particular poses special problems. Truly voluntary participation is much more difficult to obtain from persons in institutions than from community-dwelling individuals. The institution-alized person is accustomed to staff demands that are politely phrased as questions but clearly imply the expectation of cooperation. Researchers must be especially scrupulous to insure that the institutionalized aged cooperate willingly in light of the inherent conflict of interest between the investigator's need for a maximal response rate and the respondent's right to legitimate noncooperation (Reinharz, 1984).

A second issue relates to the physical or cognitive ability of impaired older persons to provide informed consent. Researchers face special dilemmas when disorientation to time, place, or person is found while interviewing an otherwise intact older person. Should the meaning of informed consent by such a respondent be questioned? As yet there are few clear directives about situations where consent of relatives or responsible persons should be obtained. The need for written informed consent according to protection of human subjects requirements makes research with institutionalized populations more difficult than with noninstitutionalized people. Some older persons who are otherwise pleased to cooperate feel that signing the informed consent form poses a special threat to them. We have often been told by potential respon-dents: "I would love to talk to you but my children told me not to sign anything." One solution to this problem is to read the consent form aloud to the participant, making a note of his or her verbal agreement to participate. Creative alternatives to traditional informed-consent procedures have been outlined by Wax (1977).

There are other factors that affect the resident's willingness to par-ticipate in research. Refusal rates may be inflated by residents' concern that their responses will be shown to staff or administration and that negative repercussions may follow. Some may be fearful that if they appear to function too well they may be discharged from the institu-tion, while others may fear that discovered impairments may result in their being moved to a location within the facility where sicker patients are found. These deep-seated, often unarticulated fears are not always amenable to investigators' simple reassurances of anonymity (Sinnott, Harris, Block, Collesano, & Jacobson, 1983; Atchley, 1969).

The researcher may find that an exploration of these issues uncovers unspoken fears, which can then be addressed openly and directly. This kind of discussion, when conducted on an individual basis, may increase the proportion of persons who are willing to participate in a research project, while also affording some protection against premature withdrawal from the project after consent has been given. Understanding resident fears may also provide important clues about the dynamics of the institutional milieu that gave rise to such fears.

Recommendations for dealing with residents' concerns about the interview situation include the suggestion that interviewers engage respondents in casual conversation before undertaking the formal portions of the interview. To do so, the researcher should be willing to spend time with the resident beyond that which is necessary to obtain data. Interviewers should also carefully explain the aims of their research and make sure that residents realize that the information provided will be used only with all identifying information removed. Older persons often feel that their responses are no longer valued by anyone, and they may be pleased when researchers stress that their opinions are being solicited so that experts in aging may have a first-hand view of particular issues or needs gained directly from the older person's perspective.

The importance of establishing good rapport in an atmosphere of mutual respect and trust cannot be overemphasized. Once again, the use of field workers who have a stake in the research outcome (Roth, 1966) is of immense value if routine and uninterested administrations of interview questions are to be avoided. We believe that this orientation to data collection leads not only to richer data, but also to increased validity and reliability of results.

Researchers also must be aware that their very presence in the facility is intrusive. They may be resented by staff who consider outsiders as being "underfoot" or as agents of surveillance. A special set of problems is created when researchers stumble into observing abuse of residents, poor service, or work habits that negatively affect patient care. Difficult decisions must often be made by researchers regarding reporting fortuitously observed problems to administrators or supervisory staff. In our own research we have typically discussed such problems with research staff, developed a consensus about handling them, and always aimed to err on the side of protecting individual patient needs even if it might jeopardize staff cooperation. Thus instances where residents consistently reported being unable to obtain proper assistance with bathing or personal hygiene without tipping staff were brought to the attention of administrators. Conversely, we try to avoid meddling in organizational problems. Thus staff abuse of patients is always reported, while other conditions that do not directly endanger residents, such as inefficiency, are considered as best left in the domain of institutional staff and administration (Kayser-Jones, 1981).

IMPLICATIONS OF THE INSTITUTIONAL CONTEXT FOR VALIDITY OF DATA

Selection of Residents as Subjects

Foremost among the challenges of quantitative institutional research is drawing a valid and meaningful sample (George, 1984). Published research reports based on residents of institutional facilities seldom reveal problems faced by researchers in this area. Very rarely is an investigator able to sample randomly, using a complete enumeration of all residents of a given facility. Published sampling descriptions often refer to interviews with elderly who were sufficiently intact to respond to research questions and provide informed consent. All residents fulfilling sampling criteria are reportedly included in many investigations. Such reports tell only part of the story. Access to medical records is seldom granted, in part to protect the privacy of residents. In reality, therefore, researchers are usually referred by nursing home staff to suitable respondents or provided with a list of those residents who, according to administrators or staff, either meet or fail to meet the specific study criteria as defined by the investigators. Such well-intentioned processes of nomination are fraught with biases that endanger the validity of any research. These biases reflect the professional and personal characteristics of nominators and are typically unrecognized by either staff or researchers. For example, an overrepresentation of problem patients may stem from the staff's desire to obtain data on "challenging" cases. Alternatively, expressive, well-liked or extroverted persons, who reflect well on the facility, may be nominated. Even when substantive biases are absent, there are likely to be problems of recall by staff. In one project we wanted to interview all persons who had spent less than six months in the institution. We were graciously given a list of all such residents by the office staff of an enthusiastically cooperative institution. Certain that they remembered all recent arrivals, they failed to consult their records. Only after interviewing several residents who had been in the facility for over a year did we discover the problem! When sampling criteria call for exclusion of certain diagnostic categories (e.g., terminally ill patients), additional difficulties are introduced in achieving common criteria among researchers and staff.

In an effort to deal with sampling issues, researchers should consult records to obtain a sampling list whenever possible. Researchers should also refrain from the temptation of work-saving shortcuts offered by staff (e.g., "We can tell you quickly which residents see the psychiatrist regularly"). If staff judgments must be relied upon, it is useful to obtain nominations and ratings from more than one staff member. Finally, it is also very useful to build questions into the interview that verify sampling criteria. Researchers may benefit from asking each respondent how long they have been in the nursing home or whether they are seeing a psychiatrist to verify sampling information obtained from staff.

Factors Affecting Residents' Responses to Research

Many contextual issues affect the responses residents living in institutions give to research questions. Motives for participation or their absence affect responses. When staff members coax or pressure residents to participate, biased responses may be evoked. Similarly, staff members who participate in research only to please their superiors or to take a break from unpleasant chores are not very likely to invest themselves in research tasks such as rating residents or environments. Reluctance of residents to express concern and dissatisfaction to outsiders has been noted above. This problem has been documented by Carp (1983), who found that high levels of satisfaction are almost uniformly portrayed by institutionalized elderly, even in facilities that are not characterized by high-quality care according to outside observers.

In some instances the residents direct their dissatisfaction to the researchers instead of to the facility. Researchers represent a far safer target for resident or family complaints than do staff, who have jurisdiction over the day-to-day lives of patients. Forthright, nondefensive, and prompt responses to even minor negative feedback can go a long way toward reducing problems in this area. Making written information about the research project available to staff, respondents, and families may avert problems. Researchers should also reflect on whether they are threatening or demanding and thus deserving of these complaints. Complaints sometimes also come from patients who feel excluded from a study. Speaking to residents not included in a given project helps defuse these feelings of rejection and attendant antagonism toward the research. Complaints also provide useful data about the institutional context. They may represent an important glimpse into concerns and dissatisfactions of residents that are often hidden behind the veil of social desirability when formal interviews are conducted (Carp, 1983).

Different kinds of problems affecting responses are posed because of the vulnerability of persons typically found in nursing homes or other institutions. Impoverished responses (especially to open-ended questions or projective tests) can reflect fatigue and illness. Institutionalized aged persons often have short attention spans and may not be able to respond to lengthy, structured interviews (Kahana, 1981; Sinnott et al. 1983).

Multiple and potent medications taken by institutionalized elderly persons pose another set of often unrecognized problems to researchers. There is little information on alterations in mood, cognitive functioning, or even cooperativeness resulting from medications taken for physical and/or mental problems by respondents. The impact of these issues on the validity of responses requires further study.

Contextual Issues Related to Interpretation of Data

Contextual issues play a particularly important role in the interpretation of data obtained from residents or staff in long-term care institutions. Quantitative studies in these settings typically provide information on the behaviors, cognitive functioning, and physical and mental health of elderly residents (Kahana, Kahana, & Young, 1984) or on attitudes and behaviors of institutional staff (Kahana & Kiyak, 1984). The institutional setting is considered implicitly or explicitly to influence the personal characteristics that are being investigated. Yet few studies demonstrate how contextual issues have been systematically examined to gain a better understanding of the institutional milieu.

While quantitative or survey researchers may not gain the in-depth familiarity with context that participant-observers acquire (Becker, 1958), many useful observations of the environmental context are likely to be made in the course of conducting research. Field observations made during quantitative research may then be related to the conceptual underpinnings of the research and to qualitative data obtained in the course of the study. Spontaneous comments by residents and staff may provide a useful adjunct to understanding and interpreting data obtained during a structured interview (Becker, 1958).

A "sociology of knowledge" perspective provides a framework for understanding the relationship between social context and personal definitions (Annandale, 1985). Accordingly, the resident's experience of the institution will differ markedly from that of a nonresident, be it a staff member or researcher. Careful attention to contextual and qualitative cues can provide quantitative researchers with insights about the resident's experience. For example, in one of our studies the respondent portrayed satisfaction with the frequency of visitation by her children. During the interview the phone rang; the resident's son was calling. In speaking to her son the resident complained bitterly about loneliness and abandonment. This discrepancy was reported in the interpretations of data where residents' satisfaction with family involvement was considered.

If such insights about a respondent's feelings are to be gained, researchers will need to spend time conversing informally with the respondent about the issues that surface in a natural situation. The presence of other setting members may elicit behaviors and statements that are more accurate reflections of characteristic modes of responding by the resident than are behaviors shown when only the interviewer—who may be received as a guest—is present (Becker, 1958). On the other hand, the guest or stranger can evoke the setting member's true feelings, which typically cannot be expressed to other setting members.

It is common practice for anthropologists and sociologists to reflect on the very nature of their relationships with their informants and the context of their field work (Gallaher, 1971; Powdermaker, 1966). Yet in social gerontological research, and especially in studies with a generally quantitative focus, the nature of these relationships is seldom made explicit. An indication in research reports about observed openness or resentment by respondents may provide important contextual data that will assist in interpreting findings. Self-disclosure is likely to be greater in situations where the respondent is eager to interact with the researcher rather than reluctant or resentful.

Diversity in perspectives of different institutional informants should also be considered in interpretation of data. Annandale (1985) has delineated the factors responsible for varying views of patients among staff of geriatric care facilities. Her analysis suggests that the work roles and degree of involvement with patients by physicians, social workers, and nurses lead to divergent impressions of patients. Thus studies that employ staff ratings of participants are well advised to consider each profession as a separate data source rather than combining ratings indiscriminately. Divergent views and attitudes by staff may also lead to conflicting expectations of patients and may provide a useful context for understanding differing patient reactions to different groups of professional staff.

FUNCTIONAL INTEGRATION OF INSTITUTIONALIZED AGED: AN ILLUSTRATION OF QUALITATIVE FACTORS IN QUANTITATIVE RESEARCH

The role of contextual issues in quantitative research in institutional settings can be illustrated in an actual study conducted by the authors. It should be noted that when the authors initiated this study they were concerned with implementing a rigorous, quantitatively oriented, quasi-experimental research design. In completing field work for the study, the potential and relevance of contextual considerations became increasingly apparent. Because of their importance both in the conduct of the study and the interpretation of findings, the investigators decided to focus on, rather than minimize, these issues in their presentation of research. For this reason we can describe the "natural history" of a field research project conducted in an institutional setting, focusing on staff and patient responses to various aspects of the study.

Our hope in summarizing contextual influences along with quantitative findings in this research is that other researchers conducting quantitative studies will be encouraged to recognize and describe contextual factors rather than omit them in disseminating findings of research in institutional settings (see Becker, 1958). We would like to see publishing practices changed in this regard.

The study explored the differential effects of functionally segregated and integrated therapy programs for mentally impaired residents of a home for the aged. In addition, it posed questions about the modifiability of cognitive and behavioral functioning of deteriorated patients through environmental manipulation and therapeutic programs. The very small number of programs designed for the cognitively impaired aged in most institutions attests to the commonly held belief that the regressed behavior of these patients represents deteriorated brain functioning and hence is not amenable to therapy (Vladeck, 1980). Yet there is growing evidence that, in spite of brain damage, there is considerable functional variation in behavior (Barnes & Raskind, 1984; Eisdorfer, 1984; U. S. Department of Health and Human Services, 1984). Recent successes reported by various therapeutic programs for the impaired aged suggest that some improvement in functioning may be possible despite considerable organic involvement (Crovitz, 1979; Poon, 1984; U. S. Department of Health and Human Services, 1984). Institutionalized aged persons are often segregated according to the degree of their mental impairment. It is often argued that such segregation benefits both impaired and well-functioning residents, since programs can be specially tailored for the needs of each group when they are segregated (Morris, 1960; Butler & Lewis, 1977). It is also argued, based on a sort of contagion hypothesis, that the well elderly should be protected from "contamination" by the more deteriorated residents. Finally, homogeneous groups are thought to present less complexity and fewer problems in management.

These factors are exemplified by the reluctance of some long-term care facilities to accept patients diagnosed as having senile dementia of the Alzheimer's type (SDAT) and by the recent development of special Alzheimer's units within institutions (Buckwalter, 1985; Brody, Feinstein, Eisdorfer, & Mather, 1984). In some cases, these units are being designed and implemented without prior consideration of the psychological impact of such segregation on residents and staff. Our study addressed the mental health implications of conducting therapy groups in which residents were either segregated or integrated according to degree of cognitive impairment.

Methods

The study was conducted at a professionally oriented, Jewish, nonprofit home for the aged, which typically housed residents on different floors, based on the degree of their physical and mental impairment and the amount of nursing care they required. The sample consisted of 54 cognitively impaired residents. To arrive at diagnoses of cognitive impairment, patients residing on floors of the home designated for the cognitively impaired were tested using the Kahn, Pollack, and Goldfarb (1961) mental status questionnaire. They ranged in age from 65 to 85 years; and all but one had lived in the home for at least a year. The 54 subjects (80% female) constituted the entire population of the two mentally impaired wards of the home. These wards were designated as "intermediate" (residents maintained independence in some activities of daily living and could carry on sustained conversations) and "impaired" (many residents were incontinent, unable to eat and dress independently, and often were unresponsive to conversation). Twenty residents from a self-care ward that housed cognitively intact elderly were also included in the study as volunteers for the integrated therapy program.

The 54 cognitively impaired residents were randomly divided into two groups: those who were to receive therapeutic programs in the form of daily recreational, occupational, and re-motivation therapy sessions, and those who were to receive no therapy. Residents in the therapy group attended one or two programs daily for an eight-week period. The group of residents receiving therapy was further divided into either functionally integrated or segregated therapy programs. The 20 "well" residents attended daily therapy sessions with the cognitively impaired patients, thereby creating a functionally integrated, heterogeneous group. The segregated group consisted only of impaired residents. The therapy programs were identical in format for both the integrated and segregated groups.

Measures

A variety of psychosocial measures was used to obtain baseline and post-treatment data on all participants. These included Kahn, Pollack, and Goldfarb's (1960) mental status questionnaire (MSQ), indices of self-care behavior, and global clinical measures of change in adjustment as rated by nursing, recreational, occupational therapy, and social work staff. Ratings were obtained for resident alertness, anxiety, mood, dependency, confusion, and sociability.

Results

Data analyses were designed to explore the effects of therapeutic programs on institutionalized elderly persons with varying degrees of cognitive impairments to compare the relative effectiveness of functionally segregated versus integrated therapy programs, as well as to compare the changes seen in the "severely impaired" versus "intermediate" groups of impaired residents.

The proportion of residents who improved on the MSQ, self-care behavior, and measures of adjustment was generally greater for the therapy group than the controls. For example, MSQ scores improved for 38% of the residents participating in therapy as compared to 17% of the controls. In considering outcomes based on participation in integrated or segregated therapy groups, consistent differences were also observed. Scores on all three sets of measures were better at posttreatment for patients in the integrated therapy groups than for those in the segregated group. These results were not statistically significant, although they reflected a consistent trend. Finally, in comparing the intermediate and impaired ward residents, it was found that the impaired group improved significantly more on the MSQ ($p < .05$) than did the intermediate group.

Consideration of contextual issues sheds further light on these data. The staff of professional groups (occupational therapy, recreational therapy, and social work) were found to rate subjects more improved than did nursing staff. Thus while, 14, 8, and 11 residents in the therapy group were rated as improved by occupational therapy, recreational therapy, and social work, respectively, only 5 were rated as improved by nursing. It is possible that nursing used different criteria from other disciplines in evaluating functioning. However, the behavior of residents may have been more closely observed by nursing staff, and thus their ratings may have been more accurate. In either case, this discrepancy has important implications for considering staff evaluations when they are provided by only one discipline. These findings confirm Annandale's (1985) observations about important differences in the perspectives of different staff on resident well-being.

Discussion of Contextual Issues

In this study, we attempted to use an experimental and quantitative approach in an effort to learn about the impact of functionally integrated or segregated therapy sessions on resident well-being. Understanding and interpreting findings of this study must involve a careful consideration of contextual factors that influenced the conduct of the study and that have implications for interpretation of our findings. As a matter of fact this context cannot be meaningfully separated from data obtained and conclusions drawn from the study.

While every effort was made by the investigators to obtain staff cooperation, it became evident as the study went on that the staff resented the added chore of bringing therapy patients to program areas on a daily basis. This resentment was often taken out on patients participating in the therapy by limiting services to them. It also resulted in frequent errors in bringing residents to integrated versus segregated programs (these errors were always corrected by research staff). Interestingly, aides, nursing staff, and professionals displayed markedly different attitudes toward residents on the one hand and toward the therapy program on the other. Aides appeared most negative, while professionals were most favorable, toward the therapy program. Understanding and altering these differences in attitude presents an important and often unreported challenge to all therapy programs. The importance of considering the ecology and organization of both patient and staff environment in organizing therapy programs was clearly underscored in this study.

Careful observation of the attendance of well-functioning residents who volunteered to attend functionally integrated activities supports the notion that the well elderly often fear contagion by the more impaired. Volunteers did not attend programs consistently and often expressed fear of associating with confused residents. This fact may have diminished the effectiveness of functionally integrated programs. In addition, it may well be that if the proportion of impaired-to-well residents were reversed—that is, a few impaired residents were to be integrated with a large group of well-functioning ones—fear of contagion would be diminished and the benefits of integrated programs to the impaired residents would be enhanced.

While there were no significant differences in the effects of functionally heterogeneous versus homogeneous therapy programs, the study shed light on the complex forces operating that may have cancelled out potential positive effects of integration. First, the mentally impaired aged who were assumed to be a relatively homogeneous group in this sample represented enough diversity to provide a semblance of integration even in the segregated groups. Second, the volunteers recruited for programs did not participate with either regularity or enthusiasm. This in itself is a valuable finding and points to an important area for future study. How does functional integration affect alert residents? Is their fear of contagion simply uninformed prejudice, or is it a founded belief? An intriguing clue to this question was found when the investigators compared volunteers who dropped out or attended irregularly to volunteers who continued to participate regularly in the program. Volunteers who dropped out showed some signs of cognitive impairment on their MSQ measures, while those who remained in the program portrayed no signs of impending cognitive impairment. Thus it is possible that interaction with the cognitively impaired is potentially threatening to older persons who are experiencing mild signs of cognitive deficit.

As an interesting epilogue to the study, its effects on the nursing home and its staff should be noted. Prior to the study, no programs were offered to meet the needs of impaired residents because of a reported shortage of staff and the generally held view that "they can't be helped; they don't even answer when you call their names." Yet in the course of the study several cases of dramatic improvement among apparently "hopeless" patients were observed by all. By the end of the study, one woman who had been habitually taciturn, with a facial expression of anguish, and who had refused involvement in all activities, occasionally smiled and began to respond to conversation. Subsequent to the study several key staff members recognized the potential benefits of treating the cognitively impaired and continued to involve them in programs with the more responsive residents who had participated in our research. An extensive remotivation program for the cognitively impaired residents was ultimately initiated in the home.

CONCLUSION

This chapter emphasized the impact of contextual issues on quantitative studies of institutionalized elderly. The authors aimed to illustrate the pervasive role of contextual influences in the conduct of every phase of the research process. Contextual issues were broadly defined to encompass diverse facets of the research enterprise. Nevertheless it is important to note that a more formal interpretation of context as "environment" is also useful and necessary in institutional research. Specifically the physical, social, and organizational milieu of institutions must be described and analyzed if researchers are to consider their data in its full relevant context. Accordingly, researchers should classify institutions based on physical environmental factors, policies, staff attitudes, and behaviors. Consideration of quality of care should incorporate all of the above issues along with an understanding of the fit, or congruence, between needs and contextual/environmental characteristics (Kahana, 1981).

Quantitative research undertaken in institutional settings must attend to contextual influences that go beyond traditional survey researchers' concerns about sampling or instrumentation. Researchers must recognize that the institutional context, in fact, permeates every phase of the research enterprise, rendering all institutional research a "field study." Once the pervasive role of context is recognized, the meaning of many traditional "controls" must be altered and the influence of strong social forces and ethical considerations must be acknowledged (Rowles, 1986).

The investigator's sensitivity to situational and organizational factors increases the likelihood that the research will be meaningful as well as scientifically sound (Kahana & Felton, 1977). Furthermore, an openness to pursuing cues regarding dynamic forces operating in the institutional environment can enhance validity and expand the parameters of research among the institutionalized elderly. In addition to the importance of understanding and working within the organizational context in which research is conducted, recognition of contextual factors insures obtaining valid data and arriving at meaningful interpretations of the data collected. The specific issues discussed in this chapter were illustrative rather than exhaustive. Nevertheless, examples demonstrated that contextual influences are pervasive and salient to every stage of designing, conducting, analyzing, and interpreting an empirical study. Better understanding of these issues and greater willingness by researchers to share information about contextual issues are likely to improve the meaningfulness of our investigation into the complex world of institutional living for the elderly.

REFERENCES

Annandale, E. (1985). Work roles and definitions of patient health. *Qualitative Sociology, 8*(2), 124–148.

Atchley, R. C. (1969). Respondents vs. refusers in an interview study of retired women. *Journal of Gerontology, 24*, 24–27.

Barnes, R., & Raskind, M. (1984). Long-term clinical management of the dementia patient. In J. P. Abrahams & V. Crooks (Eds.), *Geriatric mental health*, Orlando, FL: Grune & Stratton.

Becker, H. S. (1958). Problems of inference and proof in participant observation. *American Sociological Review, 33*, 652–659.

Brody, E. M., Feinstein, P., Eisdorfer, C., & Mather, J. (1984). Roundtable discussion—examining health care policy: Strategies for the future care of the Alzheimer's disease patient. In J. E. Hansan (Ed.), *Proceedings of the National Conference on Alzheimer's Disease: A challenge for care* (pp. 69–82). Memphis, TN: The Hillhaven Foundation.

Buckwalter, K. (1985). Personal communication.

Butler, R. N., & Lewis, M. I. (1977). *Aging and mental health: Positive psychosocial approaches.* St. Louis: C. V. Mosby.

Carp, F. M. (1983). The effect of planned housing on life satisfaction and mortality of residents. In V. Regnier & J. Pynoos (Eds.), *Housing for the elderly: Satisfactions and preferences.* New York: Garland.

Crovitz, H. (1979). Memory retraining in brain-damaged patients: The airplane list. *Cortex, 15,* 131–134.

Gallaher, A., Jr. (1964). Plainville: The twice studied town. In A. J. Vidich, J. Bensman, & M. R. Stein (Eds.), *Reflections on community studies* (pp. 285–311). New York: John Wiley & Sons.

George, L. (1984). The institutionalized. In E. B. Palmore (Ed.), *Handbook on the aged in the United States* (pp. 339–354). Westport, CT: Greenwood Press.

Goffman, E. *Asylums.* (1961). New York: Doubleday & Company.

Hoover, K. (1984). *The elements of social scientific thinking.* New York: St. Martin's Press.

Kahana, B. (1982). Social development in adulthood and aging. In B. Wolman (Ed.), *Handbook of developmental psychology* (pp. 871–889). New York: Prentice-Hall.

Kahana, B., & Kahana, E. (1970, August). Changes in mental status of elderly patients in age integrated and age segregated hospital milieus. *Journal of Advanced Psychology, 75*(2), 177–181.

Kahana, E., & Coe, R. M. (1969). Self and staff conceptions of institutionalized aged. *The Gerontologist, 9*(4), 264–277.

Kahana, E., & Felton, B. (1977). Social context and personal needs: A study of Polish Jewish aged. *Journal of Social Issues, 33*(4), 56–74.

Kahana, E., Kahana, B., & Young, R. (1984, August). *Social factors in institutional living.* Paper presented at the annual meeting of the American Psychological Association, Toronto, Canada.

Kahana, E., & Kiyak, A. (1984). Attitudes and behavior of staff in facilities for the aged. *Research on Aging, 6,* 395–416.

Kahn, R. L., Pollack, M., & Goldfarb, A. I. (1961). Factors related to individual differences in mental status of institutionalized aged. In P. Hoch & J. Zubin (Eds.), *Psychopathology of aging* (pp. 104–113). New York: Grune & Stratton.

Kayser-Jones, J. (1981). *Old, alone and neglected: Care of the aged in Scotland and in the United States.* Berkeley, CA: University of California Press.

Lawton, M. P. (1980). *Environment and aging.* Monterey, CA: Brooks/Cole.

Mishler, E. G. (1979). Meaning in context: Is there any other kind? *Harvard Educational Review, 49*(1), 3–21.

Morris, R. (1960). Expansion of cooperative relationships between hospitals and nursing homes. *Public Health Report, 75,* 1110–1114.

Poon, L. W. (1984). Memory training for older adults. In J. P. Abrahams & V. Crooks (Eds.), *Geriatric mental health* (pp. 135–151) Orlando, FL: Grune & Stratton.

Powdermaker, H. (1966). *Stranger and friend: The way of an anthropologist.* New York: Norton.

Reinharz, S. (1984). *On becoming a social scientist: From survey research and participant observation to experiential analysis.* New Brunswick, NJ: Transaction Books.

Roth, J. A. (1966). Hired hand research. *The American Sociologist, 1*(4), 190–196.
Rowles, G. D. (1986). Personal communication.
Sinnott, J. D., Harris, C. S., Block, M. R., Collesano, S., & Jacobson, S. G. (1983). *Applied research in aging: A guide to methods and resources.* Boston: Little, Brown and Company.
U. S. Department of Health and Human Services. (1984). *Alzheimer's disease: Report of the secretary's task force on Alzheimer's disease.* Washington, DC: Author.
Vladeck, B. C. (1980). *Unloving care.* New York: Basic Books.
Wax, M. L. (1977). On fieldworkers and those exposed to fieldwork: Federal regulations and moral issues. *Human Organization, 36*(3), 321–328.

12

Research as Process: Exploring the Meaning of Widowhood

Phyllis R. Silverman

When people marry they rarely consider that the statement "til death do us part" will one day become a reality for one of them. With only 8% of the current cohort of elderly having never married, it is obvious that most elderly people have been or are still married. Among the elderly there are primarily two populations: those who are already widowed and those who are yet to be widowed. Since women continue to outlive men and since the median age at which a woman is widowed is 49 (Osterweis, Solomon, & Green, 1984), most of the older population who are already widowed are women. According to the 1980 U. S. Census, 50% of all women over 65 are widowed and by the time they are 70 the number increases to 66%. Men who are widowed tend to remarry, so that only 18% of all men over 65 are widowers. The ratio of widows to widowers is 5:1, so that the option to remarry is often not available to women. To understand the experience of older women, then, it is essential to look at what being widowed means to them.

Grief in contemporary society has been medicalized and treated as if it were an illness for which the proper treatment will bring a cure (Osterweis et al., 1984; Silverman, 1986). In this model bereavement is seen as something alien, not as an expected part of the human experience. Expressions of grief are seen as symptoms, and grief is often seen as time-limited. In fact, DSM III, the American Psychiatric Association manual for making psychiatric diagnoses, states that grief that continues beyond three to six months can be an indication of psycho-pathology or, at the least, an inappropriate mourning response (Oster-weis et al., 1984). The focus in treatment is on severing ties with the past, perhaps emulating the practices of other cultures with elaborate tie-breaking rituals and ritual specialists who guide people through these periods (Rosenblatt, Walsh, & Jackson, 1976). Typically these rituals separate the widowed from their past by breaking the habits of daily interaction with their spouses (VanGennup, 1960). Rosenblatt and his colleagues point out that rituals of this sort do not exist in contemporary western society (1976). The role of caretaker to the bereaved has been assumed by health practitioners, thereby reinforcing the association of grief with deviance.

Gender differences between the way men and women mourn have received little attention. However, because it is popularly expected that men should respond to the stress of the death of a loved one with more restraint, their mourning behavior is more circumscribed (Silverman, 1986). Women are seen as more emotional, and their grief is seen as permeating more aspects of their lives (Silverman, 1981). If the appro-priate response to mourning requires giving up the past, for a woman focusing on the death of a spouse to give up the past means to give up the role of wife. The role of wife typically defines a woman's position in society. If she defines herself through her relationship to her husband, in giving up the past she leaves herself without a socially accepted position in that society. From cross-cultural studies of other societies we learn that there were rituals that followed those of tie-breaking. These facilitated the widow's reentry into society. This reentry was often marked by remarriage, e.g., levirate marriage as prescribed in the Bible (the custom of marriage between a man and his brother's widow). In other societies, women were prohibited from remarrying, e.g., the child brides of India who lived out their lives as their husbands' widows. The woman's primary role, either as wife or as widow, was through her relationship to a husband, dead or alive. Older women who were not expected to remarry often were cared for by their children, so that their position in society continued to be defined through their relationship to others, never in terms of themselves. Such rituals for reintegrating women into contemporary society are nonexistent, thus leading to difficult consequences for women. Older women who were socialized to know themselves almost exclusively through the role of wife acquire a stigmatized position (Silverman, 1981). In the words of an 80-year-old American widow: "When I was married I was someone, now I am nobody." With little guidance, widows must relinquish the active role of wife and find new roles for themselves (Lopata, 1973, 1979).

Neither the ritual of the past nor the treatment model of the present provides sufficient guidance to enable women to respond to their needs as widows. In our mobile, open society, women's roles are in flux and are being examined anew. A more appropriate framework for understanding women as widows may be one that recognizes widowhood, like marriage, as a stage in the life cycle, as a period of transition requiring the widow to make an accommodation to the changed circumstances of her life (Marris, 1974; Silverman, 1986). This may require that she find a new identity and a new place for herself in society regardless of her age. This chapter describes my attempt to understand what is involved for widows who must make a shift in their identity.

THE ORIGINS OF A RESEARCH PROBLEM

My own research with the widowed has extended over two decades. It began when I was employed by the social psychiatrist Gerald Caplan to develop a program of preventive intervention for newly widowed people thought to be at high risk for developing serious emotional problems. I developed the widow-to-widow concept and created a project using that name to demonstrate how it could work (Silverman, 1966, 1969, 1970, 1986; Silverman, MacKenzie, Pettipas, & Willson, 1975). In this project experienced widows reached out to new widows and befriended them in a mutual help exchange. The offer of help was unsolicited, and over a three-year period several hundred women were reached. Following the completion of the original experiment, we ran a widowed telephone line and then sponsored formal workshops for the widowed. This work has served as the model for an extensive network of widow-to-widow programs throughout the United States and abroad and has been my natural laboratory for studying the problems of the widowed over these years.

In 1965, when I began this work, bereavement was seen by psychologists and psychiatrists as a crisis that could be resolved in six weeks (Lindemann, 1944; Caplan, 1963). The widowed women with whom I was working gave me a chance to hear about the subjective, experiential side of widowhood. They quickly disabused me of the six-weeks notion. They told me that it takes about two years "to get your head screwed on again so that you can look to the future" (Silverman et al., 1975). They were not comfortable with the concept of recovery, although they could not clearly articulate what was wrong with it. They reported asking themselves what they were doing wrong, since they did not feel better for a long time after the death and could not reconstitute their lives as they had lived before. They reported that people, especially those who have not yet experienced a grief, kept telling them they should have been able to "get back to normal already." In the first paper I wrote on this topic (Silverman, 1966) I suggested that the concept of transition, which focuses on accommodation, not recovery, might reflect more correctly what they experienced. Widows do not give up the past; rather they change their relationship to it. The important role that defined their lives—wife—was no longer relevant, and therefore their habits of daily living had to change. Nevertheless, the past informed the present and in some way remained a part of it. As I came to understand widowhood, the widowed developed a new perspective on their loss so that the pain and sadness were no longer the guiding force in their lives, and with time they developed new roles (Silverman, 1981, 1986). In this initial work, my epistemological position was already being established. I did not study women to test a theory but rather listened to the women in order to develop a grounded theory of their experience. After my initial "discovery" of transition or change as the key experience of widowhood, my subsequent study of widowhood has focused on the nature of change associated with the death of a spouse and the interventions that make change easier to achieve.

DEVELOPING A RESEARCH STRATEGY

In describing most research efforts, emphasis is on the logical, objective methods leading to reliable and valid data. Most researchers attempt to remain objective, outside the research process and the subject matter studied. This chapter, by contrast, is an addition to the literature on research methodology that questions the use of this paradigm as the only way to approach science. The metaphor of the dispassionate scientist manipulating variables in the laboratory may not be an accurate description of scientific work. In his description of the work of physicists, S. M. Silverman (1979) notes that most researchers are guided by two belief systems: a public belief system and a private belief system. The public belief system asserts that logical, rational forces are the only factors that affect research. Thus these are the only factors scientists will acknowledge in their work. The intuitive, experiential factors that inform ideas and make meaning out of experience are not acknowledged as having legitimacy in this process (Keller, 1983).

Silverman feels that most new knowledge emanates from the "gut" of the researcher, and only afterwards is it framed in the accepted language of science. Kaplan talks about these modes as the logic of discovery and reconstructed logic (1964). Similarities can be found between this view of the influence of private beliefs and what Clinchy and Zimmerman (1985) in a study of college age women call "connected knowing." Connected knowing is the ability to acknowledge and use personal experience to inform and guide scholarly activity. This is in contrast to what they call "separate knowing," where the sources of knowledge are external to the individual. Reinharz (1984), in her development of the concept of experiential analysis, makes a strong case that meaningful research has to use both connected and separate epistemologies. Perry (1981) describes the research enterprise as a journey into making meaning out of the observations, concerns, and understanding of the researcher. In my research I draw on both modes of thinking.

My own person is very much a part of my research, and my research is a part of me. They are not separate. I do not approach this work as an outsider unable to imagine the experience of the people I study. Rather, this subject has evoked my interest because it touches my personal life. For one, I am a married woman. As I look at widowhood, I am studying a role I may occupy in the future. None of us who are involved with others will escape bereavement. Since I share in the human condition, I am subject as well as object in this study. Furthermore, I recognize that my research provides me with a way of coping with the fact that people die, by allowing me to reframe my understanding of grief as an occasion to create opportunity out of adversity.

Just as the research changes over time, so does my experiential reference point. The phase of my research I am describing in this chapter coincides with my growing consciousness about how my experience as a woman is different from that of a man. I increasingly prize the pleasure inherent in the caretaking roles of wife and mother and am less critical of myself for not aspiring to be autonomous. At the same time, I am beginning to understand some of the ways women are demeaned by others and by ourselves when we are valued *only* in relationship to men or as we compare well to them. I have also found a community of women with whom I can share my experiences and learned that I was not alone in the way I felt. While I still agree with Sullivan (1962, Frontispiece) that "we are all more simply human than otherwise, more like everyone else than different," I no longer believe that accommodation to widowhood is the same for men and for women. By valuing the difference between us, I feel I am expanding my vision of the human capacity.

Time itself has become less compartmentalized for me. For example, my research has become an ongoing inquiry whether or not I am involved in a formally funded project. I simply shape the size of the research questions to the resources I have available. I also do not compartmentalize my resources. For example, one of my resources is my husband, S. M. Silverman, a research scientist, keeper of our home computer and constant source of help in my research efforts. Personal commitments as a woman, wife, and mother have compelled me to shape the way I do my work in consideration of these other contingencies rather than in pretending that they do not exist. I have taken advantage of opportunities created in my nonresearch roles—as professor, speaker, wife, mother—to develop new perspectives on my thinking and to gather data. As I proceed I am both connected to the data and separate from it.

SEARCHING FOR A LANGUAGE TO DESCRIBE THE SELF

The phase of my research described in this chapter began in 1979 when I started writing *Helping Women Cope with Grief* (1981). In this book I described how women deal with three types of losses. At this point I had read Gilligan (1979) and Miller (1976), and my thinking was for the first time informed by feminist thinkers. Women's sense of self, these writers were saying, seemed to depend on their ability to be involved with others and maintain their connectedness to others. In men, autonomy is prized. Their focus is on their ability to be separate from others and get the job done, rather than to maintain relationships. Gilligan's and Miller's thinking helped me make sense in a new and positive way of some of my own experience as a professional and thus heightened my interest in looking at women's experience as different. At the same time they provided me with a theoretical framework to analyze the data I had collected for this book about the loss of relationships. I suggested that to cope, women needed linking relationships to maintain a connection between the past and the future. From my data I could see that coping with their bereavement led women to develop a greater sense of autonomy, competence, and effectiveness (Silverman, 1981). I could not avoid asking myself what it means "to have a greater sense of autonomy." The definition of autonomy I found in the dictionary suggested that it means to be independent of others. I was implying that these women's growing sense of competence was associated with a decrease in reliance on others. Based on my own experience, a growing sense of competence did not decrease my dependence on or connectedness with others. Instead, my connectedness persisted and changed.

Nor did the word *autonomy* describe appropriately these women's increasing comfort and self-reliance. Rather, I sensed a growing mutuality in the women's relations with others that represented change rather than separation.

I was also concerned that the concept of a growing sense of autonomy not be taken as an indicator of good accommodation to loss. To do so would be to imply that self-reliant men were not as upset as women when bereaved. More important, I rejected the implication that men needed people less than women did. More accurate language was vital to describe how men and women relate to others, how their involvement with others can change after bereavement, and how this change differs for men and women.

Shortly after I finished writing *Helping Women Cope with Grief*, I was invited to join a network of women scholars interested in women's epistemology. The Women's Educational Development Network grew out of a study of women's educational development conducted by Belenky, Clinchy, Goldberger, and Tarule (1986). Their research used a model of cognitive development devised by Perry (1970) in his study of male undergraduates at Harvard University. The study was designed to see whether or not the Perry model applied to women. At the same time, a colleague gave me an article to read by Robert Kegan (1979), who was trying to integrate the work of Piaget and Kohlberg with psychodynamic thinkers in the Freudian tradition.

Perry had studied learning patterns in college-aged men, while Kegan (1983) applied the concepts of cognitive development to emotional development. Kegan was interested in the way people experienced themselves in relationships with others. Each researcher had articulated stages that people go through as they learn and as they make meaning out of the ways they relate to themselves and to others.

I wondered if the stages they described would apply to the widowed, allowing the researcher to elaborate on their learning styles as well as on the means they use to cope with their loss. After all, to cope is in part to learn. During a critical transition in a person's life, stress emanates in large part from the fact that prior means of coping are not appropriate or effective in the new situation. People in transition need to learn new skills and acquire new information that would enable them to develop coping strategies appropriate to the new situation. While coping with bereavement occurs outside a classroom, it is still an educational process. Cognitive theory about learning styles and associated stages of development might well apply. For the first time I had a language for looking at the widowed from a developmental point of view, permitting me to describe the continuum of change they might be going through.

All of these theories converged in my mind and required continuing work before I could formulate a meaningful integration. For example, Perry talks of the dualist thinker who takes things literally, who thinks linearly and who responds to the expert as authority (1970). Kegan (1983) talks of people who are embedded in others, who rely on others for legitimation of their own feelings, and whose sense of self requires others for approbation and permission. Are these authors describing different aspects of what is really one developmental stage? What about women's development? If women's needs for others are more highly developed than men's, so that women know themselves primarily through their relationships (Miller, 1985), does this mean that most women are limited to immature ways of thinking and relating to others? Gilligan (1979) notes that women simply have a different way of thinking.

The problems inherent in applying these ideas increased when I considered that Kegan's next stage of development describes a greater mutuality. Is this the progression toward mutuality I was describing in my book and the difference for women to which Gilligan is alluding? Again, more questions were posed than answers were available. In addition, according to developmental theory, people are supposed to move, albeit haltingly, from one stage to the next in a forward progression as they age. They are not supposed to move back to an earlier stage. Is it possible to be "in" several stages at the same time? Is it possible that as a result of the impact of acute grief, for example, people return to being more dualistic and more concrete? In the words of one widow: "I needed someone to tell me how to move, how to put one foot in front of myself and then what to do next." Do they then move to the next stage as they begin to acknowledge the impact of their loss and take responsibility for dealing with it?

It was also important to ask if women of different age cohorts exhibit different developmental stages. Learning styles and character formation cannot be separated from opportunities and socialization patterns provided by environments. A popular stereotype of the elderly is that personal growth may not be a realistic goal. The question of whether *all* change was developmental had to be addressed. Still another question was whether, in giving up a role and adapting to a new one, people could change *without* moving ahead on the developmental spectrum.

In the spring of 1983 I had an opportunity to take a course with Robert Kegan. The course influenced some of my thinking, as reflected in the questions above. In addition, I learned that he did not see differences among men and women in his conceptual schema. He talked about "the need for others" in both sexes and felt that the quality of relationships changes for both and develops in the same direction. I was

not satisfied that there are no differences in male and female development. It is true that both sexes have similar needs for others in the long
run (Erikson, 1963; Levinson, 1978), but according to Erikson, a key
issue for young men is autonomy. If Gilligan (1979) is correct, young
women do not separate themselves from others in the same way. These
differences could affect how men and women make meaning out of
their marital relationships, which in turn affects what happens when
the marriage ends. More important, perhaps, I also learned that no one
was looking at what happened when death ended a relationship, nor
were most theorists looking at the meaning of death and survivorship
as it affected development, except in children (Kastenbaum, 1977).

NEW RESEARCH OPPORTUNITIES

In the winter of 1982–83 I was invited to participate in a workshop
sponsored by the Councils on Aging in New England. There I met the
director of the Arlington Council on Aging in Massachusetts, Scott
Plumb. The council sponsors a very active widow-to-widow program
for people over 65. We talked about the work of the group and its
ability to remain active over a period of five or more years. I asked why
the group was successful in contrast to other organizations in the
Greater Boston Area that had not survived over time. We talked about
how Plumb, in his role as administrator, provided continuity for the
organization but still allowed the members to run the program. To
learn more about how members saw the program, he suggested I come
and talk to the participants.

I had once submitted a formal proposal to the National Institute on
Aging to evaluate the impact on elderly widows of participation in a
widow-to-widow program, using Plumb's program as the experimental
group. The proposal was not funded. Both Plumb and I were disappointed to have lost this opportunity. I had also arranged for a graduate
student at Boston College's School of Social Work to do her master's
thesis using members of this program as subjects. Now we were proposing something I could do on my own time without funding. I began
interviewing members of the widow-to-widow program. This seemed
like a good opportunity to explore my new ideas about development
with real people. Consequently, I prepared a few questions on how
members saw themselves prior to their widowhood and how they had
changed. More of the members were willing to be interviewed than I
had anticipated, primarily women over the age of 70. Since my time and

resources were very limited, they suggested I write down a few questions and they would answer them and send them back to me.

I began to consider whether some of the questions that Belenky and associates (1986) had used in their study could be used to gather more systematic data from the members of the Arlington program. Other members of our Women's Educational Development Network had worked with these questions and had created standardized codes, so that I could categorize widows on a developmental scale, at least after their bereavement. These scores might reveal something about how they involved others in their lives, how much they depended on others for their sense of self, and the extent of their ability to act on their own behalf. The questions I chose were: how would you describe yourself to yourself, and would this have been different before your spouse died? what recent important decision did you make? how were other people involved in your decision to act? and, again, would it have been different if your spouse were alive?

I also recognized that in order to use any data I gathered, I would need to know something about the age of the respondent, when his/her spouse had died, the couple's family composition, and their educational background. It became an occasion to think through what I would want to know from a widowed person in order to understand how they had changed and to understand how their affiliation with a mutual help organization affected this accommodation. I added questions about what was most difficult, what was easiest, how they had changed, how they got involved in a mutual help group, and what they felt they got out of their affiliation. I asked them about themselves and about decisions they made. As a result, the questionnaire ended up as a six-page document. I showed this questionnaire to several members of the Arlington group. This was not what they had had in mind when they asked me to put a few questions down on paper. They looked at the questionnaire and decided it was too complicated. They could not handle this much writing.

I then conducted a few face-to-face interviews with members of the organization who were in leadership positions. My original question about what kept the organization going was answered in part. The role of the professional in providing continuity was essential, but it was also clear that the widowed people who were the leaders of this program felt a good deal of support and permission from Plumb and his staff to carry out the work of the organization on their own. It was also clear that the change that had occurred in these individuals was in the direction of greater self-reliance and self-confidence. Advanced age and even some physical disability had not inhibited the development of these men and women. My teaching schedule, however, became too heavy to allow me to do any more interviews.

I was left with a questionnaire for which I had no audience. In the spring of 1983 I was invited to be the keynote speaker at the tenth anniversary of To Live Again (TLA). This is a mutual help organization with branches in northeastern Pennsylvania and southern New Jersey that had used my early work as a model for their program. In corresponding with the anniversary planning committee, I asked if their committee might be willing to respond to my questionnaire. When they agreed, I sent 12 copies of the questionnaire—I got back 10. The completed questionnaires showed me that it was possible for people to answer the questions and that the data could be rich and valuable. Lois Zachery, a member of the Women's Education Development Network, looked at the responses to some of the questions without seeing the face sheet and was able correctly to identify men and women and the newly widowed. She encouraged me to proceed with wider distribution of the questionnaire, but I had no funds to support this effort. I would have to depend upon people's good will to return any questionnaires that were distributed. TLA stated that they were willing to go forward with a wide distribution to their chapters. They felt that individuals would return the questionnaire to me on their own.

I took 500 questionnaires to the anniversary meeting. During my talk I announced what I was doing and asked people to respond to the questionnaire when it was distributed at their chapter meetings. I was most disappointed when only 48 were returned during the next few months. I have no idea how they were distributed and what instructions were given beyond what I wrote on the face sheet. In retrospect it would have been better to give out the questionnaires to the 500 people in attendance at the meeting and to ask them to respond and return them to me within the week.

My disappointment was assuaged when I read the responses on the questionnaires that were returned. People had taken the time to write in detail how they felt. They tried to answer my queries about their coping strategies. The proportion of men who responded was the same as the proportion of widowers found in the widowed population as a whole. My initial reaction was to quantify the responses to see if I had any statistically significant findings. However, this was inappropriate because the low response rate made it unlikely that the sample would be statistically representative of the population. In addition, there was no comparison group of people who were not affiliated with TLA. I turned instead to examining the *meaning* of what people had written. I could identify trends in how the respondents' sense of self was affected by their bereavement. I could look at the nature of change and how members believed affiliation with the group affected this change.

Another opportunity to distribute additional questionnaires presented itself. The Widowed Person's Service (WPS), an affiliated program of the American Association of Retired People, sponsors a network of Widowed Persons Associations around the United States. The program has an annual meeting in the fall of every year, attracting members from all over the United States. Their programs are modeled after the widow-to-widow program. I mentioned the questionnaire to Ruth Lowensohn, administrator of the Widowed Person's Service program in Washington, D.C. She said that they would be glad to distribute it to participants at their annual meeting in Florida in October 1984. They would collect the questionnaires at the end of the meeting and return them to me. I received another 50 completed questionnaires representing about one-fourth of the conference participants. I now had 108 questionnaires.

ANALYZING THE DATA

Cathy Quinlan, a secretary at the Massachusetts General Hospital Institute of Health Professions, where I am on the faculty, was taking a statistics course as part of a graduate program in management at this time. She was looking for data she could use for a class exercise and approached me for advice. I allowed her to use my questionnaires, asking her to focus on one or two questions that might reveal differences between men and women. The questions I chose pertained to "what was the most difficult to manage once you were widowed," "what was the easiest," "what remained difficult over time," and "what became easier over time." Quinlan developed a code for the face sheet data and for the items I requested. She sorted the data and found differences in the responses of men and women.

In the fall of 1984 I received an invitation to address the First International Congress of Associations for the Widowed, to be held in England in April 1985. I decided this would be a good audience for my new data on widowhood as a period of growth and change. Since all the participants represented mutual help organizations, I believed they would have a vested interest in learning if affiliation in an analogous organization was helpful in accommodating to loss. This became my "excuse" to analyze my previously collected data despite the lack of financial support to cover my costs.

I quickly learned that it is very difficult to analyze open-ended questions on 108 questionnaires. At the same time, I was learning to use my home computer, an Osborne 1. My husband, eager to test the limits of this first generation of microcomputers, was willing to assist me. We decided to code the data in a quantitative way. To do this, I expanded on the codes Quinlan had developed and developed new codes by making lists of responses to particular questions and giving the same number to responses that appeared to have similar meaning. In order to analyze the questions derived from the study of women's educational development, I consulted with members of the Women's Educational Development Network. Zachary agreed to help me when she completed her own doctoral dissertation in the fall of 1985. My husband used database management software (d-Base II) that allowed me to set up a record for each questionnaire and count different sets of circumstances. I entered the coded data into the computer.

Holding age, sex, and length of time widowed constant, I was able to examine how responses clustered. Instead of seeking statistically significant associations, I sought frequencies or clusters that might reflect a pattern that characterized this population on one dimension after another (for a discussion of the use of computers to analyze qualitative data, see Conrad & Reinharz, 1984). Once I identified a pattern in the data I then found quotes from the questionnaires to illustrate this pattern. Examples are presented below. The absolute number of responses was also important. In other words, I had to keep in mind that a phenomenon appearing in similar *proportions* among men and women, despite large differences in absolute numbers, did not signify difference. There were five widows for every widower among the respondents. My approach to the analysis of these data grew out of the data I had available; just as the data grew out of the resources I had available.

"In Search of New Selves: Accommodating to Widowhood" (1987) is the paper I wrote. The paper begins with an examination of the demographics of the respondents, i.e., 90 female and 18 male respondents. These numbers accurately reflect the ratio of widows to widowers in the widowed population as a whole. The majority of people who answered were between the ages of 50 and 70, although the age range was very wide: for men, 41 to 71; for women, 36 to 83. Most respondents had been widowed for about a year and a half, some as little as two weeks. Twelve of the women over 70 had been widowed for more than 10 years. Most of these women had initiated the programs in their communities. Annual incomes ranged from minimal Social Security benefits to upward of $35,000. Education, too, was wide ranging. While many were college graduates, most had simply finished high school and some people had not gone past eighth grade. This distribution made me confident that the responses reflected the experiences of a range of membership in these mutual help organizations.

DIFFERENCES BETWEEN MEN AND WOMEN

Immediately after their spouse's death there are great similarities in the reactions of widows and widowers. Perhaps this is the "simply human" period (Sullivan, 1962). Both men and women focused on their pain, their loneliness, and their feeling of aloneness. Some expressed relief at the end of their spouse's suffering after a long illness. Differentiation between men's and women's responses clearly emerged within two or three months after the death. It was then that their ability to make decisions began to be important. None of the widowers stated that making decisions was a problem, while widows constantly mentioned that this was one of their worst problems. In the words of one widow:

> "At first I did not want to choose to do anything alone. I fought against making any choices."

The women wrote about this difficulty in terms of their inexperience in making decisions on their own. One widow recalled her behavior when her husband was alive: "I deferred to my husband's decisions." None of the widowers described themselves as deferring to their wives. However, in many instances widows and widowers characterized decision making as a shared activity. The women experienced discomfort when they had to act on their own. If they grew in widowhood, one of the strengths they developed was the ability to decide:

> "I had to get used to taking responsibility for making my own decisions."

> "Making important decisions for myself was a new concept to me. I now voice my own opinions and I am sometimes surprised that I am doing this— right or wrong."

> "Now I think and I decide."

The following quotes contrast the views of a widow and widower about their ability not only to decide but to act at all. A young widower of three months described himself as:

"Quiet, but very strong in coping and handling financial affairs, in making decisions."

A 36-year-old widow of six months wrote:

"I was happy, excited by life. I was queen of the shopping mall. My husband adored me, my family protected me. They try to do that now, but it doesn't work. I feel like MUSH."

The widower seems able to act in spite of his pain and his loss. His prior experience in managing his life serves him well. He toughs it out and finds continuity in his role. Women, on the other hand, don't have that prior learning in acting easily on their own behalf. A widower of six months described his life:

"I haven't changed too much. I am a self-assured individual. I know what I want and make plans to accomplish my goals—a little bit at a time. I've had to develop a new support system and I've learned to be independent—self-reliant and self-sufficient (especially around the house)."

A widow of 49, widowed for five years, recalled that prior to her husband's death:

"I did not do many things on my own, but did most things with my family in mind and could not do some things I wanted to, was not encouraged to go out alone."

These women had little sense of their selves outside of the role of wife. The women need a whole new identity: "I thought you had to be married to be happy."

Men did not talk of their loss in terms of losing the role of husband. Perhaps they did not see it as a role at all, or at least not as a self-defining one. They wrote, as did the women, of their loneliness, their need to share their lives. However, their sense of who they were was not dependent upon their relationship to their wives. While their lives may be different now, for most of the men, the way they experienced themselves did not change. As a result of the loss, men felt cut off from people, not from themselves. They talked about their need to "get out more." They talked of the need for companionship. They talked of possibly remarrying:

"Just a guy looking for a wife and not being a dreamer. I am looking for someone in my generation, with similar interests and reasonably good health."

Many focused on developing their social skills. One man talked about trying not to get so uptight in large social situations, and another was concerned with being less of an introvert when among people. One man said: "I am trying to be more understanding of people's problems." Another noted that he was "much more tolerant of others." The direction of change they made seemed to bring them more in touch with their own feelings, to acknowledge their pain and their tears, and to get in touch with the needs of others.

"I am determined to live out my years in a mood of kindness to others. If I find the right person I will marry again."

For the women, change was in the direction of a growing independence. They began to discover other selves, roles beyond that of wife.

"I was very content to stand in my husband's shadow. Now I am learning that I represent only me."

"There was the slow realization that I am really independent and that while I love and am loved by many people, no one really cares what I do on any given day. They have confidence in me—I do in myself, and slowly I am trying to shed fear, guilt and overconcern about what other people think. I am working on many facets of what I hope will be changes in lifestyle and personal growth."

These widows talked about becoming more centered in themselves, more in touch with what they want. Widows talked over and over again about the new found independence and freedom they were enjoying: "I have a freedom I never had before."

"I am a happy single person, independent and enjoying it. I wouldn't say that I wasn't independent before, but I still depended and leaned on my husband."

Change was born of necessity:

"Yes, I experienced a growth that would not have been possible before, if I had continued to be a "submissive" partner. In fact I would not have "stepped out." This does not mean that I felt liberated in losing a partner, but this is what has happened as a result."

Some women did not feel that they had lived in their husband's shadow. They had been able to speak up and they shared in decision making. Nonetheless, they too felt the need to change. They wrote about a different sense of self:

> "It has always been easy for me to express myself. However, now there is a different reason . . . to express the victories that can be gained in the grief process, and the new life that can come out of it."

Simply put, the widows began to achieve an autonomy they had not known before. They became more comfortable with themselves and learned skills needed to live alone successfully:

> "My kids tell me I have grown and expanded as a person. I know I am more generous, accepting, and sensitive than before. While I enjoy others, I also appreciate my solitude and am content in what I am."

> "I am a young widow, although not age-wise, independent, alone, but happy."

I would describe these women's relationships as characterized less by dependency than by a new mutuality. A developmental leap seems to have taken place. They still needed people and were involved with others but in a different way:

> "I have become more independent in all areas. I enjoy my ability to decide what my goals are. I probably am closer to my children and grandchildren than I would have been had my husband lived. I am also more community conscious and involved in several volunteer groups."

This material may be evidence for two important points: that widowhood is a developmental period in the life cycle, and that men and women change in different directions. The men seemed to be more *in search of others*. They became more appreciative of relationships as an important contributor to their well-being. Women, by contrast, were more *in search of themselves*. They developed self-confidence, assertiveness, and an independence they had not known before. Widowhood seemed to force on them the freedom to develop. Women developed a new appreciation of themselves, and men developed a new appreciation of others. The new relationships each sex developed seemed to allow for interdependence and mutuality rather than distance or dependency. They seemed to find new excitement in their lives, in their appreciation of the new dimensions of themselves that they had discovered, in their new involvements in volunteer community projects, and in the widowed groups to which they belonged.

IMPACT OF A MUTUAL HELP EXPERIENCE

I also wanted to know how the respondents evaluated the impact of their experience in their mutual help organizations on the way they coped with their widowhood. The following quote reflects what most people thought:

> "TLA has given me a good feeling of belonging. I have so many new friends, I feel as if I have known them all my life, though I only met them 10 months ago. TLA has lightened my fears and feelings, helped me overcome the fifth-wheel syndrome; given me a means to help others by understanding and listening and sharing myself; and to have an active social life."

The group was a social arena in which members felt cared about and had the opportunity to care for others. Since the main thrust of my analysis was on the differences between widows and widowers, I wondered if the mutual help experience was different for women and men. I assumed that women coping with the situation of giving up a relationship needed access both to new relationships and to new learning opportunities. To try simply to replace the lost relationship with a new one of the same sort would mean exchanging a past dependency for a new one. In *Helping Women Cope with Grief* I proposed that relationships available in a mutual help exchange can be seen as linking opportunities (Silverman, 1981) or, in Goffman's words (1963), as a bridge between the past and the future. In a sense they are transitional relationships with functions similar to transitional objects (Winnicott, 1953).

The questionnaires were filled with responses from women who seemed to support this view:

> "The wide range of ages and interests means there's someone and something for everyone who all have widowhood in common."

> "First it made me feel I wasn't the only one in the same situation. Secondly, it made me more outgoing and inclined to offer whatever I could to help others."

Based on the analysis in the prior sections of this chapter, we might hypothesize that a man would not require such linking relationships when accommodating to the death of his wife. On the contrary, my respondents included both widows and widowers valuing the helping opportunities available to them. Men and women had similar needs for peers and valued the relationships available in a mutual help group.

What was different was the goal of the help. A widower of several years said: "Men need help admitting their feelings." Women needed help in developing their confidence:

"Not only did WPS occupy my time and my mind. I began to feel that I can do things on my own."

"It gave me permission to be a different person. It made me feel and understand that there is no written creed that says you have to be married to be happy."

The helping process was not different for men and women. An equal proportion of similar answers was found in both groups. The need to share feelings was emphasized, even though some of the men admitted this was not easy for them. Women wrote about feelings more easily.

"I often wonder how I would have survived. The first year all we did was share our feelings and emotions every step of the way."

"They wouldn't let me run away. They let me cry . . . and finally I believed them when they said it would get better."

As a result of talking, people developed a sense of optimism, of hope:

"I began to see from others who had coped, who looked happy and had made it, that I had something to look forward to."

In addition to expressing feelings, they found the information they received valuable. They learned about benefits, and about the grief cycle.

"The lectures were helpful and the grief workshop was very good. Widowed people need a perspective on what is happening to them."

In this kind of atmosphere being widowed was acceptable. Since they were not alone with their pain, they did not have to hide their feelings or put up a front. They could even find some pleasure:

"TLA came along at the right time to help me get involved in new friendships. It kept me connected to others. My friends had disappeared and every other group I went to were couples."

"I became much less selfish with my time for others. I became much more understanding of the problems of the newly widowed."

When asked to comment specifically on what they got out of being a member, half of the respondents talked of getting a feeling of being needed from helping others and thus acquiring a purpose in life. There were no differences on this question in the responses between the sexes. Almost all the respondents commented on the feeling of being needed as a consequence of being involved, not as a reason for involvement. The role of helper provided a valuable and meaningful way of being connected to others and to themselves: "In helping others I helped myself."

NEXT STEPS

In preparing the paper for presentation in England I began to value the data I collected even more than before. While I had identified a direction of change, I had not been able to clearly connect my findings to existing theories of adult development. I needed more data. I decided to take the questionnaire to England. By this time I, too, had changed. I was ready to be more assertive in my approach to data collection. The conference sponsors, The Cruse Club of England, duplicated the questionnaire for me, and I asked the conference participants to fill it out before I presented my paper so that their response would not be influenced by my thinking. When I was present to get the data, I got a response rate of 80%. All but one of the participants were women. They came primarily from Great Britain and Western Europe, with a representative group from Australia and North America. Those who were bilingual helped their friends by translating the questions, which they answered in either French or German. Others helped to translate the answers as well. Answering the questionnaire became a community project. The informal feedback was very positive. Some women and the lone widower reported that they had gained a new perspective on their widowhood; they saw this as a learning experience. All of this encouraged me to continue to collect data in this way. I now had 100 new questionnaires; about 12 of them would need to be translated before I could use them.

I still needed more data from men to explore the idea of differences more fully. In England I met Genevieve Ginzburg from Arizona, president of a large widow-to-widow program in which many widowers were active. She agreed to distribute the questionnaires to her membership. I called the Widowed Person's Service and asked Lowensohn if they could again distribute the questionnaire at their 1985 annual meeting. Like many researchers, I was pursuing these sources of data knowing that my current work commitments would leave me almost no time to work with the data on my own. But I did not want to let these opportunities pass.

In August 1985 the University of Massachusetts Gerontology Center issued a request for proposals for a small grant to be awarded to researchers who would become Community Fellows of the Center for the 1985–86 academic year. I submitted a proposal to hire a research assistant who would analyze the new data and complete the analysis of the original data. I was awarded the fellowship. My daughter, Nancy Silverman Tobi, a graduate student in sociology, is my research assistant. She is working at home on our family computer and, like me, is blending her professional and personal lives. This research position allows her to be gainfully employed on a part-time basis while she is at home caring for her new baby. Under the terms of the fellowship the data had to be presented in the form of a publishable paper by May 1986, and we met that goal (Silverman, in press).

CONCLUSION

There is, in fact, no conclusion to this chapter. The research is in process. Just as I do not think it is possible to recover from grief but think instead that people are irrevocably changed by the experience, so, too, I know I do not end a research project, but rather am changed by it. My thinking is usually informed in a different fashion from before, leading me to a new phase of study. The past becomes prologue. In essence I am saying that my self as a researcher is not separate from my self in other roles as a living, interacting, changing person. The same rhythm that guides my life guides my research. I seem to have no need to compartmentalize my life in such a way that my professional self is separate from my personal self. In the early days of the women's movement, women were counseled not to mention their families or in any way make them part of the workplace. Women's experience was not legitimated. Instead, we were encouraged to emulate what, for a lack of a better term, can be called a male model of research, which usually was assumed to be disembodied quantitative research. I could never comfortably follow this model. I was a "closet" qualitative researcher. I felt stigmatized by my inability to conform and make what seemed to me unproductive distinctions. My experience as a wife and mother informed my work. I could not deny the strong connections (see Martin, 1985, for a further discussion on the impact of women's reproductive function on their ways of knowing). As the women's movement has matured, it has begun to search for more appropriate paradigms to guide research (Sampson, 1978; Keller, 1983; Unger, 1981). These efforts have to be joined to the sociological traditions of qualitative research described by Reinharz (1984), which have been marginal to mainstream social science for too long.

Two different views of the world are involved here, reflecting the distinction I described earlier between connected and separate knowing. Qualitative research involves connected knowing, while quantitative research subscribes more to separate knowing as a way of thinking. In the latter case we see the scientist in his sterile laboratory manipulating and controlling variables. This is the logical positivist's view of the world, following a logical, linear model in which knowledge is cumulative and everything is knowable by reducing it to its simplest elements.

In the former paradigm we see the scientist interacting with her data, as if to get inside to see how it works (Keller, 1983). The qualitative researcher is a participant in the work. Her/his interest is in describing and understanding relationships. The search is not for ultimate truths. Nor is truth achievable because these researchers are aware of how interdependent phenomena are. Kuhn (1970) describes various paradigms that have been employed in science over the centuries. He suggests that the way scientists approach data is not independent of their worldview and is, in part, a result of the way they are socialized. This would support the notion that the scientist's gender will affect his/her choice of research paradigm.

This chapter is an example of how my position as a woman influenced my epistemological position, not only in defining research questions but also in *how* I researched them. As I write I realize it also influenced how I *understood* the data I gathered. The popular view of how to deal with bereavement is to ask the mourner to let go of the past, to literally break his or her ties to it. Is this a reflection of a male view of the world that places emphasis on separateness, on externalizing experiences? Widows seem to have a hard time adhering to this model. Instead they talk of changing their relationship to the past, of reconnecting to themselves. Instead of tearing themselves away, they seem to add new relationships and new roles to their lives. The focus is on connectedness. A research paradigm that is not sensitive to these issues would lose them. The medical model using recovery as the goal misses it completely.

I have said repeatedly that I am not comfortable with dividing these ways of knowing or meaning-making into a male–female dichotomy. What becomes clear is that there is more than one way of knowing. The debate should not be between qualitative and quantitative research or along male–female lines. As widowers in my study seemed to move toward using a connected model of knowing, so, I think, science has to move in the same direction to accept that there are many ways of knowing.

REFERENCES

Belenky, M., Clinchy, B., Goldberger, N. & Tarule, J. (1986). *Women's ways of knowing: The development of self, voice and mind*. NY: Basic Books.

Caplan, G. (1963). Emotional crisis. In A. Deutch & H. Fishman (Eds.), *Encyclopedia of mental health* (Vol. 2). New York: Franklin Watts.

Clinchy, B., & Zimmerman, C. (1985). *Growing up intellectually: Issues for college women* (Working Paper No. 19). Wellesley, MA: Wellesley College, Stone Center for Developmental Services and Studies.

Conrad, P., & Reinharz, S. (Eds.). (1984). Computers and qualitative data [Special issue]. *Qualitative Sociology, 7* (1 & 2).

Erikson, E. (1963). *Childhood and society*. New York: Norton.

Gilligan, C. (1979). Women's place in man's life cycle. *Harvard Educational Review, 49,* 431–446.

Goffman, E. (1963). *Stigma*. Englewood, NJ: Prentice-Hall.

Gorer, G. (1965). *Death, grief and mourning*. London: Cresset Press.

Kaplan, A. (1964). *The conduct of inquiry: Methodology for behavioral science*. San Francisco: Chander.

Kastenbaum, R. (1977). Death and development through the life cycle. In H. Feifel (Ed.), *New meanings of death* (pp. 18–45). New York: McGraw-Hill.

Kegan, R. (1979). The evolving self: A process conception for ego psychology. *Counseling Psychologist, 8*(2), 5–34.

Kegan, R. (1983). *The evolving self*. Cambridge, MA: Harvard University Press.

Keller, E. F. (1983). *Reflections on gender and science*. New Haven, CT: Yale University Press.

Kuhn, T. (1970). *The structure of scientific revolutions* (2nd ed.). Chicago: University of Chicago Press.

Levinson, D. J. (1978). *The seasons of a man's life*. New York: Knopf.

Lindemann, E. (1944). Symptomatology and management of acute grief. *American Journal of Psychiatry, 101,* 141–149.

Lopata, H. Z. (1973). Self-identity in marriage. *The Sociological Quarterly, 14,* 407–418.

Lopata, H. Z. (1979). *Women as widows, support systems*. New York: Elsevier.

Marris, P. (1974). *Loss and change*. New York: Pantheon Books.

Martin, J. R. (1985). *Reclaiming a conversation*. New Haven, CT: Yale University Press.

Miller, J. B. (1976). *Toward a new psychology of women*. Boston: Beacon Press.

Miller, J. B. (1985). *The development of women's sense of self* (Working Paper No. 12). Wellesley, MA: Wellesley College, Stone Center for Developmental Services and Studies.

Osterweis, M., Solomon, F., & Green, M. (1984). *Bereavement: Reactions, conse-quences, and care.* Washington, DC: National Academy Press.

Perry, W. (1970). *Forms of intellectual and ethical development in the college years.* New York: Holt, Rinehart & Winston.

Perry, W. (1981). Cognitive and ethical growth: The making of meaning. In A. Chickering (Ed.), *The modern American college* (pp. 76–116). San Francisco: Jossey-Bass.

Reinharz, S. (1984). *On becoming a social scientist.* New Brunswick, NJ: Transaction Books.

Rosenblatt, P. C., Walsh, P., & Jackson, D. A. (1976). *Grief and mourning in cross-cultural perspective.* Washington, DC: HRAF Press.

Sampson, E. (1978). Scientific paradigms and social value: Wanted—A scientific revolution. *Journal of Personality and Social Psychology, 36*(11), 1332–1343.

Silverman, P. R. (1966). Services for the widowed during the period of bereave-ment. In *Social Work Practice* (pp. 170–189). New York: Columbia University Press.

Silverman, P. R. (1969). The widow-to-widow program: An experiment in preventive intervention. *Mental Hygiene, 53,* 333–337.

Silverman, P. R. (1970). The widow as caregiver in a program of preventive intervention with other widows. *Mental Hygiene, 54*(4), 540–547.

Silverman, P. R. (1981). *Helping women cope with grief.* Beverly Hills, CA: Sage.

Silverman, P. R. (1986). *Widow-to-widow.* New York: Springer.

Silverman, P. R. (1987). In search of new selves: Accommodating to widow-hood. In L. A. Bond and B. M. Wagner (Eds.), *Families in transition: Primary prevention programs that work.* Beverly Hills, CA: Sage.

Silverman, P. R. (in press). Widowhood as the next stage in the lifecycle. In H. Z. Lopata (Ed.), *Widows: North America.* Durham, NC: Duke University Press.

Silverman, P. R., MacKenzie, D., Pettipas, M., & Willson, E. (Eds.), (1975). *Helping each other in widowhood.* New York: Health Sciences Publishing.

Silverman, S. M. (1979). The clouded crystal ball: Comments on geophysical predictions. In R. F. Donnelly (Ed.), *Solar-terrestrial predictions proceedings* (Vol. II) (pp. 722–733). Washington, DC: National Oceanic and Atmosphere Administration.

Sullivan, H. S. (1962). *Schizophrenia as a human process.* New York: W. W. Norton & Co.

Unger, R. K. (1981, August). *Through the looking glass: No wonderland yet.* Presiden-tial address to Div. 35, American Psychological Association, Los Angeles, CA.

VanGennup, A. (1960). *The rites of passage.* Chicago: University of Chicago Press.

Winnicott, D. W. (1953). Transitional objects and transitional phenomena: A study of first not me possessions. *The International Journal of Psychoanalysis, 34,* 89–97.

13

Ethnographic Research
on Aging

J. Kevin Eckert

The ethnographic case study, with its emphasis on participant-observation and holism, has had a strong influence on the anthropological study of old age. Numerous ethnographic accounts are available of the daily lives of older persons living in urban hotels (Eckert, 1980; Siegal, 1978; Stephens, 1976; Teski, 1979), retirement communities (Jacobs, 1974; Johnson, 1971), apartments (Hochschild, 1973), senior high-rises (Francis, 1984; Jacobs, 1975; Ross, 1977), and nursing homes (Gubrium, 1975; Kayser-Jones, 1981) or using senior centers (Hazan, 1980; Myerhoff, 1978).

The methods employed in much of this research are qualitative and include extended residence in the community, meticulous record keeping (census taking, map making, minute behavioral descriptions), casual and serendipitous observation, informal and formal intensive interviewing, and first-hand participation in as many life events as possible. In most cases the researcher enters the field alone rather than as a member of a research team. The researcher also targets observations on key individuals and events with the assumption that the "community" is more or less homogeneous and representative of some larger whole. This assumption may be linked to the kinds of settings studied, i.e., well-defined and bounded social niches. In this sense the method is extremely well suited for identifying significant patterns of cultural behavior in terms of a local setting.

However, there are shortcomings in some of these studies and their approach. Many ethnographic studies lack an attempt by the ethnographer to test or verify hunches using research routines whereby a hypothesis can be disproved. While propositions and hypotheses are advanced with considerable descriptive supporting evidence, they are typically not presented in a manner permitting falsification. As Pelto and Pelto suggest (1978), ethnographic research should develop clearer standards for potential falsification. Operations essential for falsification include the careful definition, observation, and measurement of concepts and the specification of research operations.

When information about selection procedures of informants, settings, and other units for analysis are omitted, generalizability is impaired. For example, studies that focus on one senior citizen center, one hotel, or one apartment building are severely limited in what they can tell us about life beyond those settings. In such cases the researcher must be cautious about generalizing to other settings that may appear similar. Without a sampling strategy to select interviewees within a setting, even description of the setting itself must be questioned. My point is that researchers must be explicit about how settings and/or interviewees are selected and must understand the strengths and weaknesses of different sampling strategies. Both nonprobability and probability sampling have their place in ethnographic research. In my view, ethnographically oriented studies will increase our understanding of aging to the extent that these issues are addressed. In the following discussion an ethnographic research process will be presented that blends both qualitative and quantitative research. The goal is to preserve the insights and understanding derived from qualitative/experiential approaches while enhancing the ability to replicate, verify, and generalize findings.

THE ETHNOGRAPHIC RESEARCH PROCESS

It is uncommon for anthropologists to present in detail the processes and methods used in conducting ethnographic studies. In comparison with studies involving single research strategies (i.e., experiments), ethnographic studies frequently involve multiple methods applied in a complex yet logical order. The design of research processes in ethnographic studies goes unnoticed and unappreciated, since anthropologists typically summarize their approach with such phrases as "traditional ethnographic methods" or "participant-observation."

Figure 13-1 illustrates the overall ethnographic research process developed in an eight-year longitudinal study of older hotel dwellers

Figure 13-1

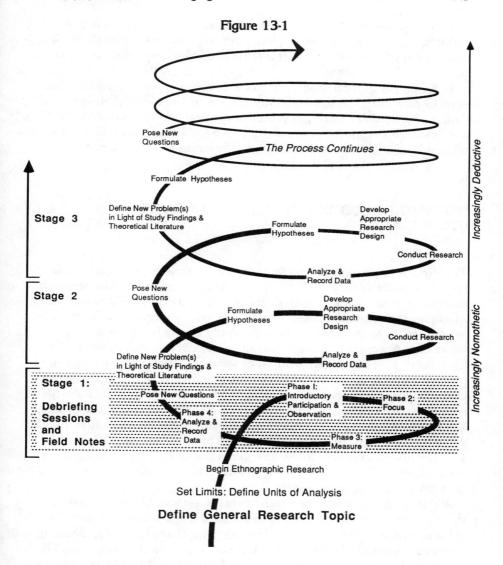

living in an urban area undergoing revitalization and development. The project was called the "Unseen Community: Old Nonwelfare Poor in Urban Hotels." Visually, Figure 13-1 appears as a spiral. As the research process moves through time, the procedures used and questions asked become increasingly focused. At the beginning stages of research, exploration, detailed description, and understanding the social organization of the setting are of prime concern. As the research process unfolds, greater emphasis is placed on explanation through testing specific hypotheses related to relevant theoretical constructs and questions.

The following discussion presents a processual history of the "Unseen Community" study, with illustrations of the kinds of insight and data it produced. The process presents a logical and reasonably systematic research design for community based field studies. I will draw on my study, *The Unseen Elderly* (1980), to illustrate this diagram.

DEFINING THE COMMUNITY AND SETTING THE STUDY LIMITS

The first step in conducting any research project is to formulate a specific research problem and related research questions. The research problem posed at the onset of Stage 1 is usually quite general. For example, the general problem might be the description of a unique setting, issue or population. While a study might focus on any one of these dimensions, it could include all three. For example, the "Unseen Community" study began with an observation that became a research problem. It was observed, in the process of conducting another study, that old people who lived in center-city hotels in San Diego, California, were poor but refused welfare (SSI) even when they were eligible for it. While the downtown environment appeared harsh, the older hotel dwellers seemed to be doing well in spite of immense odds (Bohannan, 1981). This observation led to the general research question: how do these older adults who live in single hotel rooms adjust and survive in a changing urban environment?

A critical issue in any research involves setting limits and defining the study population or units for examination and analysis in meaningful and precise terms. In the "Unseen Community" study, defining community required immediate attention. How could "community" be conceptualized and what meanings could be attached to it? Community can be conceptualized from two quite different points of view, that of the "outsider" (the etic perspective) or that of the "insider" (the emic perspective). Outsiders (typically researchers, planners, or service providers) define community on the basis of conceptual divisions dictated by political, social, or scientific objectives. Such definitions tend to be couched in the language of objectivity and precision, divorced from the culturally specific meanings and implications present in any naturally occurring situation.

Insiders' definitions of community, on the other hand, are based on the set of perceptions and models residents themselves hold. The differences between insiders' and outsiders' perceptions can be quite distinct. For example, the Stage 1 ethnography of residents living in hotels showed that different perceptions of the downtown area existed, depending upon whether one lived within or outside the area (Eckert, 1980). Many older hotel dwellers regarded the downtown as "home" and perceived the several blocks surrounding their hotels as providing them with an infrastructure of supportive services and opportunities for activity.

In contrast, city planners, the media, and the general public perceived the area to be a "skid row" or "Tenderloin." Deteriorating buildings, pawn shops, massage parlors, pornographic book stores, cheap hotels, vagrants on street corners, all reinforced their negative perceptions. In general, outsiders disapproved of the area and perceived it as blighted and a detriment to the city. From the outsiders' viewpoint, little attention was given to the heterogeneity of people who lived in and used the area. Old people who lived quietly in hotels were not differentiated from those who were more visible and actively troublesome (e.g., drifters, winos, vagrants). All were seen as somehow deviant, transient, and contributing to the area's "blight" and problems. From this point of view, the approach to the problem was simple: refurbish old buildings, build new ones, and move out the undesirables to other less visible areas of town.

Three themes continually reappear in the literature on community: the idea of territory or place, the idea of group membership or "we feeling," and the idea of social organization or structure (Ross, 1977). Each theme can be understood from the viewpoint of the insider or the outsider. For example, city planners rely heavily on community as place when they assess property values, plan services and projects, and conduct studies. Typically, community is defined as an aggregate of blocks or census tracts for which various sorts of data are tabulated. For this research the formal study area consisted of a 16-block area targeted for redevelopment and investment as a downtown retail, entertainment, and residential complex.

Community as place can also be defined from the point of view of those who live in it. Here the concept of community becomes individualized and akin to what we typically call "neighborhood"; it can be an apartment building, a street, a cluster of houses, or a named locale. This particular view of community has been very important in ethnographic studies of the elderly, since it represents the immediate context in which daily life unfolds and to which meanings and feelings are attached. This has much in common with what Rowles calls "geographical experience," i.e., the totality of an individual's involvement within the spaces and places of his or her life (Rowles, 1978, p. 18).

Intimately connected with the insiders' view of community as place is the notion of community as engendering a sense of "we feeling" or group identity and cohesion. This definition emphasizes those factors that allow people to view themselves as similar or dissimilar to others. Community as "we feeling" focuses attention on cultural or subcultural factors (e.g., shared ethnic identity, age, social status, or language) that cause a group of people to interact with each other in overlapping social networks, to share common interests, outlooks, and problems, and to participate in common institutions. A typical goal in ethnographies of old age is to uncover factors that engender group identity and cohesion and relate these to quality of life or well-being.

Finally, community can be defined as a collection of institutions with physical, personal, and social components. These institutions form the social structure and organization of an area and again can be viewed from the insider's or outsider's point of view. In the study of older hotel dwellers, key institutions providing structure for hotel life included the hotels, local restaurants, public transportation, the police, and hospitals (Eckert, 1980). While outsiders identified some of the same institutions as important, the meanings they attached to them were different from those of insiders who used them. The most obvious difference concerned the hotels themselves. Outsiders viewed them as depressing, dirty, and dangerous places, while residents viewed them as "home." Older residents saw local restaurants as critical for survival, while outsiders saw them as substandard "greasy spoons." Therefore, in any ethnographic field study, the researcher must be clear about what is meant by "community." In attempting to describe community as completely as possible, both internal and external perceptions should be taken into account.

STAGE 1: DESCRIPTION AND EXPLORATION

After the general problem has been determined and the units of analysis and study boundaries have been demarcated, ethnographic research is ready to begin. This stage is typically descriptive and exploratory, i.e., the researcher is not testing precisely defined hypotheses. Instead, data collection is aimed at generating insightful propositions relevant to the general problem under study.

The ethnographic stage of research is best suited to situations in which the researcher desires to make sense of an ongoing process that cannot be predicted in advance. Therefore, the first stage is designed so that the researcher can make initial observations and develop tentative general propositions. After formulating tentative propositions, the researcher makes further focused observations. On the basis of those observations, propositions are modified and refined (Babbie, 1979). The strongest features of the initial ethnographic phase of research are (1) the continual feedback of new information and insights to either corroborate previous observations and/or guide future observations and (2) the interplay between the worldview of insiders (the emic perspective) and outsiders (the etic perspective).

If the researcher is to gain access to the insider's beliefs, attitudes, and behaviors, it is necessary to become immersed in the "community" under study. Involvement may range from full-time living and participation in the setting to living outside the study area and remaining uninvolved (Spradley, 1980). In the "Unseen Community" study it was desirable to live in the study area and participate extensively in everyday life. Because I moved into a typical downtown hotel and lived there for one year, I was forced to challenge ethnocentric outsiders' notions about hotel life and residents. After living in a hotel for several months, I was offered a job as a desk clerk, which provided a legitimate and highly visible work role. Living and working in a hotel facilitated my being accepted and trusted by older residents. Since older people in the area viewed "the young" in hostile terms (i.e., they referred to them as "hustlers," "welfare bums," or "druggies"), my working and living there provided a steady personal exposure that allowed trust in me and subsequent rapport to develop.

Intensive round-the-clock involvement as a hotel desk clerk revealed the rhythms, benefits, and drawbacks associated with hotel life. The role of researcher-as-resident-and-desk-clerk required learning rules and norms necessary for successful adjustment to hotel life, rules that applied to residents of all ages. Continual involvement with persons living and working in the downtown area and observation of everyday life provided the opportunity for intuitive understanding of the insider's perspective and serendipitous discoveries that would not appear using less participatory research methods.

Participating in hotel life and becoming familiar with residents, hotel staff, and other functionaries in the downtown environment enhanced the reliability of the data collected. First-hand observations were made of what people actually did and were evaluated in relationship to what they said they did. It was possible to cross-check and reevaluate what people said and did over time. For example, older hotel dwellers frequently referred to themselves as "loners" and as persons who "minded their own business and didn't bother anyone." However, these very same people, when observed over time in daily activities, had cordial and friendly relationships with other residents, hotel staff, and shopkeepers. While they were self-proclaimed "loners," they engaged in social interaction on a regular basis and had social networks to support their needs.

Extensive participant-observation and informal interviewing allowed me to construct grounded survey instruments to be used with a larger randomly selected sample of hotel residents. Involvement with older hotel dwellers prior to the construction of interview questions accomplished several tasks. First, the meaningfulness and relevance of the questions asked were greatly enhanced. Second, categories of questions essential for understanding hotel life were discovered. For example, it was learned that an individual's functional capacity was a critical element for successful hotel adjustment. Therefore, questions pertaining to activities of daily living were added to the survey instrument. In this way the survey instruments that were eventually developed asked questions relevant to the lives of older hotel residents.

Bohannan (1981) has detailed the steps followed in field work and data analysis in the "Unseen Community" study. His discussion builds on the general outline of stages in participant-observation presented by Ross and Ross (1974). To summarize briefly, the Stage 1 study progressed through four related phases.

Phase 1

Phase 1 involved introductory participation and observation. The central task during this phase was to learn about the community—who were the actors in the setting, where did they go, and what did they do. For example, hotels were found to have two distinct categories of residents, those who were permanent and those who were transient. There was minimal interaction between these two groups. Permanent residents could be divided into several groups: the older retirees, the middle-aged unemployed, and younger welfare recipients. The hotel staff could also be divided into distinct categories: the manager, desk clerks, and housekeepers.

Another important task during the first phase of ethnographic research is to become comfortable in a set of roles acceptable to oneself and those being studied. This task is not always easily achieved, and it is not uncommon for several roles to be tried before a compatible one is found. For example, in the "Unseen Community" study my role changed through time. I began my research as an observer who lived in the area. I presented myself as a research associate of a local research institute. As time progressed, and as I became part of the social setting, my participation became more direct. When I became a hotel desk clerk, I was thrust into the normal flow of hotel social transactions. In the role of desk clerk I was able to establish relationships with several long-term residents of the hotel, as well as become acquainted with all the employees of the hotel. In this position I observed and participated in transactions with the police, vice squad, community mental health workers, and other social service personnel. This sort of direct participation in the lives of older hotel residents allowed me to observe the social structure and organization of the hotel.

Several methods were used to collect data during Phase 1. Considerable time was spent simply identifying and observing key behavioral settings where older retirees spent time—hotel lobbies, TV rooms, restaurants, and park benches. When I spent time in these settings, I informally interviewed the persons who used them. Extensive field notes were kept that recorded as much as possible about all aspects of life in the downtown area.

At regular intervals varying from one to three weeks, depending on need, I would get together with Paul Bohannan, the principal investigator for the study, and review my field notes in detail. As noted by Bohannan (1981), the need to explain the situation to the principal investigator made for greater detail than could be achieved in written notes. The task of the principal investigator was to ask probing questions. Sometimes, through the process of sharing experiences and responding to questions, whole new dimensions were discovered for investigation. These *debriefing* sessions were tape-recorded, subsequently transcribed, and then meticulously annotated and indexed. Categories that emerged during this process were a combination of emic and etic topics. For example, an emic category of "friendship" emerged on the basis of what people said about their relationships. An etic category called "sociality" differentiated among types of observed social interactions. Categories were created as the field work and preliminary analysis progressed.

Phase 2

The second phase of ethnographic research began approximately four months after entering the field when I noted extensive repetition in observations (see Glaser & Strauss, 1967). This phase represents a narrowing of focus on key items that emerged during Phase 1. For example, several themes came up over and over again in the initial stage of field work. Medical problems and responses, social organization, food, and psychological adjustment were all issues that had to be explored in greater detail. During this phase, observations and informal interviews focused on each of these issues.

Formal life-history interviews with key informants, e.g., hotel residents, desk clerks, maids, and others, were also begun at this time. The life-history interviews followed a uniform outline that included such general questions as early life experiences; marital, work, and health histories; life events and stresses; experiences with hotel living. The interviews were conducted in a conversational format, tape-recorded, and then transcribed.

Phase 3

Phase 3 emerged when it became essential to learn precisely *how many* did what, when, and where. The development of a sampling strategy that allowed for greater representation of older hotel residents and a contextually relevant interview schedule became critical concerns. During this phase we administered three structured interviews to a panel of 82 residents, a sample derived from all men over the age of 50 living in 12 hotels (for details of sampling procedure and findings, see Erickson and Eckert, 1977; Eckert, 1980). The first questionnaire dealt with sociality, security, and other important topics garnered from participant-observation. The second and third focused on health, social networks, and supports. Bohannan (1981, pp. 41–42) clarified the relationship between these methods:

> The questionnaires offered us hard data about the categories and ideas that had turned up in the participant observation. None of the quantitative material we obtained by means of survey research techniques could have been obtained through observation alone, although the questions or their suitability could not have been determined without the observations. One needs both.

Phase 4

The fourth phase in the ethnographic study involved analysis and synthesis of the different types of information obtained from the various methodologies and sources utilized. Quantitative numerical data collected through panel interviews were enriched by direct observations made by the field worker, life-history interviews, daily diaries, and informal interviews.

The four-year ethnographic study of the downtown redevelopment area, its hotels, and residents taught us a great deal, including the fact that hotels provided the basic social structure and served as an important source of social support for older residents. When an individual rented a room, he/she also received housekeeping services. The hotels provided furniture, linens, heat, telephone, and considerable security. Hotel desk clerks, maids, and other residents were an important part of the social support system. Not only hotels, but also the larger urban environment, provided an infrastructure of needed goods and services, thus making the downtown a practical alternative for some portion of the elderly population. The older hotel residents themselves were found to be very independent and self-reliant individuals in reasonably good functional health, a prerequisite for positive adjustments to hotel life. Since much of daily life was lived within the bounds of an area targeted for redevelopment, we hypothesized that the forthcoming demolition of much of the area would affect them significantly and harshly.

STAGE 2 OF THE ETHNOGRAPHIC RESEARCH PROCESS: HYPOTHESIS TESTING AND EXPLANATION

In the process of doing ethnography it is common for questions to emerge that have theoretical significance, can be formally stated as hypotheses, and can be tested. While ethnographers frequently state that one of the goals of ethnographic description is to generate hypotheses, they do not often follow through with the research necessary to test these propositions. I believe, however, that a key component of the ethnographic research process is to follow through in testing the relevant propositions that emerge from in-depth ethnography. In this case a central goal was to determine the short-term effects (approximately eight months) of involuntary relocation on the health, social networks, activity patterns, and psychosocial adjustment of older persons living in hotels within the community we studied. The second stage of research sought to answer a naturally emerging question left unanswered in the first stage ethnography. In broad terms, we sought to test hypotheses related to the stresses associated with forced environmental change among the elderly. This question fit into a large theoretical literature on relocation stress and in that sense was more nomothetic than idiographic. Since formal hypotheses were formulated and tested, our research design became deductive rather than inductive.

However, even in the second stage of study a strong ethnographic perspective was maintained. This perspective called for the description of the processes and procedures associated with relocation. Initially, relocation was viewed simply as the voluntary or involuntary move of persons from one type of living environment to another. However, as the Stage 2 study progressed, it became evident that relocation as implemented in this case was a far more complex process. For example, while the relocation process could be classified as involuntary (i.e., the city condemned hotels and forced the residents to move), relocatees were given a choice in selecting their postrelocation housing. Thus, their sense of control was not completely obliterated. Since they could remain in the downtown environment and relocate into similar hotels, they could retain some control over their environment. The process of relocation as it unfolded was multifaceted and complex rather than uni-dimensional and simple.

Stage 2 in the anthropological research process was closely related to Stage 1. In fact, the questions that Stage 2 research sought to answer were derived from insights gained in the previous ethnography. Fur-thermore, the focus of the research, a specific population living in a bounded geographic locale and with whom we were familiar, remained the same. Rapport and familiarity with the population accounted for a very low interviewee refusal rate. In addition, biases associated with sample loss could be eliminated on the basis of previous data and insights from Stage 1 research.

In Stage 2 research there is less need for generating conceptual description and greater need for measuring responses to specific re-search questions related to past findings and/or theoretical issues. To address such issues quasi-experimental research designs must be imple-mented. For example, Stage 2 of the "Unseen Community" project utilized a nonequivalent control group design (Brim & Spain, 1974). Older adults forced to move from downtown hotels were compared with a matched group living in contiguous hotels who were *not* forced to relocate. This design was the most powerful and appropriate for a naturally occurring relocation process over which we could exert no control. The method of data gathering was a structured one-hour interview to obtain information on physical health status, functional status, basic demographic characteristics, and general attitudes con-cerning the environment and relocation.

In the "Unseen Community" project, Stage 2 research found that characteristics of the relocation process, such as financial assistance and allowing relocatees to move into other local hotels, coupled with characteristics of the relocatees themselves, such as dispersed social networks and good functional status, helped to explain a lack of negative short-term health effects. The findings from the Stage 2 research resulted in posing a new research question, namely, what would be the longer-term impact of forced relocation on the health and well-being of older hotel dwellers? We suspected that those persons forced to relocate might experience a delayed reaction to the move as their rental assistance money was spent and the availability of decent and affordable rooms decreased. Through continued observation and interviewing, we found that while other hotel rooms in the downtown area were offered to the relocatees in the short run, environmental changes were so extensive that older persons living on fixed resources were beginning to complain about high rents, lack of inexpensive restaurants to eat in, and few shops in which to buy essential goods. To explore the question of longer-range effects, we proposed a third-stage study—one that would address this question as well as assess the physical changes in the downtown area over an eight-year period of time.

STAGE 3: THE LONGER-TERM EFFECTS OF DISPLACEMENT AND RELOCATION ON THE URBAN ELDERLY

The third stage in the research process sought to assess the longer-term (24–28 months) impact of involuntary relocation and large-scale environmental change on the health and well-being of older persons living in urban residential hotels. This study was more tightly focused than Stage 2 and was aimed at understanding in greater depth and detail the process of relocation. It extended the quasi-experimental research design and survey methods used in Stage 2.

This stage answered the questions: how does forced relocation affect the physical and mental health and functional status of relocatees? Our expectation that relocatees would experience a delayed decline in health was not supported. In general, neither those forced to relocate nor those in the matched comparison group experienced significant changes in physical, functional, or emotional health in the longer term. Qualitative understanding of the process of relocation, nature of the environmental change, social services available to older residents, and their personal characteristics, learned through in-depth longitudinal study, helped to interpret the quantitative findings.

CONCLUSION

The multistage ethnographic research process has several basic advantages when compared to single research designs. First, the initial stage allows for the discovery of grounded theory, emic concepts, and categories. As such, this increases the validity of the research questions asked and enhances operationalization of concepts during later, more deductive stages of investigation. Second, the ethnographic research process emphasizes the complementary nature of qualitative and quantitative methodologies. The question is not either this method or that method, but what approach is most appropriate to examine a particular question at a particular point in the research process. Finally, the ethnographic research process draws attention to qualities inherent in all good research, i.e., the careful definition of concepts, strategies for organizing observations (sampling), and specification of research operations so as to enhance replicability. In the research process I have described, Stages 1 through 3 were tightly intertwined, feeding back information and insight one into the other. Initial inductive and idiographic strategies melded into increasingly deductive and nomothetic strategies. The observational and qualitative data informed and guided the efforts to quantify and test given hypotheses.

The ethnographic research process is a systematic and holistic process of discovery and, at its best, should be ecologically sensitive, i.e., it should consider the older individual in his or her primary group(s), functional locale, and "community." The approach provides process data rather than the typical snapshot supplied through one-shot survey interviews. The longitudinal nature of the design allows for the cross-checking and rechecking of what people say and do. This fact increases the reliability and accuracy of the data. Similarly, the use of multiple methods and strategies (or designs) serves to alleviate the weaknesses inherent in any single design. Furthermore, the initial descriptive stage in the research process optimizes the investigator's sensitivity to the perceptions and feelings of the population being studied. This reduces the likelihood of making erroneous assumptions and conclusions about the group, as might occur when adopting an etic perspective *a priori*.

REFERENCES

Babbie, E. (1979). *The practice of social research*. Belmont, CA: Wadsworth Publishing Co.

Bohannan, P. J. (1981). Unseen community: The natural history of a research project. In D. A. Messerschmidt (Ed.), *Anthropologists at home in North America* (pp. 29–45). New York, NY: Cambridge University Press.

Brim, J. A., & Spain, D. H. (1974). *Research design in anthropology: Paradigms and pragmatics in the testing of hypotheses.* New York: Holt, Rinehart & Winston.

Eckert, J. K. (1980). *The unseen elderly.* San Diego, CA: The Campanile Press.

Erickson, R. J., & Eckert, J. K. (1977). The elderly poor in downtown San Diego hotels. *The Gerontologist, 17*(5), 440–446.

Francis, D. (1984). *Will you still need me, will you still feed me, when I'm 84.* Bloomington: Indiana University Press.

Glaser, B., & Strauss, A. (1967). *The discovery of grounded theory.* Chicago: Aldine.

Gubrium, J. F. (1975). *Living and dying at Murray Manor.* New York: St. Martins.

Hazan, H. (1980). *The limbo people.* London: Routledge and Kegan Paul.

Hochschild, A. (1973). *The unexpected community.* Englewood Cliffs, NJ: Prentice-Hall.

Jacobs, J. (1974). *Fun city.* New York: Holt, Rinehart & Winston.

Jacobs, J. (1975). *Older persons and retirement communities.* Springfield, IL: Charles C. Thomas.

Johnson, S. K. (1971). *Idlehaven.* Berkeley, CA: University of California Press.

Kayser-Jones, J. (1981). *Old, alone and neglected: Care of the aged in Scotland and the United States.* Berkeley, CA: University of California Press.

Myerhoff, B. (1978). *Number our days.* New York: Simon & Schuster.

Pelto, P. J., & Pelto, G. H. (1978). *Anthropological research: The structure of inquiry* (2nd ed.). Cambridge, England: Cambridge University Press.

Ross, J. K. (1977). *Old people, new lives.* Chicago: University of Chicago Press.

Ross, J. K., & Ross, M. H. (1974). Participant observation in political research. *Political Methodology, 1,* 63–88.

Rowles, G. D. (1978). *Prisoners of space?* Boulder, CO: Westview Press.

Siegal, H. A. (1978). *Outposts of the forgotten.* New Brunswick, NJ: Transaction Books.

Spradley, J. (1980). *Participant observation.* New York: Holt, Rinehart & Winston.

Stephens, J. (1976). *Loners, losers, and lovers.* Seattle, WA: University of Washington Press.

Teski, M. (1979). *Living together.* Washington, DC: University Press of America.

14

Combining Qualitative and Quantitative Data in the Study of Elder Abuse

Karl Pillemer

Researchers in the field of aging have successfully employed designs that combine the collection of quantitative and qualitative data (Connidis, 1981, 1983; Marshall, 1981). Connidis (1981) offers evidence that including qualitative components in a survey design can, among other benefits, allow for elaboration of answers to closed-ended survey items; provide needed context in which quantitative data can be interpreted; and suggest novel strategies of inquiry within the ongoing research project. Despite such valuable work, there are still few descriptive accounts of the efficacy of multiple-method designs in the study of aging. Because of the potential of increased research costs, investigators will wish to be reasonably certain of the value of combining methods before they undertake such designs.

The goal of this chapter is not to offer a general justification for developing triangulated designs; such arguments have been presented eloquently elsewhere (see Denzin, 1978). Instead, my aim is to provide three detailed examples from a recent study that demonstrate concretely the utility of a multiple-method approach. Using data from a study of physical abuse of elderly individuals, I will demonstrate how research insights can be obtained by combining quantitative analyses of closed-ended interview questions with qualitative data obtained from open-ended questions on the interview protocol and from tape-recorded follow-up interviews.

BACKGROUND OF THE STUDY

While domestic maltreatment of the elderly may not be a new phenomenon (see Stearns, 1986), it has come to the attention of the public as a "social problem" only recently. Since the late 1970s, a number of exploratory studies have been carried out on elder abuse and neglect (Block & Sinnott, 1979; Lau & Kosberg, 1979; Douglass, Hickey, & Noel, 1980; Sengstock & Liang, 1982; Phillips, 1983; Wolf, Godkin, & Pillemer, 1984). These studies have verified the existence of elder abuse and have provided some preliminary data on the nature of the problem. However, the methodological limitations of most of these studies have been such that we still know relatively little about elder abuse (Pedrick-Cornell & Gelles, 1982; Johnson, O'Brien & Hudson, 1985).

In order to overcome some of these methodological weaknesses and thereby contribute to the knowledge base on domestic violence against the elderly, I undertook a case-control study of victims of physical elder abuse. The study was an exploratory one, in that it proposed and tested multiple hypotheses based on five theoretical explanations of why elder abuse might occur. These five explanations are:

1. *Intra-individual dynamics.* This theory relates abusive behavior to characteristics of the abuser, such as mental illness or alcoholism.

2. *Intergenerational transmission of violent behavior.* This theory emphasizes a "cycle of violence," in which persons who are exposed to violence as children employ identical techniques in their later relationships with others.

3. *Dependency.* One variant of this theory attributes abuse to the excessive dependency of the old person, which becomes a source of stress for caregivers, who then respond with violence. An alternative theory has also been proposed, which argues that the dependency of the *abuser* is a predictor of abuse.

4. *External stress.* This view holds that factors beyond the internal dynamics of the family can produce stress for individuals, which in turn increases the likelihood of abuse. Such factors include stressful life events and chronic economic stress.

5. *Social isolation.* There is some evidence that families in which abuse occurs tend to have weaker social networks. The presence of an active social network is thought to be a deterrent to abuse.

Each of these areas was addressed in the research project. However, in this chapter I am not concerned with providing a general overview of the study findings, but rather with offering concrete examples of the utility of combining qualitative and quantitative methods to investigate the theories listed above. Findings related to the last three theoretical issues will be presented below, but only within this specific method-ological discussion. Readers interested in the complete set of findings are referred to a more detailed report on the project (Pillemer, 1986).

METHODOLOGY

This study took place in the context of an ongoing research project—the evaluation of three Model Projects on Elderly Abuse, funded by the Administration on Aging. These sites, located in Massachusetts, New York, and Rhode Island, offered casework services to elderly (aged 60 and over) victims of maltreatment. In the three-year course of the demonstration, the Model Projects intervened in over 300 cases of physical and psychological abuse, financial exploitation, and neglect. As a component of this evaluation, a special study of a sample of physically abused old persons was conducted.

In order to improve on previous research efforts in this area, the study had several important features. First, it focused only on one type of maltreatment: physical abuse. As others have noted (Pedrick-Cornell & Gelles, 1982), conceptual problems result from lumping together cases of abuse and neglect; acts of commission differ substantially from acts of omission. The sample contained only old persons who had experienced one or more acts of physical abuse, defined as "the inflic-tion of physical pain, injury, or physical coercion." This act could range from throwing an object at the other person to assaulting him or her with a knife or gun. Such acts were measured using the Conflict Tactics Scale, developed by Straus (1979).

Second, the study did not rely, as most others have, on professional accounts of maltreatment, but instead involved direct interviews with victims. Third, the study included a matched control group of non-abused elderly. Without such a control group, it is impossible to isolate factors that are associated with elder abuse. It is necessary to contrast the characteristics of the abused group with persons who are not maltreated, in order to establish characteristics unique to abusive fami-lies.

An attempt was made to interview all of the physical abuse cases at the three Model Project sites in which the staff were actively involved at the time of the study. In some cases this was impossible, due to the unwillingness or incapacity of the clients. As a result, roughly two-thirds of the active cases were actually interviewed at each site. A control group individually matched on sex and living arrangement was selected from the nonabused caseload of the Massachusetts site, a large, multiservice provider of home care to the elderly.

One additional aspect of the design needs to be noted. The interview with the abuse victims contained questions that dealt with the relationship between the abuser and the abused. In the control interviews, these questions were asked about a member of the household who occupied the same relationship to the control elder. Thus, if the abuser in one case was an oldest child, the control elder's oldest child became the subject of questions.

I conducted all the interviews, which lasted 60–90 minutes, in person. As noted earlier, a major goal of this project was to integrate quantitative and qualitative components in its design. For this reason, the interview contained both closed-ended and open-ended questions. Various scales were used to test quantitatively hypotheses derived from the five theories of elder abuse. Many opportunities were also provided to the respondent for qualitative description, and the responses to these items were recorded in detail. Thus, a scale of stressful life events was employed, but only after the respondent had been asked: "what do you find stressful in your life right now? what do you tend to worry about?"

This qualitative approach was carried further in tape-recorded interviews with seven individuals, which I conducted as follow-ups to the first interview. While relatively unstructured, the follow-up interview focused on the respondent's description of the abusive episodes and the history of his or her relationship with the abuser. Each of these interviews lasted approximately 90 minutes and was transcribed. The interviews provided additional insight into the dynamics of the abuse situations.

The study sample consisted of 42 physically abused elders and controls. In both groups, 39 respondents were women and 3 were men. Incomes tended to be low, with 77% of the abuse group and 89% of the controls having incomes of less than $6,000 per year. The sample was almost entirely white (97.6% of the abuse group and 95.2% of the controls) and predominantly Catholic (71% of the abuse group and 69% of the controls). The abused elders tended to be younger (mean age, 70) than the controls (mean age, 75). This was due to the inclusion of three persons aged, 56, 57, and 59 in the abuse group. These three individuals were severely disabled, and for this reason the Model Project staff suspended the age guideline. Of the abusers and comparison relatives, 14 (33%) in each group were husbands, 14 (33%) were sons, 10 (24%) were daughters, 2 (5%) were daughters-in-law, and 2 (5%) were brothers.

In the remainder of this chapter, I provide three examples of the way in which combining qualitative and quantitative data provided insights beyond those that would have resulted from the use of either method alone. These examples relate to three of the theoretical foci that guided the study: external stress, social support, and dependency.

EXAMPLE 1: EXTERNAL STRESS

Although perhaps less dramatic than the following two examples, the findings related to stress point out the advantages of employing both qualitative and quantitative measures. External stress (as differentiated from the stress that results from interpersonal relationships in the family) has been found to be positively related to some forms of abuse. Gil (1971) was one of the first researchers to cite such stressors as poverty and unemployment as causes of child abuse. Using a stressful-life-events approach, Justice and Justice (1976) and Straus, Gelles, and Steinmetz (1980) found that child-abusing families experienced a greater number of such events than did families free of child abuse. No definitive data exist regarding whether a similar relationship holds in the case of elder abuse.

In the present study, the respondents were given a short stressful-life-events scale. They were asked whether, in the preceding year, anyone in the old person's household had died, had a close relative die, been ill or injured, been divorced, been married, been arrested, left the household, joined the household, lost a job, retired, or whether the household had changed residence. Affirmative responses for these items were tallied into a score for the number of stressful life events in the household which were then compared using a paired T-test. The average number of events in the abused group was significantly higher than in the control group (1.9 events to .4 events; $p < .01$).

On their own, these findings might lead us to believe that stress itself may be a factor in elder abuse. However, in each case in which interviewees responded that a stressor had occurred, they were asked to describe the event. Such data revealed that the responses to the life-events scale were confounded by the abuse situation itself. That is, in three of the variables, the abuser was involved in the stressful incident. In most of the incidents involving arrest, the abuser was arrested *because of* violence against the elder, rather than becoming violent at some point after having been arrested. Similarly, a number of abusers entered and left the household in the same year, because the situation had become untenable. When these three items were dropped, the differences in overall stress between the two groups were not statistically significant.

Thus, I was able to conclude that the two groups did not differ in stressful events *unrelated* to the abuser. Death or illness of household members did not strike the abusive families more frequently, nor did divorce or unemployment. Based on the combination of qualitative and quantitative findings, it seems reasonable to modify the stressful life events scale in a way that separates out abuser-related stress from truly *external* sources of stress.

EXAMPLE 2: SOCIAL ISOLATION

For two reasons, it is important to consider the degree of social isolation of a family as a possible contributor to elder abuse. First, there is a large body of literature supporting the thesis that social support acts as a moderator of life stress and facilitates coping with crises (for reviews of this literature, see Cobb, 1976; Wan, 1982). Researchers have found, for example, that social support has a positive impact on health status and health behavior. At least one gerontological research group (Zarit, Reever, & Bach-Peterson, 1980) found that support from kin reduced feelings of burden on the part of caregivers to the elderly. Social support resources may substantially strengthen the ability of families of the aged to cope with stress.

Second, social isolation has been found to characterize families in which child and spouse abuse occurs. Hennessey's (1979) comprehensive review of the literature suggests that child abusers are social isolates. Gil (1971) found that about half the parents in his study had lived one year or less in the home in which the abuse occurred; this is an indication that ties to the surrounding community are lacking. Justice and Justice (1976) note that abusive parents in their study tended to be "loners," while Gelles (1972) and Stark, Flitcraft, Zuckerman, Robinson, and Frazier (1981) reported similar findings for spouse abusers.

Nye (1979) provides a reasonable explanation for this aspect of abusive families, based on exchange theory. Violence that is considered to be illegitimate tends to be hidden. Detection of such violence can result in informal sanctions from friends, kin, and neighbors and formal sanctions from the police and courts. Thus he hypothesizes that child and spouse abuse will be "less frequent in families that have relatives and/or friends living nearby" (p. 36). The presence of an active social support network may thus have a deterrent effect on elder abuse as well, for it is a highly illegitimate behavior. For these reasons, the presence or absence of an active support network were assessed in this study.

The primary quantitative measure used to obtain information about the social support network was the Social Resources Rating Scale (SRRS), which is part of the Older Americans Resources and Services (OARS) instrument. This scale measures the quality and quantity of relationships with family and friends, as well as the availability of assistance should the person require it (George, Landesman, & Fillenbaum, 1982). The scale contains eight items, which can be grouped into five indices of social support. On two of these indices, significant differences were found between the two groups. One scale, which measures the amount of contacts, showed a difference between the groups, with the abused clients having significantly less contact. The second scale measures satisfaction with contacts. The abused elders were significantly more likely to be dissatisfied with their social relationships (a more detailed description of these findings appears in Pillemer, 1985b).

Based on these findings, the abused elders do appear to be more isolated. They tend to have fewer overall contacts and to score significantly lower on their subjective evaluation of their social situation. We might conclude that the critical issue is the *amount* of involvement of outsiders in the home: the greater this is, the less easily a relative can be abusive without incurring the costs of negative sanctions from others. Such a finding, as noted earlier, would certainly be consistent with research on other forms of family violence.

As before, however, the quantitative data present only one part of the total picture. One of the open-ended questions in the interview asked the respondents to describe the way in which the abuser had had an impact on their social relationships. The responses to this question revealed an aspect of the relationship that I had not anticipated. They indicated that being in an abusive relationship may not only be an *effect* of lack of social contact, but, rather, that the causal path may go in the opposite direction. That is, the abuser may prevent or inhibit outside social contact through threatening behavior, or the conflict in the situation may make others uncomfortable and therefore less likely to visit.

This interpretation of the abuse situation comes through strongly in the qualitative data. Many respondents identified the abuser as a major factor in diminished social contact. In some cases, this took the form of directly preventing interaction with friends and relatives. One abusive husband in the sample, for example, forbade his wife from calling her friends. Similarly, four of the mothers of abusive adult children noted that the behavior of the latter became worse when they (the mothers) were on the telephone. As one victim reported: "He makes it hard for me to talk on the telephone. He mimics me while I'm talking. Sometimes I just throw the phone down." This is serious, indeed, for the telephone is frequently the most important source of contact for the elderly.

In general, however, social contact was limited not because the abuser expressly forbade it, but because others found the erratic and antisocial behavior of the abuser threatening. As one abused wife reported:

> I'd like to be able to go out and enjoy myself, but my husband always gets drunk. Our children used to take us out, but now my son says he can't stand the sight of him. And I don't blame them for not caring, the way he acts. Even the grandchildren don't care anymore. . . . The family keeps away, and that hurts.

Similarly, an abused mother stated that "It's hard to invite people over. I'm embarrassed. He talks out of line sometimes." Another woman quit her "Friendly Club" because her daughter-in-law would "start screaming" whenever the club met in her home. In a third case, the husband's bizarre behavior frightened his young grandson so badly that the child was never brought back to the house. The abuser can thus be the key factor in reducing the elderly person's contact with the outside world. A vicious circle may then exist: persons who might be able to intervene to ameliorate the situation are driven away, which allows the abuser's behavior to worsen. This in turn leads to further isolation.

EXAMPLE 3: DEPENDENCY AND ELDER ABUSE

The previous two examples have demonstrated that qualitative data can lead to reinterpretation of quantitative findings. While the qualitative measures did not contradict the structured items, they shed new light on the meaning of the results obtained from the former. In my final example, the most striking feature of the qualitative data was its similarity to the quantitative findings (see Pillemer, 1985a, for a more detailed discussion). In this case, the interpretation of the closed-ended items was supported and expanded upon by the descriptive data. This example is treated at greater length for two reasons. First, the interplay of the two data sources is clearer here and provides an unusually good argument for combining both approaches. Second, the substantive findings are more important than the two already discussed because of their implications for understanding and intervening in situations of elder abuse.

In the literature on elder abuse, the belief that the dependency of elderly individuals is a major cause of the abuse is probably the most consistently asserted. This view has developed in large part from recent gerontological research on the strains on families taking care of elderly relatives (Zarit et al., 1980; Archbold, 1982; Fengler & Goodrich, 1979; Horowitz & Schindelman, 1980; Silverstone & Hyman, 1976). Based on such findings, a number of researchers have assumed that the growing dependency of an elderly person increases the likelihood that he or she will be abused.

Davidson (1979), for example, links abuse to the "crises" created by the needs of an elderly parent for care. Steinmetz (1983) has been perhaps the major proponent of this view, arguing that families undergo "generational inversion," in which the elderly person becomes dependent upon his or her children for financial, physical, and/or emotional support. This situation places the caregiver under severe stress. Similarly, King (1983, p. 8) claims that the "dependency [of the elder] is the most common precondition in domestic abuse." Thus the dependency of an old person is frequently cited as a major risk factor in maltreatment.

This form of dependency does not provide an adequate explanation of elder abuse. Many of the elderly are dependent on their relatives (Kulys & Tobin, 1980). Why are some of these dependent elderly abused and others not? Since abuse occurs in only a small proportion of families, no simple, direct correlation between the dependency of an old person and abuse exists. Indeed, some preliminary research findings indicate that an important cause of abuse may be the reverse: that is, the dependency of the *abuser* on his or her victim may lead to abuse. Wolf, Strugnell, and Godkin (1982) found a "web of mutual dependency" between abuser and abused. In two-thirds of their cases, the perpetrator was reported to be financially dependent on the victim. Phillips (1983) reported that the abused elderly in her study were no more impaired than a nonabused comparison group, and Hwalek, Sengstock, and Lawrence (1984) found the financial dependency of the caretaker to be a significant risk factor in elder abuse.

The theoretical issue raised by these findings is an important one: why would the continued dependency of an adult child or spouse upon an elderly person be associated with physical abuse? A persuasive explanation of this phenomenon can be developed from exchange theory. In his attempt to apply exchange theory to aging, Dowd (1975) asserts that "intrinsic to the concept of exchange is the notion of power." He continues: "The partner in a social exchange who is less dependent on that exchange for the gratifications he seeks enjoys a power advantage" (p. 587). This advantage can be employed to make the exchange partner comply with one's wishes. If we add to this observation Goode's (1971) point that people do not choose to use overt force when they have other resources at their disposal, then the hypothesis that the dependency of the elderly person breeds abuse can be questioned. If someone already holds much power over another, why would he or she resort to force? If the abused is severely dependent, then the abuser would have a wealth of options to force that person to comply: violence would not be necessary.

An explanation based on the family violence literature helps resolve this issue. In an attempt to identify common features of family abuse, Finkelhor (1983) notes that abuse can occur as a response to perceived powerlessness. Acts of abuse, he notes, "seem to be acts carried out by abusers to compensate for their perceived lack or loss of power" (p. 19). Thus, spouse abuse has been found to be related to a sense of powerlessness, and the physical abuse of children "tends to start with a feeling of parental impotence" (p. 19). In elder abuse, this perceived power *deficit* may be a more important factor than the notion that the abuser holds much power in the relationship. In such a situation, the abusive individual feels that he or she lacks control and seeks to restore power (Finkelhor, 1983, p. 19). Having few resources with which to do so, the person then resorts to violence.

In summary, at the outset of this study, it was thought that dependency might play an important role in elder abuse. However, it was impossible to predict who was depending on whom in these abusive relationships. Does an elderly person come to make excessive demands on caregivers, as the prevailing view holds? Does the abuser strike out in response to excessive demands made by a dependent elderly relative? Or are the abusers themselves excessively dependent on the victim, with unrealistic expectations of what the latter can provide? The study attempted to shed light on these questions.

Using quantitative measures I asked: are the abused elderly more physically impaired and in poorer health than the controls? The first measure employed to test this hypothesis was the inventory of illnesses from the Older Americans Resources and Services (OARS) instrument (George, Landesman, & Fillenbaum, 1982). The abused and nonabused groups were compared on 24 conditions, ranging from arthritis and eye problems to heart disease and cancer. The respondents were asked whether they had the condition and, if so, the degree to which it interfered with their daily activities: not at all, a little, or a great deal.

No significant differences ($p < .05$) were found between the groups on any of the illnesses, with the exception of glaucoma; even on that condition, the difference was slight. To explore this issue further, an index was constructed from the 24 illnesses with the following coding: does not have condition = 0; interferes not at all = 1; interferes a little = 2; interferes a great deal = 3. The scores for each individual were tabulated and a paired T-test was performed. No significant differences were found between cases and controls on this illness scale.

Much research has shown, however, that diagnostic condition is not as reliable an indicator of the vulnerability of the elderly as is functional impairment. That is, to what extent is the individual unable to carry out basic functions essential to daily living regardless of the presence or absence of disease? Some researchers have categorized these functions as personal activities of daily living (ADLs—bathing, dressing, ambulation, etc.) and instrumental activities of daily living (IADLs—food shopping, cooking, cleaning, etc.). Many instruments exist to assess functional status. For this study, the Index of Functional Vulnerability (IFV), which was developed at the Hebrew Rehabilitation Center for the Aged in Boston, Massachusetts (Morris, 1982), was selected.

The hypothesis that the dependency of the victim leads to abuse would indicate that the abused elders should be more impaired on each item of the IFV than are the controls. Test for differences between the groups, however, found that this was not the case; in fact, the *reverse* actually held in some instances. No significant differences were found in the following variables: needing help or having great difficulty with meal preparation; being healthy enough to walk up and down stairs without help; using a walker or wheelchair at least some of the time to get around; being able to identify the correct year; the number of days on which the person went outside of his or her dwelling in the past week; being able to feed oneself; or being unable to pursue desired activities because of poor health.

These data indicate that abused elderly were not more functionally impaired than the controls in many critical ADLs. In addition, the abused group was found to be significantly *less* impaired than the control group in certain areas. The abused individuals were less likely to need help or to have great difficulty with taking out garbage (45% in the abuse group to 71% of the controls; $p < .05$) and were more likely to report that they were healthy enough to do ordinary housework (62% to 38%; $p < .05$).

Despite these findings, it could still be argued that while those in the abused group are not more impaired in general, they may be more dependent specifically on the abusers. We must ask: do abused elders depend more on the abuser (rather than other potential helpers) than do the controls on their comparison relative? In one measure, respondents were asked whether there was someone who would care for them if they became seriously ill or disabled. Those who answered affirmatively were asked to identify the most likely helper. These responses were then coded as "helper is abuser/comparison" or "helper is other." The abused group was much less likely to name the abuser as the person they would be most likely to depend on for help (26% to 63%; $p < .01$).

In a more direct measure of the dependency of the elder on the abuser or the comparison relative, the respondent was asked directly: "people depend on each other for many things; how much do you depend on (abuser/comparison) in each of the following areas?" Respondents were asked to answer "entirely dependent," "somewhat dependent," or "independent," in each of these areas: housing, cooking or cleaning, household repair, companionship and social activities, financial support, and transportation. No significant differences were found in five of the six areas. A difference was found in financial dependency, but the abused group was more likely to be *independent* than the control group (69% to 48%; $p < .05$).

When all of the above measures were taken into consideration, the hypothesis that the impairment and dependency of an elderly person led to physical abuse was called seriously into question. None of the data tended even slightly in that direction: either no significant differences were found or the abuse group was *less* dependent than the controls. Based on the exchange perspective outlined earlier, the alternative hypothesis must be explored: that the dependency of the abuser on his or her victim is a critical predictor of abuse.

The principal quantitative measure employed to assess the extent to which the abusers or comparison relatives were dependent on the elderly respondents was a dependency index identical to that just discussed, with the questions reversed. That is, the respondent was asked: "how much does (abuser/comparison) depend on *you* in these areas?" The abusers were found to be significantly more dependent on the elderly in four areas: housing, household repair, financial assistance, and transportation. I was thus led to conclude that the abuser's dependency was a more important factor than that of the victim.

The qualitative data were entirely consistent with the quantitative findings. If anything, the general portrait of abusers as persons with strong dependencies on their victims was even clearer from the qualitative than from the quantitative data. After a number of careful readings of my notes on each respondent, as well as the transcripts of the tape-recorded interviews, it became possible to categorize the cases into three groups, according to what appeared to me to be the salient features of the dependency relationship. In eight cases, the question of dependency did not appear to be particularly salient. Issues of imbalanced exchange did not surface to a great degree in the interviews and did not seem to be important in explaining the maltreatment. In seven cases, the respondents' increased impairment had led to heavy responsibilities for the caretakers, which in turn led to heightened stress in the relationship. The abuse in these cases was thus linked to the increased dependency of the elder. In the remaining 27 cases, however, the victims supported dependent persons who maltreated them.

A few examples will help to illustrate this type of relationship.

- An elderly woman had lived with her son for six months. "He drank all the time. You never knew how he was going to come home. He wouldn't work, wouldn't pay rent." She supported him throughout this period.
- The daughter of one victim moved in with her and has never contributed in any way to her mother's support. "I support *her*. She has epilepsy and is on disability. She's supposed to give me $50.00 a month but she never does. She even stole a $25.00 gift certificate I won. We haven't gotten along ever. It's only nice when she's not here."

An interesting variant in this category was five cases in which wives were abused by severely disabled husbands they were caring for. For example:

- A frail woman, living in an elderly housing project, had had a stable relationship with her husband. He developed Alzheimer's disease and needed constant supervision. "He would beat me pretty bad, choke me. He grabbed me and said 'I'll kill you.'"

These case descriptions, like the quantitative findings presented earlier, call into question the image of the elder abuser as a usually stable, well-intentioned individual who is brought to violent behavior by the excessive demands of an old person. In these examples, the abusers appear as persons with few resources who are frequently unable to meet their own basic needs. Instead, they are heavily dependent individuals: sometimes children who have been unable to separate from their parents; sometimes disabled or demented spouses; sometimes alcoholics. Rather than being powerful in the relationship, they are relatively powerless.

The data presented here raise an important question: if the abused elder frequently holds a good deal of power in the relationship, why does he or she not get out of it? That is, why does the victim submit to abuse rather than force the abuser to leave? If we assume that people weigh the rewards and costs of any situation, we can posit either that remaining in an abusive relationship provides rewards of some kind or that leaving the relationship appears to carry too many costs. What, then, might these rewards and costs be? Definitive data were not obtained on this question, but the open-ended responses shed some light on it.

By far the most commonly given reason for staying with an abusive dependent relative stressed the formal relationship and indicated that no other choice was really available. Such responses included the following:

"I was brought up to take care of your own. Where else is he going to go?"

"You can't throw your children out."

Thus norms and generalizations were invoked that the elder person chose to live by.

Other victims elaborated on the relationship tie by expressing worry over what the relative (most often an adult child) would do without them.

"We take him back because he don't have no other place to go."

"I can't put her out. Where can I put her? I haven't got the heart. She couldn't support herself."

A few spouses cited a desire to reciprocate for past kindness.

"He's my husband. He'd do the same for me."

"I wouldn't leave him because he was a good husband when he was well."

In some cases, the victim reported that he or she would lose concrete rewards if the abuser were forced to leave. Loneliness was one consequence.

"He's all I've got in the world."

"Having her live here helped because I'm afraid of crime. It's better not to get the reputation of living alone."

Concern about grandchildren was another fear. One elderly woman was unwilling to put out her daughter-in-law for fear that she would be kept from the grandchildren:

"I lived with her for my grandchildren's sake. I didn't have the heart to say get out. I just couldn't do it. . . . I'd miss the kids. I'd be worried about the kids. At least I felt that while they were here I could see them . . . that's my main thing now, my grandchildren."

In this example, the qualitative data serve three important functions. First, on a basic level, they provide a sense of the day-to-day interactions in which dependency relationships are worked out. As such, they make this form of relationship more "real" to a reader of the research than the structured items themselves. Second, these measures provide independent information on reasons why older people choose to stay with dependent, abusive relatives. Future research can explore such issues in a more systematic fashion based on the information obtained in this study. Perhaps most important, the findings regarding dependency are both in opposition to previous research and counterintuitive. The quantitative results on their own might not be entirely convincing; however, in concert with the comparatively rich qualitative description, the findings have intuitive appeal. Thus, although the data obtained from open-ended questions do not lead to a radical reinterpretation of the quantitative findings, they increase our understanding of the findings and can guide future research.

CONCLUSION

In this chapter, I have attempted to support the idea of using multiple methods in the study of aging. I offered three examples in which the inclusion of qualitative components in an interview schedule provided important information concerning physical abuse of the elderly. The inclusion of such items did not depend on a major increase in the level of effort or cost. To be certain, some funds were needed to transcribe the tape-recorded interviews. But the relative gain in valuable insight into this perplexing problem was, I believe, well worth the cost and effort. Future investigators into the aging family would do well to consider such multiple-method designs.

REFERENCES

Archbold, P. G. (1982). An analysis of parent-caring by women. *Home Health Care Services Quarterly, 3*(2), 5–26.

Block, M. R., & Sinnott, J. D. (1979). *The battered elder syndrome: An exploratory study.* College Park, MD: University of Maryland, Center on Aging.

Cobb, S. (1976). Social support as a moderator of life stress. *Psychosomatic Medicine, 38,* 300–312.

Connidis, I. (1981). The stigmatizing effects of a problem orientation to aging research. *Canadian Journal of Social Work Education, 7*(2), 9–19.

Connidis, I. (1983). Integrating qualitative and quantitative methods in survey research on aging: An assessment. *Qualitative Sociology, 6*(4), 334–352.

Davidson, J. L. (1979). Elder abuse. In M. R. Block & J. D. Sinnott (Eds.), *The battered elder syndrome: An exploratory study* (pp. 49–55). College Park, MD: University of Maryland, Center on Aging.

Denzin, N. K. (1978). *The research act.* New York: McGraw-Hill.

Douglass, R. L., Hickey, T., & Noel, C. (1980). *A study of maltreatment of the elderly and other vulnerable adults.* Ann Arbor, MI: University of Michigan, Institute of Gerontology.

Dowd, J. J. (1975). Aging and exchange: A preface to theory. *Journal of Gerontology, 30*(5), 584–594.

Fengler, A. P., & Goodrich, N. (1979). Wives of elderly disabled men: The hidden patients. *The Gerontologist, 19*(2), 175–183.

Finkelhor, D. (1983). Common features of family abuse. In D. Finkelhor, R. J. Gelles, G. Hotaling, & M. Straus (Eds.), *The Dark Side of Families: Current Family Violence Research* (pp. 7–28). Beverly Hills, CA: Sage.

Gelles, R. J. (1972). *The violent home.* Beverly Hills, CA: Sage.

Gelles, R. J., & Straus, M. A. (1980). Stress and child abuse. In H. Kempe & R. E. Helfer (Eds.), *The battered child* (3rd ed.) (pp. 86–103). Chicago: University of Chicago Press.

George, L. K., Landesman, R., & Fillenbaum, G. G. (1982). Developing measures of functional status and service utilization: Refining and extending the OARS methodology. Durham, N.C.: Final Report to NRTA/AARP Andrus Foundation.

Gil, D. G. (1971). *Violence against children: Physical child abuse in the United States.* Cambridge, MA: Harvard University Press.

Glaser, B. G., & Strauss, A. L. (1967). *The discovery of grounded theory: Strategies for qualitative research.* Chicago: Aldine.

Goode, W. J. (1971). Force and violence in the family. In S. K. Steinmetz & M. A. Straus (Eds.), *Violence in the family* (pp. 25–43). New York: Dodd, Mead.

Hennessey, S. (1979). Child abuse. In M. R. Block & J. D. Sinnott (Eds.), *The battered elder syndrome: An exploratory study* (pp. 19–32). College Park, MD: University of Maryland, Center on Aging.

Horowitz, A., & Schindelman, L. W. (1980, November). *The impact of caring for an elderly relative.* Paper presented at the annual meeting of the Gerontological Society of America, San Diego, CA.

Hwalek, M., Sengstock, M., & Lawrence, R. (1984, November). *Assessing the probability of abuse of the elderly.* Paper presented at the annual meeting of Gerontological Society of America, San Diego, CA.

Johnson, T. F., O'Brien, J. G., & Hudson, M. F. (1985). *Elder neglect and abuse.* Westport, CT: Greenwood Press.

Justice, B., & Justice, R. (1976). *The abusing family.* New York: Human Sciences Press.

King, N. R. (1983). Exploitation and abuse of older family members: An overview of the problem. *Response to Violence in the Family and Sexual Assault, 6*(2), 1–15.

Kulys, R., & Tobin, S. (1980). Older people and their "Responsible Others." *Social Work, 25*(2), 138–145.

Lau, E., & Kosberg, J. (1979). Abuse of the elderly by informal care providers. *Aging,* September–October, 10–15.

Marshall, V. W. (1981). Participant observation in a multiple-methods study of a retirement community: A research narrative. *Mid-American Review of Sociology, 11,* 29–44.

Morris, J. N. (1982). Massachusetts elderly: Their vulnerability and need for support services and the role of the commonwealth's home care corporations. Boston: Hebrew Rehabilitation Center for the Aged.

Nye, I. F. (1979). Choice, exchange and the family. In W. R. Burr, R. Hill, F. I. Nye, & I. L. Reiss (Eds.), *Contemporary theories about the family* (Vol. II) (pp. 1–41). New York: The Free Press.

Pedrick-Cornell, C., & Gelles, R. (1982). Elderly abuse: The status of current knowledge. *Family Relations, 31,* 457–465.

Phillips, L. R. (1983). Abuse and neglect of the frail elderly at home: An exploration of theoretical relationships. *Journal of Advanced Nursing, 8,* 379–392.

Pillemer, K. (1985a). The dangers of dependency: New findings on domestic violence against the elderly. *Social Problems, 33*(2), 146–158.

Pillemer, K. (1985b). Social isolation and elder abuse. *Response, 8*(4), 2–4.

Pillemer, K. (1986). Risk factors in elder abuse: Results from a case control study. In K. Pillemer & R. Wolf (Eds.), *Elder abuse: Conflict in the family* (pp. 239–263). Dover, MA: Auburn House.

Sengstock, M. C., & Liang, J. (1982). *Identifying and characterizing elder abuse.* Detroit, MI: Wayne State University, Institute of Gerontology.

Silverstone, B., & Hyman, H. K. (1976). *You and your aging parent.* New York: Pantheon.

Stark, E., Flitcraft, A., Zuckerman, D., Robinson, J., & Frazier, W. (1981). *Wife abuse in the medical setting: An introduction for health personnel.* (Monograph Series, Vol. 7). Rockville, MD: National Clearinghouse on Domestic Violence.

Stearns, P. (1986). Old age family conflict: The perspective of the past. In K. Pillemer & R. Wolf (Eds.), *Elder abuse: Conflict in the family* (pp. 3–48). Dover, MA: Auburn House Publishing Company.

Steinmetz, S. (1983). Dependency, stress, and violence between middle-aged caregivers and their elderly parents. In J. I. Kosberg (Ed.), *Abuse and mal-treatment of the elderly* (pp. 134–149). Littleton, MA: John Wright PGS.

Straus, M. A. (1979). Measuring intrafamily conflict and violence: The Conflict Tactics (CT) Scales. *Journal of Marriage and the Family, 41*, 75–88.

Straus, M., Gelles, R. J., and Steinmetz, S. (1980). *Behind closed doors: Violence in the American family.* New York: Doubleday.

Wan, T. T. H. (1982). *Stressful life events, social support networks and gerontological health.* Lexington, MA: Lexington Books.

Wolf, R. S., Godkin, M. A., & Pillemer, K. (1984). *Elder abuse and neglect: Report from three model projects.* Worcester, MA: University of Massachusetts Medical Center, University Center on Aging.

Wolf, R. S., Strugnell, C. P., & Godkin, M. A. (1982). *Preliminary findings from three model projects on elderly abuse.* Worcester, MA: University of Massachusetts Medical Center, Center on Aging.

Zarit, S. H., Reever, K. E., & Bach-Peterson, J. (1980). Relatives of impaired elderly: Correlates of feelings of burden. *The Gerontologist, 20*(6), 649–655.

15

The Use of Qualitative Methodologies in Large-Scale Cross-Cultural Research

Charlotte Ikels
Jennie Keith
Christine L. Fry

This chapter[1] describes and analyzes the trials and tribulations as well as the rewards of participation in a large-scale cross-cultural research project known as Project AGE[2]. Many who value qualitative data about human experience might consider large-scale comparative study a utopian enterprise. We do not consider our goal of comparable qualitative data utopian, in the sense of unrealistic or impossible, but we have learned to view this enterprise as utopian in another sense. Utopian experiments place great emphasis on the processes as well as the products of social interaction; collaborative and qualitative research must do the same. Research combining these two elements requires continuous negotiation of the competing demands of appropriate comparison and ethnographic validity. Although the creation of a research design that includes both goals is essential, the effort to keep them in balance must be a central activity throughout the lifetime of the project.

The intense demands of field work may make the requirements of the original comparative scheme seem too rigid. The goals of comparison may make tempting a standardization of interview or observation protocols that obscures cultural realities. The demands of collecting qualitative data may be particularly problematic in the context of what we have learned to call the "quantitative imperative." In a research enterprise that combines quantitative and qualitative data collection, collaboration on the former is easier. It is easier to create the quantitative instruments and easier to keep score of how well the project is doing in using them. More time-consuming decisions and less quantifiable progress in the qualitative domain may take on lower priority by default.

IMPLEMENTATION

Goals

Broad consequences of growing old in various sociocultural settings have been hypothesized by other researchers in two distinct ways, but at the time (1979) when Project AGE was being contemplated, these generalizations were, with rare exceptions (Myerhoff & Simic, 1978), based on secondary data not collected with age issues in mind or on first-hand, but noncomparable, case illustrations.

According to the first hypothesis, modernization has a curvilinear relationship to the status of the old. Earlier stages of modernization have a negative effect, but in later stages the old do better as supports such as pensions and improved health care appear (Cowgill & Holmes, 1972; Cowgill, 1974). During the negative phase, rapid social change undermines the benefits of seniority and accumulated knowledge as sources of prestige for the old. Second, modernization leads to more complex social structures (greater role specialization, more stratification) that may affect old people negatively by providing alternative bases of power and prestige, particularly for the young, and by producing great discontinuities across the life span.

The second broad hypothesis about factors affecting the old and the aging process focused on cultural values. Culture areas were contrasted in terms of their respective treatment of the old with, for example, China (Hsu, 1981) and Japan (Palmore, 1975) ranking high, the Western world, low. Certain U.S. populations, such as blacks or Hispanics, were also characterized as more respectful or supportive of the elderly than the white middle class (Clark & Mendelson, 1969; Trela & Sokolovsky, 1979). The effects of cultural values were often eloquently described but seldom explained. The unanswered questions remained: why and how do certain cultures value old age, and what are the mechanisms through which cultural values operate?

Project AGE was conceived to evaluate these two broad types of hypotheses. The individual team members viewed participation in Project AGE as an opportunity to contribute to the development of an empirically based theoretical framework that would place their own research in a broader context. Fry and Keith articulated the variables of theoretical interest, proposed means of operationalizing these variables, and suggested data-gathering strategies that could be utilized in a wide variety of cultural settings. They also planned to function as the project coordinators, as well as to carry out their own research in their respective sites. Fry's home institution, Loyola University of Chicago, served as the contracting party for the National Institute on Aging and disbursed the project's funds to the home institutions of the other project investigators.

Site and Team Selection

Eight interdependent clusters of variables (labeled in our theoretical framework as social system, norms and expectations, roles and status, resource control, generational relations, economy and demography, health and functionality, and well-being) were selected for study, although some, such as the social system variables, were considered more independent than others. Given the primacy of social system variables for the development of the theoretical framework (which will not be dealt with in this chapter), it was essential that the sites selected for investigation vary systematically in terms of scale and subsistence pattern. Consequently, the planners decided from the beginning that the sites should include a broad range of social systems from small-scale hunting and gathering societies to herding, horticultural, agricultural, and industrial societies. In addition, individuals selected for participation in the project were expected to have already demonstrated a theoretical interest in aging or age-related issues and to have conducted research in a site appropriate for inclusion in the study. In short, the team members were expected to be experienced field workers sufficiently knowledgeable about their sites that methodological problems could be raised and dealt with prior to their departure from the United States.

Despite the restrictions the above criteria imposed on recruitment, assembling such a team was not an impossibility. Maintaining such a team, however, has been more difficult because of the vicissitudes of funding and the need for political clearance. Because of its complexity, Project AGE was divided into two phases. The first (1982–85) was a pilot phase in which the research design was adapted to three sites (two in the United States and one in a Chinese community). The second phase (1987–90) incorporates strategies and findings from the pilot and extends the comparative design to additional sites that are smaller and markedly different in subsistence patterns. Investigators assigned to the second phase could not always await their turn (sabbaticals come and go, family circumstances change) and understandably sometimes chose other options, which necessitated a second round of recruitment. Furthermore, as most anthropologists know, the host country often plays a determining role in what kinds of research, if any, it will allow to be carried out in its territory, and for this reason we had to shift the site of our Chinese component. As a result of combinations of these factors, the research sites for Phase 1 were all large-scale societies (or communities within such societies): Hong Kong; Momence, Illinois; and Swarthmore, Pennsylvania. The research sites for Phase 2 were, with one exception, all small-scale hunting and gathering, pastoral, or agricultural societies: two sites in Botswana and two in Ireland.

Development of Strategies and Instruments

Since our major objective in gathering data was an "ethnography of age," i.e., an understanding of how individuals conceptualize the life course, how norms and values shape the individual's experience of the life course, and how age as an objective feature affects social interaction, we employed a range of methods. These methods, however, had to be suitable for a variety of social settings, as well as comprehensible to individuals of varying degrees of sophistication. In short, we needed instruments and methods that would allow for the collection of comparable data at the same time that they preserved the categories that were meaningful to the informants. Our general technique for balancing validity and comparability was to agree on conceptual definitions and on measurement *strategies*, but not to use standardized instruments. For example, although the strategy chosen for measuring perceptions of the life course in each site is a sorting task, the "people" sorted are not standard, but appropriate to each context. The step-by-step strategy that produces the culture-specific items for sorting is the same in each site.

In selecting methods the investigators were guided by their knowledge of what informants were likely to tolerate, e.g., how long informants would be willing to participate in an interview, how verbal they were likely to be, how much the interview would inconvenience other members of the household. Some researchers anticipated conducting their interviews in private, in large living rooms, with verbal, unhurried informants. Others foresaw public interviews with laconic informants anxious to get on with the day's work. These contrasting expectations resulted in a mini-max strategy, the paring of the original interview schedule to the minimum so that its total length did not exceed the maximum acceptable length in the least hospitable environment. This paring was carried out before the interviewing got underway and resulted in a tight minimal format that, because of the inclusion of many open-ended questions, nevertheless allowed room for expansive informants. Thus all investigators agreed in advance on the data that had to be collected in order to meet the needs of the project but also felt that their own individual interests could be pursued once these had been met. For example, some researchers were unhappily resigned to the decision to drop a detailed set of questions on social networks from the interview schedule but were comforted by the thought that they could (at least in theory) append such questions should informant enthusiasm allow.

Four major strategies were developed for use in Project AGE: the interview schedule and an accompanying card-sort known as the Age Game, participant-observation in age homogeneous as well as age heterogeneous settings, observations of behavior in public spaces, and collection of life histories from older informants. All team members were comfortable with these approaches, although they believed site-specific modifications would be required before implementation. Throughout the project a major task for all team members was maintaining enough contact to ensure that these modifications did not diverge beyond the point of comparability.

The Age Game

The instrument we developed to explore the meaning of age and the differentiation of the adult life course is the Age Game. We have called it a "game" partly because it makes informants more tolerant of our questions, but more importantly because it is gamelike in that informants are actively involved in constructing age groups and life stages. Each informant is presented with a set of "social persona" characterized by criteria that are community specific. In Phase 1 we all used 3 x 5 cards, with English words or Chinese characters on them, to describe the social persona. In Phase 2 probably only the Irish will see 3 x 5 cards and English words. In the other sites the social persona will be represented by icons, and the media will increase in size or the ethnographer will rely more on verbal than on visual cues. In Hong Kong, where a substantial proportion of elderly female informants are illiterate, the interviewer read the cards aloud, and these informants were generally able to perform the card-sort without difficulty.

The development of the persona is carried out with the assistance of key informants in each research site. Key informants are individuals who by virtue of social position and experience have a broad perspective on their communities and can articulate the dominant values and underlying principles of social organization. Preliminary interviews with key informants representing different age groups and social classes led to the selection of the attributes to be included in the description of the social persona. In one interview informants were asked to describe their view of the stages of life and to play a version of the game "20 questions," in which the object was to guess the age of an individual by asking the researcher about the individual's attributes. Each researcher then considered the range of attributes, e.g., the attribute marital status (which was employed in all Phase 1 card decks) ranged from single, through married for the first time, separated, divorced, widowed, to remarried.

Informants were later asked to combine attributes in a "Make-A-Person" interview, which revealed culturally relevant combinations of attributes. Finally the researchers themselves generated various combinations of attributes to construct hypothetical individuals; 100 of these combinations were then presented to the key informants, who were asked to evaluate the plausibility of the combinations and to assign an age range to those deemed plausible. Combinations on which there was high informant consensus as to plausibility and age range were selected for inclusion in the final decks of 48 cards, each deck describing 24 men and 24 women. The goal was to include three individuals of each sex in each decade of life, e.g., twenties, thirties, and forties; typical and atypical individuals were described for each decade. During our later interviews, however, less sophisticated informants tended to have difficulty dealing with atypical combinations.

In the three sites of Phase 1 the attributes used in the descriptions of the social persona were similar in that marital status, stage of domestic cycle, living arrangement, and nature of labor-force participation were all mentioned by key informants; but there were also differences. Home ownership, for example, took on tremendous significance as a life-course marker in Momence. Thus persona in the Momence card deck are frequently described as renting, as still paying off the mortgage, or as having paid off the mortgage. There are clear expectations about when these events should occur, and individuals are acutely aware as to whether or not they are "on time." In Swarthmore, on the other hand, the status of one's parents looms large. Are they still alive? Retired? Moving in with one? In Hong Kong living arrangements coupled with domestic cycle are salient less for what they tell about where a person stands in the life course than for what they tell about the quality of that person's life. The number of attributes on the Hong

Kong cards is fewer than on those of the other two sites to facilitate their use with illiterates.

Examples of cards from each deck are provided below:

Momence

A married man

Has preschool children

Is paying mortgage on home

Graduated from college

Works out of town

Swarthmore

A married woman

Has children in college

Lives with her husband whose mother has moved in with them

Works part-time in Swarthmore

Her parents are retired

Hong Kong

A married woman

Has children in middle school

Has temporary/part-time work

Lives with her parents-in-law

Following construction of the social persona, we interviewed a random sample of 200 adults (as defined locally) in each community, with an oversampling of the population aged 60 or older. The sampling frame included all adults in the community. In the case of Hong Kong, with a population in excess of five million, such a sampling frame was impractical. Furthermore, to have included all of Hong Kong as a single community would have rendered our efforts at participant-observation meaningless. Consequently, in Hong Kong four contiguous or nearly contiguous neighborhoods, which varied by socioeconomic status, constituted the sampling frame.

The informant is presented with a shuffled deck of cards and asked to sort them into groups on the basis of life stage or age. Thus the informant ponders the descriptors of each social persona, places the cards in piles in a row, and then responds to a set of questions intended to elicit the underlying dimensions of the life course that presumably guided the sorting process as well as the informant's own attitudes and feelings toward the various age groups, including his or her own. The sorting of the cards yields information that can be readily analyzed through multidimensional scaling and cluster analysis. From the placement of the persona in groups, we calculate an inter-persona distance matrix, employing an algorithm that takes into account differences between those who make few distinctions (sorted into few groups) and those who make many (sorted into many groups). From this matrix the computer then generates "pictures" of the life course in one or more dimensions. The results of the sorting from all sites are immediately obtainable, interpretable, and comparable. The data acquired through the set of questions about the age groups are, by contrast, open-ended and require intensive content analysis.

These questions explore both generally and concretely the informant's perceptions of the life cycle. Depending on age, the informant may have experienced only the first stage or may have passed through all but the last stage of the life cycle. Accordingly, evaluations of the various stages may be based on direct personal experience, on observations of others occupying the stage, or on general impressions acquired through the media or casual conversation. Informants are first asked: (1) Why are these people put together? (2) What do you call them? (3) How (or when) does one become a member of this age group? (4) What are their primary concerns? (5) What is the best/worst thing about being in this age group? (6) What is the age range of this age group? A second set of questions explores the informant's own feelings about the various groups: (1) Which group would you most/least like to be in and why? (2) In which of these groups do you know the most/least people? (3) With which of these groups do you find it easiest/hardest to get along and why? A third set of questions taps the informant's own experience with the older age groups (those containing individuals 60 years of age or older). For each older age group the informant is asked: (1) When did you last have contact with someone in this age group? (2) What did you do together? (3) How did you come to know this person? (4) Do you ever help each other out and how? Finally the informant is asked to provide a concrete example for each older age group of a person he/she actually knows who "is doing well/poorly as an older person." The development of a coding scheme able to capture the nuances of these very rich responses for comparative analysis will be dealt with below in the section on "Interpretation."

The interview schedule accompanying the Age Game also collects data on the informant's household composition, proximity to a wide range of relatives (specific to each site), education, occupation, organizational memberships, perceptions of community issues, health, functionality, and well-being. Functionality and well-being are excellent examples of concepts central to our comparative goal that required measurement strategies permitting cultural validity. We agreed on conceptual definitions of these variables, e.g., functionality is defined as the capability of performing certain activities necessary for full adult participation in the particular community and measured by a four-point scale from "cannot do this without assistance" to "have no difficulty doing this." However, discovery of the specific activities necessary for full participation in each setting was a major goal of participant-observation and key-informant interviewing. Thus the ability to drive a car is important for full participation in Momence and Swarthmore, but not in Hong Kong. In Hong Kong mobility is measured by one's ability to get around on public transportation. Literacy is essential in all three sites, but since there are so few illiterates in either of the American sites, it was not necessary to measure it. In Hong Kong, however, illiteracy is common among older women and seriously compromises their participation in community affairs; therefore, it was included as a measure of functionality.

We define well-being as the individual's assessment of his or her life compared to his or her definition of the best life possible in the community. We selected a self-rated and self-anchored definition of well-being for two reasons. A self-anchoring definition is the most appropriate for a research endeavor that includes the goal of evaluating the influence of cultural context. We expected definitions of the best possible life to be different in different communities, and the results from the first phase of Project AGE show this variation. In addition, review of the literature and consultations with specialists also made clear that subjective, self-rated definitions of well-being are widely used in gerontology (Lawton, 1972; Nydegger, 1977, 1986).

In our research, informants are shown a ladder (or flight of stairs) with six levels and are asked to place themselves on the level that corresponds most closely with their evaluation of life at the present time. This approach is an adaptation of the Cantril Self-Anchoring Ladder (Cantril, 1965), which has been evaluated positively in a comparative psychometric analysis of seven commonly used measures (George, 1981, pp. 365–374). In this review, George points out that the Cantril Self-Anchoring Ladder has "superb" population and subgroup norms, as it has been used in 12 countries and with close to 20,000 individuals. In addition, it is rated as adequate in terms of applicability to heterogeneous samples, quantification and discriminability, and validity and ease of administration. We also ask the informant to evaluate his or her life as it was 5 to 10 years ago and as he or she expects it to be 5 to 10 years hence. Thus when we code the textual responses, we are able to determine whether the individual is talking about "satisfaction" with his or her entire life to date or about "happiness" at the moment. The Cantril Ladder is also readily adaptable to diverse populations. Drawings of ladders were used with American populations; flights of stairs were more comprehensible to Hong Kong informants. In Botswana, !Kung populations, though not accustomed to interpreting drawings on paper, are accustomed to reading maps sketched with sticks in the sand.

Participant-Observation in Formal Settings

Since we already had access to other works, e.g., local histories and government documents describing the salient features of the particular communities, we were relatively free to direct our attention to the collection of data focused around the impact of age. Participant-observation as a research strategy provides an invaluable means of comparing what people say with what they actually do. This comparison is necessitated not by doubts about informants' veracity so much as by the fact that much of what we are interested in learning about is not a focus of interest of the informants themselves. They are seldom in a position to comment on their own behavior, as they have made no systematic efforts to study it and are often unaware of how they may behave differently in different settings. Even when informants are aware that they modify their behavior on the basis of the characteristics of those with whom they are interacting, they may regard such modifications as natural or trivial and not worthy of note (Whiting & Whiting, 1973, p. 284).

Since we are especially concerned with the influence of age on social participation and since we hypothesize that relationships with peers are qualitatively different from relationships with individuals of different ages, we planned to observe settings in which the participants varied in terms of relative age. Specifically, we sought age-homogeneous and age-heterogeneous settings in which to observe ordinary interaction, and our goal was to locate settings in the same neighborhoods in which we did our interviewing. Thus in all three of the Phase 1 sites we were able to locate organizations whose members were all elderly. We noted the characteristics of the formal and informal leaders of such organizations as well as the topics of interest, the manner of discussion, and the motives for participation of the ordinary membership. A major difference among the communities is, of course, the extent to which elderly residents participate in formal organizations; in Momence and Swarthmore such participation is not unusual, whereas in Hong Kong it is the rare elder who involves him/herself in affairs outside of the household. We were also able to locate age-heterogeneous organizations, churches, social clubs, or community affairs and interest groups in all the communities and, as in the case of the age-homogeneous organizations, observe them over a period of several months. Our presence was noted by the people whom we were observing, who were aware of the general nature of our study but not of our specific hypotheses. Many of these individuals offered to share their own observations with us, and some eventually came to function as volunteer assistants.

Observations in Public Spaces

We also wanted to learn about the relative visibility of the elderly in the various communities. What kinds of opportunities do people have in everyday life to encounter the elderly? What are the elderly likely to be doing? How different are their public activities from those of people of younger age groups? Are older people more likely to be in same-sex groupings than younger people? Are they relatively more likely to be found in peer groups than younger people? Do people of different ages share the same space simultaneously, or do they use it on a time-sharing basis? Do people of different ages congregate in entirely different public spaces?

In order to answer these questions we decided on two strategies: spot observations and time-lapse observations of interaction in selected public spaces. Our first task was to discover the range of public spaces from which we would select target sites. We wanted sites that were comparable across the various communities but also representative of the particular communities. Utilization of public spaces varies by time of day as well as by time of year, so it was necessary to observe the sites at several different times of the day as well as at the time of the year when people were likely to be making use of them, i.e., during the summer rather than the winter. In addition, high-density communities such as Hong Kong are characterized by intensive use of public spaces and facilities compared to the less dense communities.

We chose to observe in parks, restaurants, libraries, post offices, grocery stores, pharmacies, and "sitting out" areas. Since Hong Kong is in many ways a bicultural community with a traditional and a modern "Westernized" sector, we chose sites from both sectors. For example, we observed a traditional herbalist's shop as well as a modern pharmacy selling cosmetics and prepackaged pharmaceuticals, a traditional noodle shop as well as a modern snack shop. For the spot observations we drew maps of each site and filled in the locations of individuals or groups of individuals as soon as we arrived at the site, noting the age and sex composition of groupings as well as their joint activity.

The time-lapse observations required that we observe interaction over a 15-minute or longer interval. Some of these observations were carried out in the same sites as above, e.g., restaurants, but others were carried out in new sites, such as bus stops, crosswalks, and subway trains. These latter sites provided opportunities to observe the interaction of people under stress, particularly in Hong Kong. Who stands patiently in a queue for a bus? Who attempts to cut the queue? With what result? Who leads a pack of nervous pedestrians into the crosswalk in the face of oncoming traffic? Who assists whom in crossing the street? Who offers a seat to whom on a crowded train? All of these measures are attempts to discover the unspoken rules underlying the public code of courtesy and whether age and sex are significant variables in the operation of this code. In other communities this code could be studied in drinking behavior in pubs, in the distribution of food at informal gatherings, or in seating or viewing arrangements at public ceremonies.

Collection of Life Histories

The life histories are intended as both amplifications of the lives of the older people in our interview sample and sources of data on issues that cannot be obtained in a one-to-two hour interview or from the informal observations that come from living in the community. Specifically, we are interested in learning the pathways that older people took during the course of their lives and how these previous experiences shape their evaluations of their current lives. To what extent did they follow or violate a cultural script as they matured and grew old? How much control did they expect to have over their own lives? What were their goals at different stages of their lives and how did they reach them? How do they account for the failures or disappointments in their lives? Fate? Injustice? Personal flaws? Historical events beyond anyone's control?

The problems inherent in the collection of life-history data have been dealt with at length elsewhere, e.g., Frank & Vanderburgh, (1986), Langness (1965), Mandelbaum (1973), and Watson (1976). Here let us state that we are aware that any life history is inevitably a partial life history and that the particular form it takes is the result of the collaborative efforts of the researcher and the teller. The difficulty in cross-cultural research is to assure that the interests and discourse style of the informant are preserved while at the same time the theoretical issues of concern to the investigators are adequately explored. The collection of life histories is labor-intensive and consequently requires that we select from among our older informants a subsample that will reflect the range of life experiences characteristic of the older genera-tion. We feel this goal can be achieved by careful selection of 12 to 15 informants in each community, provided criteria of gender, age, size of kinship network, health status, socioeconomic status, and other com-munity-specific characteristics can be met.

To preserve the informant's biographical framework we began with a broad question about how he or she perceived his or her life: e.g., if we were going to write a book about it, what would the chapters be or what would the most important events in it be? Then the framework was progressively "filled in" during subsequent interview sessions that included questions about typical days and significant others at various stages of life. Many Hong Kong informants are not accustomed to discussions at this level of abstraction, and they were not prepared to generate spontaneously the outline of their lives. Our compromise in such cases was to propose several possible frameworks that we already knew to be familiar to them, along with a few novel ones. Thus we suggested that some people were likely to describe their lives with reference to some major personal event, in terms of the ease or diffi-culty of their circumstances, or in terms of their emotional states. Others were likely to link their lives to the places where they had lived or to historical events. Most hesitant Hong Kong informants quickly seized on the last framework.

Measuring Progress

Inventories are extremely useful in keeping track of variables and their data sources and in keeping the project focused on the problem under investigation. In doing qualitative research it is very easy to become fascinated by the data, to lose sight of the forest by concentrating on the individual trees. As the research activities shift from the early exploratory phase to the more focused phase (Keith, 1986), the creation of a variable inventory is essential. Initially the inventory is a simple list of the variables or components of the theoretical framework, along with the conceptual and operational definitions worked out in the grant proposal. The proposed sources of measurement of each variable, e.g., Age Game question 6 and life histories, should also be listed. As work progresses and operational definitions require modification or proposed sources of measurement do not yield adequate information, site-spe-cific adaptations can be tried and communicated to the coordinators and members of other teams. From the perspective of the coordinators the variable inventory is above all a check to make certain that all variables relevant to the theory have empirical indicators from each site.

Communication and Coordination

Project AGE began with a workshop in 1980, during which the researchers and several consultants discussed major concepts that would require measurement in the different cultural settings proposed for the study. The result of the workshop was a set of conceptual definitions that could be used in the various settings and, for each concept, a *strategy*, but not a standard instrument, for obtaining the data that would be valid for the cultural context. The three researchers who conducted the field work during Phase 1 met again for three days before going to their field sites and developed the basic instruments that would guide data collection. Three months into the research two team members met in Hong Kong, while the third visited Hong Kong six months later. Nearly weekly phone calls and at least three face-to-face meetings were arranged between the coordinator/field workers in the two U.S. sites. Copies of all the field notes from Hong Kong were sent to one of the coordinators, and letters and phone calls about research activities and problems were exchanged at least once a month—most often when some decision point was approaching.

In our original plan one of the researchers was to receive all the field reports and then send excerpts to everyone in order to keep field activities closely coordinated. In actuality it was impossible to meet this goal and carry out research at the same time. Consequently, our communication was patterned by the demands of the individual projects, and the inevitable lack of synchronization created stresses for everyone. In the second phase, coordination of field work will be a separate full-time responsibility.

Two different sources of communication difficulties stand out: timing and maintaining an appreciation of "emics," i.e., preserving respect for the cultural differences among the sites even when these differences make modification of instruments necessary. Because field work flows in distinctive channels around the events and institutions of any social setting, the *timing* of various research activities cannot be tightly scheduled. On the other hand, because acquiring comparable data is a central goal, decisions that can be made only in the course of field work, e.g., those about culturally appropriate measurements, must be synchronized so that the choices made in one location do not become constraining *faits accomplis* for the others.

When the Hong Kong team, for example, was ready to begin observations of public spaces, it had to send out urgent demands for the other two teams to participate in decisions about the selection of locations. When different activities are underway elsewhere, however, the other teams find it difficult to shift full attention to decisions needed by someone far away. Even when all teams make the effort to shift attention, the bases of judgment for the decisions may be shaky. What is a compelling reality at one site might be only an abstract issue at the others. Later, as the other teams prepare to undertake this activity, it may be too late to renegotiate the prior decision, since the first team has already acted on the original conclusion.

Three other problems relating to timing are especially acute for those conducting their research outside of the United States. They, like all other team members, are funded for a specific time, but unlike U.S.-based team members they are compelled to take this time limitation very seriously. A quick trip back to the field site between semesters to tidy up loose ends is simply not possible, so those working abroad constantly feel the need to be working on all fronts simultaneously. Furthermore, most of the teams conducting their research outside of the United States are working in a foreign language. All research instruments have to be translated into the appropriate language, and all interviews have to be translated into English in order to make them available to the coordinators. Time for these activities should be generously allotted.

Finally, there are occasions when fast communication is necessary, and the mails do not allow this. A request for clarification may be sent, but while waiting for the mail to turn around, the researcher tries to move forward. Three weeks later when the response arrives, it may not be what was expected, but the costs of undoing what has already been done are so high that it is not worth making the changes. To avoid this kind of timing problem we found it worthwhile to schedule telephone calls. We also found that there is nothing like face-to-face interaction to promote decision making. The most effective decisions we made were those grounded in visits across the sites. For each of the two site visits to Hong Kong we prepared an agenda of issues to be discussed and decisions that had to be made. When researchers have walked through the study neighborhoods in each others' sites, they develop a more realistic appreciation of the constraints under which the local team operates as well as the particularly interesting aspects of each setting. We also learned the need for extreme precision in long-distance communication. What is obvious to the speaker who sits with the relevant protocol or form in front of him/her is not necessarily obvious to the listener 10,000 miles away who will not see the protocol for another several weeks. Our most instructive example concerns preprinted electronically read coding sheets. It was "obvious" to one site that responses were to be recorded by the connecting of lines and equally "obvious" to another that spaces were to be filled in. This discrepancy would not have occurred had a sample marked form been exchanged; in fact, several hundred forms had to be recoded.

Visits across sites must be included in project budgets; their contribution to data quality cannot be overstated. In our second phase, visits will be made to all research communities by the coordinators. Finally, as stated above, the greatest lesson that we learned is that coordination is a full-time job. No field workers can conduct an administrative project in their "spare" time. Not only is there no such thing as spare time during field work, but the very enterprise of developing understanding of a cultural context becomes an obstacle to continuing awareness of research priorities and events in other settings.

INTERPRETATION

Setting Priorities

One of the most difficult decisions we faced upon return from our field sites was the sequencing of analysis. Not surprisingly, we—and the potential funder of our second phase—wanted to see the results of our labors as quickly as possible. The surest path to quick results was to tackle the readily quantifiable data first. Furthermore, much of this data had already been coded while the research was in progress and was ready for computer entry. The most immediately accessible data was from the Age Game card-sort, and we quickly became experts at interpreting multidimensional scaling solutions. Simultaneously we had to manage the qualitative data from the open-ended responses, our field notes, and other research protocols.

The general strategy for managing textual information was similar across the three sites, although the specifics of creating computer files varied. At Swarthmore a special BASIC program was written for the Project. At Harvard, a text-management package known as SPIRES was employed for the Hong Kong data. At Loyola, text was entered on an IBM PC using Final Word; these files were then uploaded to the mainframe as ASCII text files, where they were merged into larger files and then managed through SAS. All of these approaches allowed for moving around and regrouping the responses to the Age Game and other parts of the interview. Selected responses, e.g., all the responses of informants to a particular question about all the age groups, were then printed out. Scanning of such printouts proved very helpful in the eventual development of the coding scheme used for content analysis of open-ended responses. Following the development of this scheme selected texts were printed, and the numerical codes indicating the major themes in the texts were then written directly onto the printout. These numerical codes were then entered as data files, which were converted into SPSSX files for statistical analyses.

Priority setting during analysis was also complicated by the different interests of the researchers. Just as in the field work stage, some teams moved faster or in a different sequence from others. Whoever tackled a particular problem first developed the outline of the coding scheme for that problem. Analysts with other priorities could not simply drop whatever they were doing to evaluate the applicability of the coding scheme to their own data. These conflicts about priorities are not an inevitable result of collaborative, multisite research. In our own case we had originally planned for the coordinators to begin field work six to nine months before the Hong Kong team. Similarly, they would have entered the analysis stage six to nine months before the Hong Kong team, and decisions would have been made under less time pressure. Because of problems with the federal budget, however, the funding agency could not make money available until halfway through the originally scheduled first year, and, consequently, all Phase 1 researchers entered the field—and left it—simultaneously.

Development of Coding Schemes

Despite the tremendous effort required, we are most pleased with our success in developing a codebook, which we believe facilitates two of the key goals of our work: (1) making the data sets comparable and (2) preserving their cultural uniqueness. Much of our quantitative analysis is based on the Age Game and the accompanying interview. Some of these data are restricted in variation or were recorded using closed categories. Much, however, consists of lengthy narrative responses to open-ended questions. These latter data must be reduced through a content analysis of responses and subsequently encoded in a numerical format suitable for computer-assisted statistical analysis.

The codes discussed below are applicable to the responses to the Age Game and to much of the interview schedule, e.g., reasons for well-being and definitions of quality of life. Each code consists of six digits, of which the first digit provides "syntactical" information; the next four, thematic information; and the sixth digit, a "valence" (or evaluation of the theme by the informant). By syntactical factors we mean temporal or conditioning references made by the informant to qualify his/her response. For example, a person might say in response to the question, "What is the best thing about being in this age group?" that,

"In the past . . ." or "If their health is good . . ." or "Some people that age . . ." Each of these qualifications of the general statement can be captured by placing the applicable digit in the first position.

The thematic aspect of the code was created inductively. Prior to a face-to-face three-day marathon during which the first version of the codebook was drafted, each of the Phase 1 researchers considered the variation in responses that characterized her informants. After considerable negotiation we were able to settle upon 15 distinctive themes (and eventually hundreds of subthemes) for which we developed site-specific annotations. We then returned to our home institutions and began to apply the code to a small block of data. In this process we realized the need for more annotations and refinements and were in frequent contact. We discovered that some responses were difficult to classify (e.g., should a concern about having enough money to support the family be considered a financial matter or a family matter?) and developed a scheme of cross-references for problematic situations. We also realized that for some analytical purposes we would probably need to collapse the codes or combine codes that appeared under different themes. We are currently working with 15 themes: age, physical status, education, work, finances, nonwork activities, marriage, living arrangements, domestic life, interpersonal relationships (outside of the family), responsibility, achievement and goals, personal attributes, quality of life, and life-course development. We have what we consider a workable version of the codebook for the sites of Phase 1, but we fully expect modifications (of greater magnitude than new annotations) to be necessitated by the findings of the Phase 2 researchers. Thus the codebook will in some senses continually evolve to take account of cultural uniqueness and already coded data will require some recoding.

The final digit, expressing valence, captures the evaluations of the informant. We realized quickly that without the capability of encoding this aspect of a response we would seriously violate the informant's real meaning. The simple statement "that is the time when the children begin leaving home" may have a positive connotation to a Swarthmore parent but a negative one to a Hong Kong parent. When attempting to interpret reasons for well-being, the valence of this type of statement is critical. Determining the valence is, however, tricky. Unless the informant has indicated elsewhere how he or she feels about this particular matter, it may be difficult to assign a valence. The person who conducted the field work may be sufficiently familiar with the culture and the ways people talk about certain issues to assign a valence even when the informant has not specifically stated how he feels, but a coder with no prior experience with the culture cannot be expected to make this kind of decision. Consequently, we erred on the side of caution and assigned a neutral valence unless the informant revealed a clear evaluation. The sixth digit is also used to indicate whether a gender-specific reference is made, e.g., that something is only true or more true of males (or of females).

The coding unit was the entire answer that the informant gave to a particular open-ended question. Some informants, such as those quoted below, gave very brief responses, whereas others provided 200-word paragraphs. Our goal was to determine which themes (or subthemes) were most salient to the speaker. Consequently, computer space for each response was allocated on the basis of the number of themes (or subthemes) typical informants referenced in their answers—usually three, four, or five, depending on question and on site. The length of the answer was not a reliable guide to the number of themes referenced. One woman, for example, provided a response several paragraphs long to the question about the concerns of a particular age group. Despite its length, only one subtheme (or "subdimension") was mentioned—that of fear of divorce or desertion. In contrast, the brief answers utilized below to illustrate the application of the coding scheme referenced two dimensions in the first case and three in the second.

A 62-year-old female resident of Swarthmore who sorted four age groups stated that the best thing about being in the fourth (or oldest) age group is:

> They are able to continue living the life they want to lead (014211)/. They are seeing their family develop (009261).

The first code can be divided into three parts: (1) a syntax code of 0, meaning that the response is a simple unconditioned statement; (2) a thematic code of 1421, meaning that dimension 14 (quality of life) and subtheme 21 (freedom/autonomy) under quality of life are referenced; and (3) a valence code of 1, indicating a positive evaluation. In this case, the annotation for 14211 in the codebook is "Can do what want to; come and go as please"—a perfect fit! Similarly the second code can be divided into three parts: (1) a syntax code of 0; (2) a thematic code of 0926, meaning that dimension 9 (domestic life) and subtheme 26 (children's development) are referenced; and (3) a valence code of 1. Codebook examples of 09261 include "Seeing them grow, bloom. Maturing with your children."

A 60-year-old Hong Kong female living in the poorest neighborhood in which we interviewed responded thus when asked about the "best possible life in Hong Kong."

Not married (007110)/. Supported by parents (005240)/. No need to worry about anything (014803).

All three comments are unconditioned, therefore the first digit is 0 in all cases. Given the nature of the question, all the responses are assumed to be positively evaluated, so the coder refrained from explicitly marking them (a source of intercoder unreliability here). Furthermore, since a valence of 3 indicates absence (of the referenced phenomenon), in the case of the final segment there would have been a conflict over the choice of the sixth digit. The first thematic code (0711) indicates simply the state of being single. The second (0524) indicates financial support from parents (without specifying whether this is a blessing or an embarrassment), and the third (1480) refers to worries and stressors. With a valence of 3 the annotations of this subtheme indicate lessening worries, removal of stressors, "not a worry in the world," etc.

Units of Analysis

Since Project AGE is a comparative study of communities from different parts of the world, we must consider the kinds of variation we are dealing with and how they articulate with our theoretical model. What is to be our unit of analysis—the individuals within the community or the community itself? For hypotheses examining intracultural variation, individuals within the community are the unit. For hypotheses examining cross-cultural variation, the community is the unit. The types of data required for measurement at these two levels are quite different, although, for some purposes, community-level measures can be constructed from individual-level measurements.

Where the community is our unit of analysis, the explanatory models are essentially descriptive, with data coming from very heterogeneous sources, including systematic observations, key informants, life-history informants, public documents, and responses to the Age Game interview. On the basis of these descriptive models the communities can be ranked in terms of such variables as, for example, rate of change, clarity of age grades, and opportunities for the young. Where the hypotheses call for analyses of intracultural variation, the models are associational and derive from statistical testing of the relationships among selected variables.

One of the problems with qualitative data is that there is so much that it is difficult to see the patterns. In their book *Qualitative Data Analysis* (1984), Miles and Huberman present a number of strategies involving matrices and graphics to display the variation in the data. We use what we are calling a "Variable Display Table." For each variable the possible sources of measurement are listed, with each principal investigator summarizing the indicators from each relevant data source. With agreement on the comparative ranking of the sites on each variable, the co-directors display these data using a "Site Ordered Predictor-Outcome Matrix" (Miles & Huberman 1984, pp. 167–176). This is a matrix in which the X-axis defines the study variables and the Y-axis, the sites. The cells of the matrix then display the data for that variable across sites. On a limited basis the site-ordered predictor-outcome matrix can display the data to evaluate individual hypotheses or a cluster of hypotheses.

Congruence with the hypothesized relations supports the model that has been guiding the project; deviations indicate lack of support. Since we have a battery of both quantitative and qualitative data in hand, should one site not "fit" the projected model it will not be explained away as an aberration. Instead, the data from all sites will be reexamined and the model modified to best explain the data. For instance, we have already learned that functionality if not a single variable but several—some of which are community-specific, while others, e.g., biological capacity, are universal. As the comparative analysis progresses, we fully expect to return to the data from individual sites with new ways of looking at the variables and their operational indicators.

Dissemination of Results

Each investigator is responsible for the eventual write-up of the results of the research within his/her site, and we expect that each will publish a monograph highlighting the findings. The ethnographies of each site will be similar in organization, since parallel questions, research strategies, and analytical techniques were employed. Our plan is to publish these ethnographies as a series, each volume of which will contain the same introductory and concluding chapters relating, respectively, the theory and methods of the project and the results of the comparative analysis. The investigators are also free to publish selected aspects of their work for more restricted audiences, e.g., China specialists or political anthropologists, and are encouraged to use comparative material from the other sites with the permission of the other team members.

In addition to the individual ethnographies, the key publication resulting from this project will be a comparative volume that evaluates and modifies the initial theoretical framework. This will be an edited volume that introduces the project and research design, describes the effectiveness of the theory in accounting for the well-being of the elderly in each site, and concludes with a chapter integrating the findings. We also anticipate a number of journal articles employing data from all the sites and focusing on variables not initially emphasized in the research design, e.g., the impact of socioeconomic status on perceptions of aging, the relationship between one's view of the life course and one's current placement in it.

CONCLUSION

As we hope we have demonstrated, working with qualitative data in collaborative cross-cultural research presents both opportunities and frustrations. An enormous degree of commitment over a long period of time is essential for such a project to bear fruit. Indeed, we are still pruning our data, but we all believe that the investment is essential. We can understand the human experience of aging only with data that are both culturally valid and comparable, and these data can result only from qualitative and collaborative research.

NOTES

[1] The authors would like to acknowledge funding from the National Institute on Aging for the research on which this chapter is based. We would also like to thank Jeanette Dickerson-Putman, Patricia Draper, Anthony Glascock, and Henry Harpending for their contributions to the development of this chapter.
[2] An acronym for age, generation, and experience that has become the shorthand title for the project funded as "Age and Culture."

REFERENCES

Cantril, H. (1965). *The pattern of human concerns*. New Brunswick, NJ: Rutgers University Press.
Clark, M., & Mendelson, M. (1969). Mexican-American aged in San Francisco: A case description. *The Gerontologist, 9*, 90–95.
Cowgill, D. O. (1974). Aging and modernization: A revision of the theory. In J. Gubrium (Ed.), *Late life: Communities and environmental policy* (pp. 123–146). Springfield, IL: Charles C. Thomas.

Cowgill, D. O., & Holmes, L. D. (Eds.). (1972). *Aging and modernization*. New York: Appleton-Century-Crofts.

Frank, G., & Vanderburgh, R. (1986). Life histories. In C. L. Fry & J. Keith (Eds.), *New methods for old age research* (pp. 185–212). South Hadley, MA: Bergin & Garvey.

George, L. K. (1981). Subjective well-being: Conceptual and methodological issues. *Annual Review of Geriatrics and Gerontology, 2*, 345–382.

Hsu, F. L. K. (1981). *Americans & Chinese* (3rd ed.). Honolulu: The University Press of Hawaii.

Keith, J. (1986). Participant observation. In C. L. Fry & J. Keith (Eds.), *New methods for old age research* (pp. 1–20). New York: Praeger (A Bergin and Garvey Book).

Langness, L. L. (1965). *The life history in anthropological science*. New York: Holt, Rinehart, & Winston.

Lawton, M. P. (1972). The dimensions of morale. In D. Kent, R. Kastenbaum, & S. Sherwood (Eds.), *Research, planning, and action for the elderly* (pp. 144–165). New York: Behavioral Publications.

Mandelbaum, D. G. (1973). The study of life history: Gandhi. *Current Anthropology, 14*(3), 177–206.

Miles, M. B., & Huberman, A. M. (1984). *Qualitative data analysis*. Beverly Hills, CA: Sage.

Myerhoff, B., & Simic, A. (Eds.). (1978). *Life's career—Aging: Cross-cultural studies in growing old*. Beverly Hills, CA: Sage.

Nydegger, C. (Ed.). (1977). *Measuring morale* (Special Publication No. 3). Washington, DC: Gerontological Society.

Nydegger, C. (1986). Measuring morale. In C. L. Fry & J. Keith (Eds.), *New methods for old age research* (pp. 213–230). New York: Praeger (A Bergin and Garvey Book).

Palmore, E. (1975). *The honorable elders: A cross-cultural analysis of aging in Japan*. Durham, NC: Duke University Press.

Trela, J. E., & Sokolovsky, J. H. (1979). Culture, ethnicity, and policy for the aged. In D. E. Gelfand & A. J. Kutzik (Eds.), *Ethnicity and aging: Theory, research, and policy* (pp. 117–136). New York: Springer.

Watson, L. C. (1976). Understanding a life history as a subjective document. *Ethos, 4*, 95–131.

Whiting, B., & Whiting, J. (1973). Methods for observing and recording behavior. In R. Naroll & R. Cohen (Eds.), *A handbook of method in cultural anthropology* (pp. 282–315). New York: Columbia University Press.

PART 3
Commentary

Commentary 1

A New Climate for Qualitative Research

Anselm Strauss

The contributors to this volume reveal both the full array of qualitative research issues and the current smorgasbord of answers to them. To begin with, there are a variety of methods used: life histories, published autobiographies, interviews of various kinds done in short or long series, observations in private or public places, observations done as participants in events or organizations, observations done as outsider-researchers, and so forth. Sometimes two or three methods are used together. Sometimes they are used in conjunction with survey questionnaires or special instruments, and then qualitative and quantitative analysis is combined. The researchers may just use, or illustrate with, or urge, or advocate one method or combinations. Some simply present their findings with brief descriptions of methods (especially of data collection, rarely of analysis); others give more detailed description of steps taken, and even detail personalized experiences in the field that lend both credibility to their findings and flavor to their narratives.

They come at their research problems, too, with far from uniform positions, whether explicitly stated or not, on what is more or less desirable, or at least more valuable: "understanding" their subjects' lives, or dense description, or verifying hypotheses, or extending and clarifying extant theory, or formulating new substantive theory useful for gerontology, or answering policy or policy-informing questions. Above all they offer considerable variety, from exemplification or advocacy of a personalized approach at one extreme, to somewhat more standardized approaches on the other. However, as the editors have noted, there is a fairly uniform stance taken on antipositivistic extremism, a leaning toward inductive approaches to materials rather than deductions, or at least precise deductions, from established theories, and the like.

Social and behavioral scientists who use or are turning to qualitative methods today work in a somewhat different climate from before, albeit preceding generations certainly faced some of the same issues: how to collect better data, how to analyze more convincingly, how to build more effective theory, and so forth. Most recently, various scholarly traditions in each discipline, whether new or rejuvenated, plus various intellectual and social movements (like antipositivism and feminism), have generated an atmosphere where there is greater tolerance toward qualitative inquiries among many of the quantification people, and far less defensiveness among the qualitative researchers about their research, than was evident even five or ten years ago. Some lessons learned in earlier eras have certainly been forgotten, but thoughtful and sometimes penetratingly good articles and books are streaming nowadays from the presses, attacking problems that attend the researching of new phenomena, new kinds of populations, and at new research sites.

Both through their strengths and weaknesses the chapters in this volume raise again very important issues for qualitative researchers. They confront gerontologists no less than us all.

ANALYSIS AND DATA COLLECTION

Qualitative researchers are long on data collection, certainly in their amount of discussion and understanding of this and in descriptions of their data collecting. They are exceedingly short, however, on giving comparable attention to their analyses of data. Concern with improving data collection, and under quite new conditions, is essential but is not the issue being raised here. The issue is, when do we get down to the business of conveying just what we actually do when engaging in qualitative *analysis*? Some of us do "it" superbly well. Possibly, some teach it effectively. For the most part, however, explicit teaching is minimal, the students or research assistants learning by social osmosis and trial-and-error. What is certain is that qualitative analysis varies considerably from researcher to researcher. We need to know what these varieties are: their strengths and weaknesses, advantages and disadvantages for different kinds of data and studies. We will not know this until sustained collective attention is paid to making explicit the various analytic styles and procedures. Only then are we likely to do our analyses more effectively and quickly—and to give them more credibility. But this does *not* mean arguing exclusively for one analytic style or set of procedures.

WHAT KIND OR LEVEL OF ANALYSIS?

In the introduction to this volume, the editors refer in passing to conceptually rich description and then move to discussing a necessary balance between actors' viewpoints and the researcher's conceptual interpreting of them. But consider: there are many types of interpretation in social science. For example, even a journalistic or commonsensical description is colored by at least an implicit analysis, and often by an interpretation consciously derived from a perspective. Our anthropological, psychological, and sociological interpretations of presented descriptions, regardless of their form, are still interpretations about descriptive texts. But what if we are interpreting data so as to develop and test hypotheses, or sets of hypotheses? Whether precisely formulated or not, the hypotheses will include concepts. In the chapters of this volume, they often remain implicit rather than clearly stated, and often, too, have the status of commonsense concepts or are derived from lay usage, rather than from theory, or developed *de novo*. Also they may be formulated for policy- or practice-oriented purposes; or directed at negating lay stereotypes, rather than directed at the findings or assertions of the technical literature.

When data are analyzed (interpreted) for theoretical purposes, presumably the researcher will develop or use existing concepts, will form them into at least implicit but related hypotheses, and also present findings related to them and to the theory in which they are embedded. This means that to some degree the researcher will have attempted their verification and the establishment or modification of theory. Theory-organized qualitative research varies somewhat, of course, in how explicitly the hypotheses are formulated in the complexity of the linkages among them. In the grounded theory tradition in which I work, monographs tend to have a rather large number of interrelated concepts, which practice reflects the complexity of the qualitative analysis and the self-conscious development of theory.

Surely there is a place in social science research, including that of social gerontology, for studies that run the full range of types—wholly descriptive, hypothesis formulating, hypothesis testing, theoretical, and so forth. They are all useful, for different purposes.

SAMPLING

There has been criticism by qualitative researchers, and of course by quantitative ones, about research findings that are based on "samples of one" social units—one kind of population, one organization, and so forth—or, worse yet, findings based on studying just a few individuals, let alone case studies of one or two individuals. This sampling issue to some extent has bothered many of us.

There are two relevant points I cannot forbear making. The first is that researchers ought to understand precisely what level or kind of comprehension (description . . . theory) they are aiming at and then make this crystal clear to their readers, as well as give the rationale for their basic sampling decisions. Through such locational orientations readers can get additional indicators for judging the credibility of the presented analyses. My second point is a rather special one, pertaining to the "theoretical sampling" advocated by Barney Glaser and me (1967) for those who wish to develop genuinely grounded theories. Theoretical sampling is directed by the emerging theory; its practice means highly focused choices of sites, events, and actors to be observed, and/or interviewing done at those sites or of specific persons or around theoretically specified events. And all because of specific hypotheses that have been generated. J. Kevin Eckert's use of quasi-experiments seems close to some aspects of theoretical sampling. Perhaps the main difference is that the latter is based on coding of data from the very first interviews or field notes; then there is a feeding back of data obtained, as directed by this sampling; then there is further coding and sampling; this develops into successive coding, leading always to further sampling and data collection. This goes on continually throughout the life of the research project. The whole process is self-consciously systematic. Social gerontologists who are especially interested in developing or verifying theory, or both, might well think about using theoretical sampling in preference to the more normal selective or only partly systematic and somewhat implicit theoretical sampling reflected in various chapters in this volume.

WHY THEORY?

My own passionately held position is this: theory is cumulative but substantive findings in social science mostly are not—they tend to change when social conditions change, whether that occurs within a few years or over decades. Genuinely grounded theory is not discarded; it gets modified or refashioned, and so can both direct research efforts and profit by them. If social gerontology is to be truly cumulative, it needs theory. And if social gerontologists wish to make contributions beyond their specialty—to other specialties or to their encompassing disciplines—then some of them need to do theoretically oriented work. Why should someone like myself, an outsider to gerontology, want to read your writings, other than through curiosity about your methods or because I, too, have older friends and relatives or am myself growing older? You need to speak to social scientists like me, too!

My commentary on the work of qualitative social gerontologists has been designed to help locate these chapters in the larger analytic terrain and to encourage the authors and other gerontologists to think of themselves as both contributing to and receiving the benefits of the lively work and debate going on in that broader arena.

REFERENCE

Glaser, B. G., & Strauss, A. L. (1967). *The discovery of grounded theory*. Chicago: Aldine.

Commentary 2

Qualitative Research: Legitimacy and the Uses of the Stranger

David Gutmann

A book like this is long overdue in gerontology. It is good to find a collection of mainly young investigators who have the guts, in the face of funding priorities toward quantitative research, to move closer to their subjects instead of away from them. Faced with these loaded dice, some qualitative researchers become (understandably) defensive and boast their moral superiority over better-funded, more conventionally legitimized quantitative researchers: "our budgets may be slim, but our hearts—as opposed to those who only quantify and measure—are large with love for our informants."

To avoid the slide into defensive sentimentality, we should use the occasion provided by this volume to remind ourselves of the unique sources and uses of qualitative methods. As part of our stocktaking, we should first address the question of legitimacy and the routes to scientific respectability. We should remind ourselves that our legitimacy does not require our victimization, or even our superior capacity for loving. No: our legitimacy as a group rests on a more enduring basis—a great tradition: the seminal thinkers and investigators in the behavioral sciences came, without exception, from the naturalistic, qualitative mold. Thus, developmental psychology began with a child-watcher, Piaget. Dynamic psychology began with Freud's third ear. Finally, our sophisticated, complex consciousness of human community—and of ourselves in community—came largely from anthropologists: qualitative researchers *par excellence*, they went to the field without large grants and without "standard" instruments. They were armed only with their courage and their voracious *appetite for reality*.

Most importantly, these examples from the work of our founding fathers and mothers teach us that the power of our methods does not reside in our gender or our political situation; that power resides in the scope and clarity of our observations. In qualitative research, we typically abandon the search for an illusory certainty in exchange for a special kind of potency—the amazing exploratory powers of the eyes and of the ears. The aim is to open up the F Stops on our sight and to remove the filters that are imposed by *a priori* instruments searching for neutralized, precoded data.

THROUGH THE EYES OF THE STRANGER

Our editors' sponsorship of dedicated *looking*—the *eros* of vision—can only be applauded; but at the same time, there are spotted through this volume some assumptions about research and human nature that could lead to new blinders, to losses rather than gains in acuity. I refer to the assumption, throughout many of these pieces, that one or another form of participant-observation is the strategy of choice; and that regardless of the particular research mission, one is required—for both moral and scientific reasons—to engage with the subject in a "full" and "human" way. Despite the vicissitudes of participant-observation, the notion that one should be a buddy to one's subject, that one should break down the alienating boundaries between the subject and the investigator, is an unexamined assumption in many of these texts. I have no argument with the use of participant-observation as one legitimate strategy, but I do not believe that such "friendly" approaches exhaust the possibilities of qualitative research. Finally, these untested assumptions come not from scientific experience but from the same sentimentality that so easily infiltrates our field and so easily gets identified with it. I would like to put forward a radically different posture—that of the "stranger" rather than the "buddy." This stance can also enhance observation, and so belongs within the ambit of qualitative methods.

The following notes on the uses of the stranger in naturalistic interviewing come out of a fairly long stretch of field experience in four societies—the Navajo, the Lowland and Highland Maya of Mexico, and the Druze of the Middle East. During those years, I was simultaneously generating and testing a model of developmental change in the psychology of older men—a set of notions holding that fairly standard and predictable changes, more related to life stage than to cultural situation, to nature rather than to nurture—take place at the more unconscious or appetitive strata of personality. In this enterprise, I did not approach the subjects as an anthropologist might: I did not use them as informants on cultural practices, but as informants on themselves and on their subjective relation to cultural practices. In brief, I was more interested in data on their *inner life* than on reports of their daily comings and goings in their social worlds. My task was to generate not friendship (though I was not adverse to that outcome) but the very special and distinct state of *rapport*, the condition that comes about when a subject wants to talk about the private matters, the dangerous excitements, that are of interest to you both. I quickly discovered that I could not generate the kinds of rapport that my clinical training had taught me to recognize and appreciate through the use of standard interview instruments. For one thing, these tools are revealed, under field conditions, to be based on an egocentric illusion: namely, that the investigator's fixed procedures will "standardize" the entire situation, including the subject's understanding of and response to the interview itself. But as I soon discovered, even within high-consensus village societies, individual respondents would have grossly different understandings about my purposes and about the meaning of the interview—ranging from the suspicion that I was a government agent to the frank delusion that I had been sent by God to chronicle the history of the village before the imminent destruction of the world. Evidently, then, the "apperceptive mass" of preformed ideas that respondents brought to the interview setting was different in each case and could grossly influence, in untraceable ways, the degree of rapport and the quality of the data itself.

Clearly, the usual "standard" procedures would neither reveal the subject's apperceptive mass nor reduce its effects; it would only leave these biasing distortions planted forever in the data. Before the working alliance can be achieved, the subject's distorting—albeit to him, real—apperceptive mass should be highlighted; and he should be given a reassuring experience in terms of such concerns. In brief, the standard condition—rapport—is in each case reached *via* different and nonstandard approaches.

I soon came to realize that the apperceptive mass was mobilized and focused on me, because of my unique status: in the subject's eyes I was always the alien, the *stranger*. And as such, I furnished a projective ecology, a kind of walking Rorschach blot, for meanings that had their origins not in me but in the subject—in his own experiences with the alien, including the estranged parts of himself.

Commonsense tells us that familiarity is based on a long history of shared significant experience; therefore I could not "dis-alienate" myself in the subject's eyes by becoming a buddy, by wearing his costume, or even by speaking his language: each of these affectations would only turn me into a different version of the stranger without reducing the apperceptive mass associated with that condition. Through trial-and-error I came to realize that, since one is ineluctably the stranger, it was necessary to use rather than deny that condition. The alien, the person who does not speak the local language, is a fitting metaphor and reciprocal of that which is alien within the self. The stranger is so defined by the fact that he is not part of our consequential social system; confiding in him we run no risk of rejection, of having to live with the social reverberations of our private utterance. The stranger, even more than the friend, can be the reliable sponsor of rapport. Consequently, if I acknowledged that status instead of fearing it, I could gain special entree to the respondent's private world.

Accordingly, before I began to interview the next stranger, I did not try to diminish our differences. Instead of speaking his language, I spoke through interpreters; I did not try to dress like a traditional; and I paid no tribute to our common humanity or to the superiority of the Third World over my own. Instead, I called attention to our evident differences and turned them into the fulcrum of the interview itself. Thus I began sessions by asking the subject, despite my strangeness, to confide in me about his own life. "I realize that it is hard to talk frankly to someone that you do not know. So before I ask *my* questions, I am ready to answer any questions that you have about me." A person's questions are better than his answers as a guide to salient concerns; thus the invited interview gave me a chance to know and respond to the subject's apperceptions—and particularly his suspicions—in regard to the interview itself. The best strategy is to make explicit any suspicions that the subject brings up—directly or indirectly—in his own invited interview: "I think that you are worried about me. You think that I am an agent of the government. No man can know what is really in the heart of another, and so it will do no good for me to deny this. All I can do is ask you to talk to me and hear *my* questions. You can make up your own mind if these are the questions of a government spy."

Along the same lines, and contrary to the ethos of advocacy research, confrontation was often a good deal more effective than compliance in provoking real rapport. For example, I once interviewed 80-year-old Clyde Peshlakai, a renowned medicine man of the Western Navajo. At the outset, we spent two fruitless hours while he derided the white man for rapacious treatment of the Navajo. Full of proper liberal guilt, I grinned in pious agreement. However, my exercise in brotherhood did not provoke the like in him, but only increased his scorn for me: What kind of a man will not stand up for his own people? But finally, running out of other cheeks to turn, I became angry in my own right, interrupted Peshlakai, and told him that I could not answer for other Bellacana (white men); but for myself, I did not need anything that belonged to the Navajo. I had my own car, my own house, my own land, and my own woman. All I wanted from him was his goddamn story. Though still the stranger, I was at least no longer a poltroon. For the first time Peshlakai looked at me straight on and asked, in English, "where did you say you come from?" After that, he revealed some of the vulnerability, even depression, that underlay his brave show. His ways, the old ways, were passing now because the young men—he waved dismissingly toward his grandsons—would not learn the "rain songs, sheep songs, and grass songs" that old men know. And because I had become the legitimized stranger, Peshlakai invited me, indirectly, to become his apprentice.

This encounter was instructive in a number of ways. I learned, for example, that the stranger is not necessarily barred from community, but instead marks the first stage in relatedness. Remember that our own children first come to us as strangers; and perhaps Peshlakai saw in me the stranger-as-child, the stranger waiting to be instructed, to be made fully human. As a consequence, in later interviews, say among the Maya, I took the stance of the *interested* stranger, a naive and even stupid man, but one who *insisted* on being instructed: "You say that your life has been corn and beans. Another Maya from Pustunich would understand what you meant. But I am a *gringo* and so you must explain to me fully about these things. Now: What about corn, and what about beans?"

Confronting questions can, paradoxically, increase rapport and broaden the observational spectrum. In the field, one discovers that there are successive levels of the subject's text, each of which is revealed in response to confronting questions posed under conditions of rapport. Let me give an example, from the time when I was part of a team studying epileptiform disorders among Navajo children. Interviewing the parents of a retarded, seizure-prone daughter, I asked them to tell me about her disease. They began with a good "clinical" account, detailing the history of symptoms and their medication. While the report was plausible in the medical sense, I was not satisfied. I said that I was not an Anglo doctor and suspected that there was a different, Navajo story of this disorder. Surprised, but also a touch pleased, the parents allowed that indeed their daughter had been a victim of envy witchcraft: "We used to have wealth in sheep and horses, and an envious man did witchcraft against my daughter with this result." In his study of Navajo witchcraft, this is the sort of account that Kluckholn (1944) was typically given: the witch as distant, faceless stranger. As an anthropologist, Kluckholn was satisfied with this relatively impersonal version of Navajo sorcery. But having been trained in clinical psychology, and sensing a more intimate relationship between the purported witch and his victim, I dug further: "But many Navajo have wealth in sheep, horse, and turquoise," I said. "Why did he pick on you? What was the relationship between you?" In response, another skin of the onion was removed: turning to his wife the husband said, "It is time to tell what really happened." Now he said that the witch was in fact his father-in-law: the father of his wife and the grandfather of the afflicted daughter. He went on to explain that the grandfather had been a prominent medicine man who "went to the bad side" and became a witch. To be initiated into the sorcerer's society, he had to violate the firmest taboos and bring harm to his family. "But why," I asked, "would a good man, a healer, become a witch?" This time, the mother answered: "It wasn't his fault. But after my mother died, he married a younger woman, and my new stepmother was never satisfied, demanding things, always costing my father money. That's why he turned to the bad side and did sorcery against me and my family: it was to make more money; it was to please her."

I was (and still am) very pleased with this interview. For one thing, it bolstered my belief that universal tensions and needs can find expression through parochial human practices. In the above case, an episode of witchcraft, from the exotic Navajo culture, turns out to be yet another version of a standard human drama: oedipal rivalry between stepmother and stepdaughter. Here the victim says, in effect: "I and my family were not willfully harmed by my loving father. He was forced to it by my selfish stepmother."

More to the point, I was impressed, both then and now, by the dialectics of the naturalistic interview: the reciprocal relationship between legitimacy, confrontation, and rapport, between bluntness on the part of the interviewer and frankness on the part of the subject. In the field your real asset is not your loving-kindness, but your *legitimacy*; and your first and most vital task is to create, in the face of your evident strangeness, your own legitimacy. To repeat, you claim legitimacy by believing in the value of *passionate investigation* and by acting as though legitimacy has already been achieved. Thus the investigator disregards the usual proprieties and demonstrates instead—through challenging probes—the appetite for reality. In effect, the investigator demonstrates legitimacy *by risking illegitimacy*. Again, love is not enough: the informant does not respond to your warmth—that can be feigned or inconstant—but to a legitimacy that cannot be faked. Trusting the investigator's legitimacy, subjects become increasingly open to their own inner voices, to strange inner promptings that can acquire their own legitimacy in the course of the interview.

Finally, I do not claim that the stranger-as-investigator is superior to the advocate-as-investigator. Ultimately, there is room for both—and for other, as yet unimagined styles. I only wish to stake the claim of the "stranger" *persona* within the house of qualitative research—and to make it available to those who find that it matches their special mission and their special temperament.

REFERENCE

Kluckholn, C. (1944). *Navajo witchcraft*. Cambridge, MA: Peabody Museum.

Commentary 3

Us, Not Them: Breaking Through Denial Of Age

Betty Friedan

It seems to me from reading this book, that qualitative gerontology is the *only* way to go if we want to understand what aging is all about. I say this because I've been immersing myself in the state of the art of gerontology, and I've seen the extent to which the experience of the aging individual is not acknowledged, understood or studied. My observations about men's and women's lives before writing *The Feminine Mystique* were similar to what I think is going on now with older people. Women's experiences were denied without our even knowing we were denying them, while at the same time studies were done claiming to produce insight about women's lives without taking into account women's actual experiences.

Earlier I recognized that there was a feminine mystique. Now I am writing a book which takes on the age mystique. What I have been finding is the enormous denial of the personhood of older people. This is as true for gerontology, as it is for society as a whole. We define, we see age only as decline from youth. We seem unable to look at the experience of age in its own terms—age itself has no substance or meaning, no independent way of being defined, no values of its own. Our own exaggerated denial of our aging is the force that feeds this way of thinking about old age—as non-existent.

The denials to which we go are extreme. The terror we feel about aging is obvious: age is defined only as a problem; studies of age are done primarily in nursing homes; the study of age is the study of institutions, established on the medical model to deal with sickness, pathology; and age is seen only as decline. Gerontological studies deal primarily with the most extreme problems; the most problematic and pathological of the ways of being old. Since we don't identify with these images, we can deny our own age. Gerontologists as well speak of older people as *them*, denying their own aging. The inability to speak of *us* reflects an inability to identify with the people studied or see ourselves as aging people.

The reverse of this idea is also true. If we take our own aging experience seriously, we can identify with those we study and understand their aging in more meaningful ways. If we deny our own aging, then we cannot understand others'.

Just as women needed to learn *how* and be liberated *to* take their own experience seriously, so too we now need to find ways to take the experience of all of us as we age seriously.

In this book I found the potential for doing that. I found an attempt to depart from that tradition that separates out objects of study as *them*. Some of the authors are not fully released from the dominant mode of studying people as others, and thus they use an apologetic tone at times. They torture themselves in the effort to break loose. Even so, the book provides models for thinking about the personhood of people in age. It does this by offering us studies using empathy with people over 60 and seeing them first and foremost as people.

I'd like to comment specifically on four chapters. In Kathy MacPherson's chapter on the menopause collective we have a glimpse into a group that was defining menopause simply as a stage of life, not necessarily as a problem. The group was engaged in defining their own menopause and not having their menopause defined for them. This is a marvellous example of the need to reclaim experiences. Because the researcher was a member of the group, she could identify with the other women as people. She is a woman who is aging and from that sense of shared experience she could understand what the women were doing. But she became trapped in her own apologies about the fact that she was doing just that. What should have been a *sine qua non* for her research was something that she was so self-conscious about doing, that she became deflected from the study of her group to a study of herself studying the group.

In Phyllis Silverman's study, widowhood is thought of as a period of life, not only as a loss, but also as a period of growth and change. Because she wanted to find out what the widows themselves had to say, she has produced a study that is different, that sees women as people. Her data and observations and my own interviews suggest that widowhood can, in fact, be a period of growth as well as loss for women who have been defined and define themselves primarily as wives, a change necessary (and one permitted consciously now) to life lived in a new way that develops unsuspected personal strengths. We do not need to think of widowhood only in its medical aspects, as grief that must be ended as soon as possible so the woman can return to the kind of person she once was.

Phyllis Silverman uses an important image when describing how it is that she tries to understand the widows. She talks about connected seeing, seeing with empathy and identification. This connected seeing allows us to see things differently and see different things. Connected seeing is not simply a technique, it takes connection seriously, and takes the experience of the people we study seriously. With connected seeing we transform the approach to widowhood from the medical problem of grief, from something to get rid of, into a new issue, a new period of life. (It seems interesting that in this book, we see primarily women restive with the limits of "separate," linear, one-dimensional, *objective* ways of knowing which gerontologists have confined themselves to in the name of an obsolete, male-defined science. But I do not claim that it is only women who have the capacity for "connected seeing". Graham Rowles, Robert Kastenbaum and the other men of this book, along with the women, should stop apologizing; they are on the front edge.)

The methods of qualitative gerontology *enable* us to see the experienced reality, the personal truth of age. They enable us to get rid of the damaging, stereotypical ageist or "poor dear" images because people's experience becomes alive to us and we begin to understand what it is to be old.

For this reason I found Aluma Motenko's study of men caring for their disabled wives fascinating. She talked to the husbands about what they were doing, and while she talked with them, she did not put on the lens of "poor old people" or a feminist lens which rejects out of hand the caretaker role. Rather she gives us a wonderful picture of men thinking through the caretaker role. Instead of the denigration and martyrdom which comes about when caretaking is imposed, in these men we see, as I suggest in *The Second Stage*, the value and strengths of caretaking as a *chosen* role.

We see these men define what they are doing as a job. We see them valuing their competence in their new role, a real role that gives them opportunities for pride and self-respect. Since they have chosen this role, they are not martyrs. Since they are men, they think anything they do is important. For them, this is an important role. Women as well as men can choose the caretaker role and gain strength from it. As a feminist I recognize the mistakes we made by defining caretaking only as martyrdom. I know the mistakes we made by seeing ourselves as victims, and by drawing attention to our roles exclusively as stressful.

When we choose roles, any roles, they can give us purpose and self-respect.

To me this chapter is also a reminder that as we study roles beyond middle-age, we need to understand what those roles are by drawing on the experience of people in those roles. Old age is the age beyond the defined roles. To know what lies beyond, we cannot rely on the notions and rebellions of those who are younger.

I also want to comment on the chapter by the Kahanas and Kathryn Riley which discusses contextual factors inside nursing homes. Between the lines of their chapter I read the important piece of information that the aides were resentful of having to bring participants to new activities for therapy and energizing. We have to remember that even if our interventions are wonderful, even if we can guarantee improvement in impaired patients, it won't last. And the improvement will be less than it might have been since the aides will be resentful and will make the patients pay for it later, in some other phase of the round of institutional life. The hostility and resentment of the staff—whatever its source—is part and parcel of this disinterest and inability to see older people as people, the same problem with which I began this essay. Because this is so, *any* study claiming to demonstrate the efficacy of an intervention becomes suspect. For, given the ageism of nursing home personnel documented here, any intervention that pays attention to or arouses the patients as people will bring them alive. More important, any study presenting as fact or norm of aging the decline, deterioration and pathology of women and men in nursing homes has to be suspect: the very resentment of the staff at carrying out orders or therapy which arouses patients from doped passivity implies their basic collusion in imposed impairment.

In this volume there is an attempt to see individuals in age as human beings, as growing, developing persons. In my mind, it is the only gerontology worth doing, and helps us make sense of what is done in quantitative studies. Before and after we put the data into the computer we need to find out from older people themselves what the real story is. We have to have the ability to find out the essential elements.

We learned a lot from our break-throughs with the women's movement. And now as more and more people are beginning to live long lives, we need the same breakthrough in the study of old people as people. Only if we think of youth—not old age—as the end point of life, do we fall into the trap of not seeing the picture whole, the picture real, and the picture in its qualitatively nuanced, experienced dimensions. Qualitative gerontology, starting with the experience of real people in age, breaks through that denial and begins to confront the mysterious reality of age.

Index